Applied Medical Image Processing

SECOND EDITION

Applied Medical Image Processing

A Basic Course

SECOND EDITION

Wolfgang Birkfellner

Center for Medical Physics and Biomedical Engineering
Medical University of Vienna
Vienna, Austria

With contributions by

Michael Figl and Johann Hummel
Center for Medical Physics and Biomedical Engineering
Medical University of Vienna
Vienna, Austria

Ziv Yaniv and Özgür Güler
Sheikh Zayad Institute for Pediatric Surgical Innovation
Children's National Medical Center
Washington, District of Columbia, USA

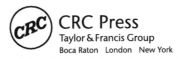

CRC Press
Taylor & Francis Group
Boca Raton   London   New York

CRC Press is an imprint of the
Taylor & Francis Group, an **Informa** business

MATLAB® is a trademark of The MathWorks, Inc. and is used with permission. The MathWorks does not warrant the accuracy of the text or exercises in this book. This book's use or discussion of MATLAB® software or related products does not constitute endorsement or sponsorship by The MathWorks of a particular pedagogical approach or particular use of the MATLAB® software.

Taylor & Francis
Taylor & Francis Group
6000 Broken Sound Parkway NW, Suite 300
Boca Raton, FL 33487-2742

© 2014 by Taylor & Francis Group, LLC
Taylor & Francis is an Informa business

No claim to original U.S. Government works

Printed on acid-free paper
Version Date: 20140114

International Standard Book Number-13: 978-1-4665-5557-0 (Hardback)

Library of Congress Cataloging-in-Publication Data

Birkfellner, Wolfgang, author.
    Applied medical image processing : a basic course / Wolfgang Birkfellner. -- Second edition.
    p. ; cm.
    Includes bibliographical references and index.
    ISBN 978-1-4665-5557-0 (hardcover : alk. paper)
    I. Title.
    [DNLM: 1. Diagnostic Imaging--methods. 2. Image Interpretation, Computer-Assisted--methods.
3. Image Processing, Computer-Assisted--methods. WN 180]

    RC78.7.D53
    616.07'54--dc23   2013047334

Visit the Taylor & Francis Web site at
http://www.taylorandfrancis.com

and the CRC Press Web site at
http://www.crcpress.com

I dedicate this book to Katharina, Joseph, Carl and Anton – the most important people in the world to me – and to my academic mentor and advisor, Helmar Bergmann – WB

Contents-in-Brief

List of Figures, xiii

List of Tables, xxi

Foreword, xxiii

Preface to the First Edition, xxv

Preface to the Second Edition, xxvii

User Guide, xxix

Acknowledgments, xxxi

CHAPTER 1 ▪ A Few Basics of Medical Image Sources   1

CHAPTER 2 ▪ Image Processing in Clinical Practice   45

CHAPTER 3 ▪ Image Representation   59

CHAPTER 4 ▪ Operations in Intensity Space   91

CHAPTER 5 ▪ Filtering and Transformations   115

CHAPTER 6 ▪ Segmentation   177

CHAPTER 7 ▪ Spatial Transforms   215

CHAPTER 8 ▪ Rendering and Surface Models   251

CHAPTER 9 ▪ Registration   297

CHAPTER 10 ▪ CT Reconstruction   339

CHAPTER 11 ▪ A Tutorial on Image-Guided Therapy   371

CHAPTER 12 ▪ A Selection of MATLAB® Commands   397

Glossary, 403

List of MATLAB sample scripts, 407

Epilogue, 413

Index, 415

Contents

List of Figures, xiii

List of Tables, xxi

Foreword, xxiii

Preface to the First Edition, xxv

Preface to the Second Edition, xxvii

User Guide, xxix

Acknowledgments, xxxi

CHAPTER 1 ▪ A Few Basics of Medical Image Sources   1

Johann Hummel

1.1	RADIOLOGY	2
1.2	THE ELECTROMAGNETIC SPECTRUM	2
1.3	BASIC X-RAY PHYSICS	3
1.4	ATTENUATION AND IMAGING	7
1.5	COMPUTED TOMOGRAPHY	10
1.6	MAGNETIC RESONANCE TOMOGRAPHY	17
1.7	ULTRASOUND	28
1.8	NUCLEAR MEDICINE AND MOLECULAR IMAGING	33
1.9	OTHER IMAGING TECHNIQUES	36
1.10	RADIATION PROTECTION AND DOSIMETRY	39
1.11	SUMMARY AND FURTHER REFERENCES	43

CHAPTER 2 ▪ Image Processing in Clinical Practice   45

Wolfgang Birkfellner

2.1	APPLICATION EXAMPLES	45
2.2	IMAGE DATABASES	45
2.3	INTENSITY OPERATIONS	46
2.4	FILTER OPERATIONS	47
2.5	SEGMENTATION	48
2.6	SPATIAL TRANSFORMS	49

2.7	RENDERING AND SURFACE MODELS	51
2.8	REGISTRATION	54
2.9	CT RECONSTRUCTION	56
2.10	SUMMARY	56

CHAPTER 3 ■ Image Representation   59

Wolfgang Birkfellner

3.1	PIXELS AND VOXELS	59
3.2	GRAY SCALE AND COLOR REPRESENTATION	63
3.3	IMAGE FILE FORMATS	66
3.4	DICOM	71
3.5	OTHER FORMATS – ANALYZE 7.5, NIFTI AND INTERFILE	73
3.6	IMAGE QUALITY AND THE SIGNAL-TO-NOISE RATIO	74
3.7	PRACTICAL LESSONS	75
3.8	SUMMARY AND FURTHER REFERENCES	89

CHAPTER 4 ■ Operations in Intensity Space   91

Wolfgang Birkfellner

4.1	THE INTENSITY TRANSFORM FUNCTION AND THE DYNAMIC RANGE	91
4.2	WINDOWING	93
4.3	HISTOGRAMS AND HISTOGRAM OPERATIONS	95
4.4	DITHERING AND DEPTH	98
4.5	PRACTICAL LESSONS	98
4.6	SUMMARY AND FURTHER REFERENCES	113

CHAPTER 5 ■ Filtering and Transformations   115

Wolfgang Birkfellner

5.1	THE FILTERING OPERATION	116
5.2	THE FOURIER TRANSFORM	128
5.3	OTHER TRANSFORMS	140
5.4	PRACTICAL LESSONS	143
5.5	SUMMARY AND FURTHER REFERENCES	174

CHAPTER 6 ■ Segmentation   177

Wolfgang Birkfellner

6.1	THE SEGMENTATION PROBLEM	177
6.2	ROI DEFINITION AND CENTROIDS	178
6.3	THRESHOLDING	178
6.4	REGION GROWING	181
6.5	MORE SOPHISTICATED SEGMENTATION METHODS	183
6.6	MORPHOLOGICAL OPERATIONS	185

6.7	EVALUATION OF SEGMENTATION RESULTS	188
6.8	PRACTICAL LESSONS	190
6.9	SUMMARY AND FURTHER REFERENCES	212

CHAPTER 7 ▪ Spatial Transforms | 215

Wolfgang Birkfellner

7.1	DISCRETIZATION – RESOLUTION AND ARTIFACTS	215
7.2	INTERPOLATION AND VOLUME REGULARIZATION	216
7.3	TRANSLATION AND ROTATION	219
7.4	REFORMATTING	228
7.5	TRACKING AND IMAGE-GUIDED THERAPY	229
7.6	PRACTICAL LESSONS	233
7.7	SUMMARY AND FURTHER REFERENCES	249

CHAPTER 8 ▪ Rendering and Surface Models | 251

Wolfgang Birkfellner

8.1	VISUALIZATION	251
8.2	ORTHOGONAL AND PERSPECTIVE PROJECTION, AND THE VIEWPOINT	252
8.3	RAYCASTING	252
8.4	SURFACE–BASED RENDERING	258
8.5	PRACTICAL LESSONS	267
8.6	SUMMARY AND FURTHER REFERENCES	295

CHAPTER 9 ▪ Registration | 297

Wolfgang Birkfellner

9.1	FUSING INFORMATION	297
9.2	REGISTRATION PARADIGMS	299
9.3	MERIT FUNCTIONS	302
9.4	OPTIMIZATION STRATEGIES	313
9.5	SOME GENERAL COMMENTS	315
9.6	CAMERA CALIBRATION	316
9.7	REGISTRATION TO PHYSICAL SPACE	319
9.8	EVALUATION OF REGISTRATION RESULTS	322
9.9	PRACTICAL LESSONS	323
9.10	SUMMARY AND FURTHER REFERENCES	338

CHAPTER 10 ▪ CT Reconstruction | 339

Michael Figl

10.1	INTRODUCTION	339
10.2	RADON TRANSFORM	340
10.3	ALGEBRAIC RECONSTRUCTION	345

10.4 SOME REMARKS ON FOURIER TRANSFORM AND FILTERING 351

10.5 FILTERED BACKPROJECTION 354

10.6 PRACTICAL LESSONS 360

10.7 SUMMARY AND FURTHER REFERENCES 368

CHAPTER 11 ■ A Tutorial on Image-Guided Therapy   371

Özgür Güler and Ziv Yaniv

11.1 A HANDS-ON APPROACH TO CAMERA CALIBRATION AND IMAGE-GUIDED THERAPY 371

11.2 TRANSFORMATIONS 372

11.3 CAMERA CALIBRATION 375

11.4 IMAGE-GUIDED THERAPY, INTRODUCTION 379

11.5 IMAGE-GUIDED THERAPY, NAVIGATION SYSTEM 381

11.6 IMAGE-GUIDED THERAPY, THEORY IN PRACTICE 384

11.7 SUMMARY AND FURTHER REFERENCES 390

CHAPTER 12 ■ A Selection of MATLAB® Commands   397

12.1 CONTROL STRUCTURES AND OPERATORS 397

12.2 I/O AND DATA STRUCTURES 398

12.3 MATHEMATICAL FUNCTIONS 399

12.4 FURTHER REFERENCES 401

Glossary, 403

List of MATLAB sample scripts, 407

Epilogue, 413

Index, 415

List of Figures

1.1   A sketch of a typical x-ray spectrum.   4

1.2   The principle of an x-ray tube.   5

1.3   An image of an x-ray tube.   6

1.4   An illustration of the Compton- and photoeffect as well as pair production.   9

1.5   The principle of computed tomography.   10

1.6   A simple sketch of a sinogram.   11

1.7   A photograph of the first commercially available CT.   12

1.8   The principle of the four CT-scanner generations.   13

1.9   A multislice CT scanner.   14

1.10 An illustration of the amount of image data produced by multislice CT.   15

1.11 A linear accelerator for radiation oncology with an imaging unit attached.   16

1.12 A cone beam CT for dental radiology.   17

1.13 Metal artifacts in CT.   18

1.14 A sketch of precession motion.   19

1.15 An interventional MR machine.   21

1.16 Differences in T_1 and T_2 MR images.   22

1.17 Effects of insufficient field homogeneity in MR.   26

1.18 Effects of dental fillings in MR.   26

1.19 A modern 7 Tesla MR machine.   28

1.20 Two B-mode ultrasound transducer.   30

1.21 Speckle in ultrasound images.   31

1.22 A 3D ultrasound transducer.   32

1.23 The principle of a γ-camera.   35

1.24 A ring artifact in SPECT-reconstruction.   36

1.25 A dual-head gamma camera.   37

1.26 A modern PET-CT machine.   38

1.27 An OCT image of basalioma.   39

1.28 Effects of ionizing radiation on a video surveillance camera.   41

2.1   Screenshot of a DICOM database patient selection dialog.   46

2.2   Various views of a CT image with different intensity windowing.   47

2.3   Sobel filtering applied to planning CT data.   48

2.4   An application of intensity thresholding.   49

2.5   An application of atlas based segmentation.   50

2.6   Interpolation of image resolution in a CT image.   51

2.7   An example of reformatting.   52

2.8   DRR - rendering for beam verification in radiotherapy.   52

2.9   Surface rendering of organs-at-risk and planned target volumes in radio-
        therapy.   53

2.10   3D visualization of reformatted slices and surface renderings.   53

2.11   Rigid registration of CT and CBCT volume data.   55

2.12   Deformable registration of CT and CBCT volume data.   56

2.13   Registration of 3D CT and 2D x-ray data.   57

3.1   A CT slice showing the pixel structure of images.   60

3.2   A CT slice and its representation as a surface.   61

3.3   An illustration of physical vs. isotropic voxel spacing in a CT volume. 62

3.4   An early example of color photography.   65

3.5   A CT slice, saved in PGM format.   66

3.6   JPG image representation.   69

3.7   Header of a DICOM file.   72

3.8   Another DICOM header.   73

3.9   An Analyze 7.5 header, viewed in a hex-editor.   74

3.10   Image data used for Example 3.7.1.   76

3.11   A DSA image, the result of Example 3.7.1.   77

3.12   A file properties dialog showing the size of an image file.   78

3.13   A MATLAB screenshot.   78

3.14   The output from Example 3.7.2.   79

3.15   The output from Example 3.7.2 saved as PGM.   81

3.16   The "Open File" Dialog of ImageJ.   82

3.17   A DICOM file as displayed by ImageJ.   83

3.18   A screenshot of 3DSlicer.   83

3.19   Importing patient data into the 3DSlicer database.   84

3.20   A screenshot of images from a DICOM volume imported to 3DSlicer.   84

3.21   Output from Example 3.7.4.   86

3.22   Eight x-ray images acquired with different dose.   86

3.23   Selection of a signal free area in an x-ray image for SNR evaluation.   88

4.1   Effects of different gray scale representations.   92

4.2   A response curve.   93

4.3   Sigmoid curves as a model for a contrast transfer function.   94

4.4   A clinical example illustrating the importance of windowing.   94

4.5   A screenshot of the effects of windowing in *3DSlicer*.   95

4.6   The shape of an intensity transfer function for windowing.   96

4.7   Effects of windowing a 12 bit image.   97

4.8	Sample intensity histograms.	98
4.9	The output from `LinearIntensityTransform_4.m`.	99
4.10	Three analog photographs taken with different color filters.	100
4.11	The analog B&W photographs from Example 4.5.2 after inversion.	101
4.12	The result of Example 4.5.2, a color composite from B&W photographs.	102
4.13	A screenshot of intensity transfer function manipulation on color images using GIMP.	103
4.14	The output from `LogExample_4.m`.	104
4.15	Non-linear intensity transforms using a Sigmoid-function.	106
4.16	The output from Example 4.16.	107
4.17	A screenshot from *ImageJ*, showing its contrast enhancement functionality.	108
4.18	Contrast enhancement in *ImageJ*.	109
4.19	A well-behaved image from Example 4.16.	110
4.20	An image with a cluttered histogram from Example 4.16.	112
4.21	Linear intensity transforms in ImageJ.	112
4.22	Intensity windowing in ImageJ.	113
5.1	The spherical aberration, an example for aberrations in a suboptimal imaging system.	117
5.2	The spot diagram of a spherical mirror.	117
5.3	Effects of smoothing an image in the spatial domain.	119
5.4	An example of the sharpening operation.	120
5.5	An example of apparent changes in brightness due to convolution.	120
5.6	Numerical differentiation examples of simple functions.	122
5.7	The effect of simple differentiating kernels.	123
5.8	An image after differentiation.	124
5.9	Illustration of four- and eight-connectedness.	125
5.10	Effects of median filtering.	127
5.11	The effects of anisotropic diffusion filtering.	127
5.12	Representation of a vector in Cartesian coordinates.	129
5.13	An illustration on how a change in unit vectors affects the components of a given vector.	130
5.14	Characteristic features of a plane wave.	132
5.15	Representation of numbers in the complex plane.	134
5.16	The principle of the Fourier transform of images with finite size.	135
5.17	A wraparound artifact in MRI.	136
5.18	Motion artifacts in MRI.	138
5.19	The power spectrum of an image.	139
5.20	M13, the globular cluster in Hercules.	140
5.21	The modulation transfer function of a spherical mirror.	141
5.22	Principle of the Hesse normal form.	142
5.23	A simple and classical example for the distance transform.	143

5.24   Output from Example 5.4.1, a lowpass-filtering operation on an image.   144

5.25   Screenshot of ImageJ for basic filtering operations.   145

5.26   Basic filtering operations in ImageJ.   146

5.27   An image after Sobel filtering.   148

5.28   Output from Example 5.4.5 showing the effects of median filtering.   151

5.29   A simple example of frequency filtering.   153

5.30   The spectra of a C major chord played on different instruments.   154

5.31   Frequency filtering effects on a rectangle.   155

5.32   A simple 2D image with defined frequencies.   156

5.33   The result of directional filtering on a 2D image.   157

5.34   An illustrative example for the convolution operation.   159

5.35   Numerical differentiation in k-space.   160

5.36   Frequency filtering on an image.   161

5.37   High-pass filtering of an image.   162

5.38   A typical PSF derived from a MTF.   163

5.39   A sharp Gaussian PSF and the associated MTF.   164

5.40   Effects of convolution in k-space.   164

5.41   Images of a point source from a γ camera at various resolutions.   165

5.42   The MTF of an Anger camera with a resolution of 64 x 64 pixels.   166

5.43   The MTF of an Anger camera with a resolution of 1024 x 1024 pixels.   168

5.44   A binary sample image used for a Hough-transform.   168

5.45   An illustration of the basic principles of the Hough transform.   169

5.46   A representation in Hough-space.   170

5.47   An image after Hough-transform.   172

5.48   A second sample image for the Hough transform.   173

5.49   The result of applying a distance transformation to the outcome of Example 5.4.10.   174

6.1   A segmentation example on a CT slice of the human heart.   179

6.2   Examples of thresholding as a segmentation method.   180

6.3   Segmentation using region growing – an example using GIMP.   181

6.4   Region growing applied to a CT-scan of the heart.   182

6.5   Two CT slices of the aorta in different orientations.   183

6.6   An example of a segmentation algorithm from ITKSnap.   186

6.7   Progress of a level-set segmentation algorithm.   187

6.8   Final segmentation results from ITKSnap.   187

6.9   A simple example of erosion and dilation.   188

6.10   An example for the Hausdorff distance applied to simple graphs.   189

6.11   An illustration of the asymmetric nature of the Hausdorff distance.   189

6.12   ROI example images from a scintigraphic camera.   190

6.13   A sample image from Example 6.8.3, a simple region growing algorithm.   193

6.14 A medical example for segmentation using region growing.   195

6.15 Another medical example for segmentation using region growing.   196

6.16 A binary phantom for 3D-segmentation.   196

6.17 The result of a simple active contours example.   199

6.18 Effects of improving the active contours example from Example 6.8.5.   201

6.19 The effect of a further refinement of the active contours segmentation algorithm in Example 6.8.5.   202

6.20 An illustration for an active contour segmentation example.   203

6.21 The result from Example 6.8.6, an implementation of erosion.   204

6.22 An x-ray of a pelvis during brachytherapy.   206

6.23 Various segmentation efforts on an x-ray image using simple thresholding.   207

6.24 Several preprocessing steps prior to segmentation in Example 6.8.8.1.   208

6.25 The output from Example 6.8.8.1.   209

6.26 Segmentation of structures in Example 6.8.8.1 using region growing.   210

6.27 Preprocessing steps for Example 6.8.8.2.   210

6.28 The enhanced CT-slice for segmentation from Example 6.8.8.2.   211

6.29 The result of Example 6.8.8.2.   212

6.30 A manual segmentation effort on an MR slice.   213

7.1   An interpolation example on a PET image.   216

7.2   A grid for bilinear intensity interpolation.   217

7.3   A grid for trilinear intensity interpolation.   218

7.4   Various types of interpolation.   219

7.5   An illustration of non-commutative spatial transforms.   221

7.6   The principle of the PCA transform.   226

7.7   An example of curved reformatting from dentistry.   229

7.8   An optical tracking system.   232

7.9   An electromagnetic tracking system.   232

7.10 A passive tool for an optical tracking system.   233

7.11 An image-guided surgery system.   234

7.12 A result from Example 7.6.1 – the rotation of 2D images.   235

7.13 Effects of changing the center of rotation in Example 7.6.1.   236

7.14 The result of NNInterpolation_7.m.   237

7.15 The output of the BiLinearInterpolation_7.m script.   239

7.16 A demonstration of the PCA on binary images.   240

7.17 The result of Example 7.6.3, the principal axes transform.   243

7.18 A few results of reformatting a 3D cone.   246

7.19 Three sample slices in original axial orientation from the CT-dataset used in Example 7.6.5.   247

7.20 A set of orthogonally reformatted slices from the pigBig.img CT dataset.   248

7.21 An oblique reformatting of the volume generated by ThreeDConvolutionBig_7.m.   250

8.1	The principle of raycasting without perspective.	254
8.2	The principle of raycasting with perspective.	255
8.3	An example of maximum intensity projection.	255
8.4	An example of summed voxel rendering.	256
8.5	An example of volume compositing.	257
8.6	A transfer function for volume compositing.	258
8.7	An example of depth shading.	259
8.8	An example of surface shading.	259
8.9	The principle of computing gradients for surface shading.	261
8.10	A comparison of rendered voxel surfaces and triangulated models.	262
8.11	A screenshot from a software for simulating long bone fractures.	264
8.12	The basic setup of the marching squares algorithm.	265
8.13	Two out of 15 possible configurations of the marching cubes algorithm.	265
8.14	The principle of Gouraud-shading.	267
8.15	A virtual endoscopy of the spinal canal.	268
8.16	The effects of perspective projection on a simple geometric shape.	270
8.17	Output from Example 8.5.2, a simple raycasting algorithm.	271
8.18	Output from Example 8.5.2.	273
8.19	A summed voxel rendering from Example 8.5.2.	273
8.20	Output from Example 8.5.3, a perspective splat rendering.	276
8.21	A perspective DRR.	277
8.22	A color-coded volume rendering.	279
8.23	A depth shading generated by a splat rendering algorithm.	282
8.24	A depth shading following the inverse square law.	282
8.25	A surface plot of an intermediate result from Example 8.5.6.	284
8.26	The result from Example 8.5.6, a surface rendering algorithm.	286
8.27	More results from Example 8.5.6.	287
8.28	Screenshot for downloading sample data for 3DSlicer.	288
8.29	Menu settings for rendering using 3DSlicer.	288
8.30	A volume rendering using 3DSlicer.	289
8.31	Another example of volume rendering using 3DSlicer.	289
8.32	A result from the `Triangulation_8.m` example, rendered in Paraview.	292
8.33	A better surface model, also rendered in Paraview.	293
8.34	Modified depth shadings for improved surface rendering in Example 8.5.9.	294
8.35	Surface rendering with additional shading effects.	295
9.1	A sample image from PET-CT.	298
9.2	An example of unregistered CT and MR slices.	299
9.3	A screenshot of the registration tool in AnalyzeAVW.	300
9.4	The volume transformation matrix as derived by the AnalyzeAVW registration tool.	301

9.5	The principle of comparing gray values in registration merit functions.	303
9.6	An intramodal example of joint histograms.	305
9.7	Histograms for two random variables.	306
9.8	A surface plot of joint histograms.	306
9.9	An intermodal example of joint histograms.	307
9.10	A second intermodal example of joint histograms.	308
9.11	A plot of Shannon's entropy from a registration example.	309
9.12	A plot of the mutual information merit function.	310
9.13	An example of PET-MR registration.	311
9.14	An edge representation of co-registered slices.	311
9.15	The distance transform of an MR image from Example 9.9.4.	312
9.16	The resulting merit function plots from Example 9.9.4.	312
9.17	A simple illustration of the Nelder-Mead algorithm.	314
9.18	An illustration of the camera calibration problem.	317
9.19	The Vogele-Bale-Hohner mouthpiece, a device for non-invasive registration using fiducial markers.	320
9.20	Three images of a spine reference-dataset for 2D/3D image registration.	322
9.21	The output of Example 9.9.1, a computation of the cross-correlation merit function during image rotation.	325
9.22	Two sample outputs from modified versions of More2DRegistration_9.m.	325
9.23	Three sample images used in the practical lessons.	326
9.24	Two simple functions to be optimized in Example 9.9.5.	331
9.25	The result of a local optimization in dependence of the starting value.	332
9.26	The result of a local optimization using a different implementation.	332
9.27	The result of a local optimization in dependence of the starting value for an inverse rect-function.	333
10.1	Principle of a parallel beam CT.	341
10.2	Normal form of a line.	341
10.3	Simple Radon transform examples.	343
10.4	Image discretization.	344
10.5	Rotation of an image after discretization.	344
10.6	Radon transform of the Shepp and Logan phantom.	345
10.7	Rotation by nearest neighbor interpolation.	347
10.8	Shape of a system matrix.	348
10.9	Orthogonal projection to a subspace.	349
10.10	Kaczmarz algorithm.	350
10.11	Minimal distance of a point to a plane.	351
10.12	Algebraic reconstructed Shepp and Logan phantom.	352
10.13	Filtering using the Fourier transform.	353
10.14	Projection slice theorem.	355
10.15	Backprojection.	357

10.16	Filtered Radon transform of a square.	359
10.17	Filtered backprojection examples.	359
10.18	Mesh of a filtered backprojection.	359
10.19	Simple backprojection.	360
10.20	Simple backprojection.	361
10.21	Simple and filtered backprojection.	361
10.22	Backprojection using the Hann filter.	362
10.23	Ring artifact.	364
10.24	Finding the ring artifact.	364
10.25	Streak artifact.	365
10.26	Several backprojections from a simple implementation of the Feldkamp-CBCT reconstruction algorithm.	366
10.27	Cone Beam Projection	367
11.1	The pinhole camera model.	372
11.2	Central projection.	373
11.3	Planar homography.	374
11.4	Calibration phantom for x-ray.	376
11.5	Software architecture for hands-on IGI tutorial.	380
11.6	Patterns for camera calibration and our LEGO^{TM} phantom.	381
11.7	Camera calibration application.	392
11.8	Tracked tool and pivot calibration application.	392
11.9	Procedure planning steps.	392
11.10	Identification of registration fiducials in image and physical spaces.	393
11.11	Navigation: physical setup and display.	393
11.12	Tracking accuracy evaluation.	393
11.13	Human computer interaction devices.	394
11.14	Remote control application.	394
11.15	Nearly collinear fiducial configuration, physical setup and display.	395
11.16	FRE and TRE are uncorrelated.	395
11.17	Point clouds for ICP registration.	396
A.1	The output of a C++ example program.	413

List of Tables

1.1 T_1 and T_2 constants in ms for various tissues for B=1 Tesla. Data from W.R. Hendee: Medical Imaging Physics, Wiley, 2002.   22

1.2   Quality factors of different radiation types in regard to radiation protection. The factors are due to interpret in the way that 1 Gy of α-radiation equals 20 Gy of γ-radiation with respect to its biological effects.   40

1.3   Symptoms from deterministic damage after whole body exposure with photons (q-factor 1).   42

1.4   Some examples of radiation exposures.   42

1.5   Some examples of x-ray exposures.   43

4.1   Typical Hounsfield units of some materials and tissue types. Data are taken from A. Oppelt (ed.): Imaging Systems for Medical Diagnostics, Wiley VCH, (2006).   95

9.1   The 2 x 2 table for our simple example of girls and boys, drinking beer or milk. The central part of this table is a joint histogram of the two properties, similar to the Figures 9.6, 9.8 and 9.9. Later in this chapter, we will illustrate the concept of "disorder" (or *entropy*) using this example.   306

9.2   An alternative 2 x 2 table for beer- or milk-drinking girls and boys. While the total numbers stay the same, this distribution shows lesser disorder since we can make quite likely conclusions about the other property from a given property.   308

11.1   Iterative Closest Point algorithm.   389

Supplementary Resources Disclaimer

Additional resources were previously made available for this title on CD. However, as CD has become a less accessible format, all resources have been moved to a more convenient online download option.

You can find these resources available here: www.routledge.com/9781466555570

Please note: Where this title mentions the associated disc, please use the downloadable resources instead.

Foreword

Applied Medical Image Processing: A Basic Course is a superbly measured introduction to the field of medical imaging. Albert Einstein is purported to have said "The grand aim of all science is to cover the greatest number of empirical facts by logical deduction from the smallest number of hypotheses and axioms". I think Einstein might have been pleased with this wonderful work by Wolfgang Birkfellner (with contributions by Michael Figl and Johann Hummel) who have adroitly tackled the challenge of "less is more" with their basic course on medical image processing. This author is intimately familiar with such a challenge, having published two similar books. As with those works, these authors have attempted to find the elusive compromise between sufficient detail and simple formulations to produce a useful reference in the field that will stand the test of time. I believe this work will meet that test.

The discipline of modern medical imaging is really quite young, having its landmark launch in the early 1970s with the development of CT scanning. With that advent, imaging became fully digital, and three-dimensional. This heralded a rich future for imaging in the healthcare industry facilitated by computers. Computers are so embedded in medical imaging that we have lost sight of them as the enabling technology which has made multi-modality, multi-dimensional, multi-faceted medical imaging possible to do and, indeed, impossible to be without. The roots of this remarkable revolution remain important. A basic understanding of the fundamental principles, tenets and concepts underlying modern medical imaging is critically important in order to advance and realize its full future potential.

That is why this book is significant and timely. It provides a cogent, not overly simplified, not excessively mathematical treatise of basic principles that the student, trainee, young scientist, and junior practitioner can readily grasp and apply. Such empowerment will inevitably lead to advancing the state of the art in medical imaging science. This will be the opportunity presented to those students whose college or university professors select this book as a basic text in their imaging courses. It will enable the diligent student who studies and peruses it to implement the principles and concepts outlined. It will permit him or her to become an active participant, contributor and perhaps even a "new Godfrey Hounsfield".[1]

The authors, based on their personal experience, have established the goal for this introductory volume to teach undergraduate and first year Ph.D. students what they need to know in order to consider and pursue a career in medical imaging, or at least to work productively with those who do. They address four specific aims to achieve this goal:

> produce an essential overview of relevant basic methods in applied medical image processing (the emphasis is on "applied", suggesting the underlying goal that the outcome have practical, useful consequences);

---

[1]Godfrey Hounsfield was a Nobel prize winner in medicine for his invention of the first CT scanner.

little prior knowledge beyond basic scientific principles is required to grasp the concepts and methods of the work;

promote hands-on learning by providing working programs that demonstrate algorithms and methods rather than mere recital of the theoretical and sometimes complex mathematical underpinnings of these capabilities; and

learning would not be constrained by need for or access to expensive software or sophisticated programming capabilities.

This latter aim is admirably met by providing in the book more than 70 scripts and examples of algorithmic code to be developed, tested, applied and learned by the student using readily available software. The extrapolation from fundamental theory and concepts to working testable code will make the learning experience satisfying and the acquired domain knowledge enduring.

The chapters in the book provide a logical, necessary and quite sufficient coverage of the basics in medical image processing. They include cogent treatments of image acquisition from multiple sources, various image formats and representations, basic image intensity-based transforms, elegant image filtering transforms, image segmentation methods (arguably one of the most challenging, complex, and important capabilities needed in medical image processing), image registration methods (to bring multi-modal images into coherent spatial alignment), rendering and surface modeling approaches to object visualization, and finally (a circular return to the beginning chapter) the closing chapter on CT reconstruction, the same basic principles used by Godfrey Hounsfield over 40 years ago to launch the era of 3D digital imaging of which this book speaks. Throughout this sequence of chapters, the references to prior relevant work, the images used to demonstrate principles and applications, and the clarity of explanation generously included throughout the text, make the learning experience not only memorable, but enjoyable.

This reviewer thinks that the authors of *Applied Medical Image Processing: A Basic Course* should be proud of their work, and derive satisfaction from its publication. It will help facilitate the ongoing, almost magical evolution of modern medical imaging. It will ground the young scientists, engineers and physicians engaged in the field with a solid foundation from which to launch their aspirations to forge and shape the promising future. I believe the book will find its way into the curriculum of science and engineering departments in reputable college undergraduate programs and in seminal university graduate programs. In addition to the matriculated students and learners, other beneficiaries will be faculty and practicing professionals who may use it as a refresher course, returning them to the basics in order to soundly develop new approaches and advances. They, like the great artist Henri Matisse, will be driven to say "I want to reach a point of condensation of sensations to make a picture". I add that they who read this book will be able to make "a truly useful picture".

Richard A. Robb, Ph.D.
Scheller Professor in Medical Research
Professor of Biophysics and Computer Science
Mayo Clinic College of Medicine

Preface to the First Edition

Given the rapid evolution of radiological imaging in the past four decades, medical image processing nowadays is an essential tool for clinical research. Applications range from research in neuroscience, biomechanics and biomedical engineering to clinical routine tasks such as the visualization of huge datasets provided by modern computed tomography systems in radiology, the manufacturing of patient-specific prostheses for orthopedic surgery, the precise planning of dose distributions in radiation oncology, the fusion of multimodal image data for therapy monitoring in internal medicine, and computer-aided neurosurgical interventions.

For more than a decade, we have been working as scientists in this vital field of research at various institutions and hospitals; and still, it is a fascinating subject. We have also taught the subject of medical image processing to undergraduate and graduate students of medical physics, biomedical engineering, medicine and computer science; our audience usually also was at least interested and some students even shared our sense of fascination.

However, besides our own enthusiasm, we always felt a little bit unsatisfied with the available textbooks on the subject of medical image processing. Some of them we found very formal, others were discontinuous due to the fact that they were written by a multitude of authors; some are not very useful as an introduction since they are too specialized, and a few are of little use at all.

On the other hand, there are a number of good introductions to image processing in general, but the requirements of the medical community differ in some important aspects; above all, we do not deal with images in a common sense since most of our imaging machines acquire their data outside the visual spectrum. Furthermore, many modern imaging methods are three-dimensional. The problems of handling voxels and 3D datasets, spatial transforms in 3D, and data fusion are usually not being dealt with to a sufficient extent in these works.

Based on our own experience, we came to the conclusion that an introductory textbook for undergraduate and first year Ph.D. students should have the following features:

It should give an overview of the relevant basic methods in applied medical image processing.

It should assume little prior knowledge beyond basic applied mathematics, physics and programming.

It should be tangible; rather than giving theoretic derivations, it would be nice to demonstrate how things work in real life.

It should be accessible. The use of expensive software or highly sophisticated programming techniques is to be avoided.

You hold the outcome of such an effort in your hands. Whether we met our own demands is to be judged by you. If you find errors – quite likely, there are a number of them – or if you have suggestions for improvement, we would be grateful if you would point those out to us. Have fun!

Wolfgang Birkfellner, Michael Figl, and Johann Hummel

Preface to the Second Edition

Four years after completing the first edition of our textbook, which resulted from a series of lectures given by us in courses at the Medical University of Vienna as well as other institutions, we now present a second edition of our work. The general outline and the topics of the book have stayed the same, but with growing experience in using the teaching materials presented here, we felt that a little update would be warranted. We've come up with a few additional MATLAB® examples, for instance on using color (Examples 4.5.2 and 8.5.4), on advanced histogram-based image intensity operations (Example 4.5.6), on signal processing using Fourier series (Example 5.4.6.2) and on cone beam computed tomography reconstruction (Example 10.6.5).

Beyond that, we have added a few examples where two popular, freely available 2D and 3D image processing programs, *ImageJ*[2] and *3D Slicer*[3] are used to illustrate how the algorithms and methods discussed are used in "real" software – Examples 3.7.3, 4.5.7, 5.4.2 and 8.5.7 are the result of this effort.

Aside from additional examples and various changes in the text, which mainly give additional illustrative examples and clarifications, we have also written two new chapters for this edition. Chapter 2 was added to give a connection between the algorithms and methods presented and the application of these methods in clinical software from radiology, nuclear medicine and radiotherapy. And our friends Özgür Güler and Ziv Yaniv were kind enough to add Chapter 11 – an image-guided therapy tutorial that allows for 3D tracking of a stylus using a webcam and for "image-guided surgery" on a widely available "patient". We are proud to have this exceptional piece of work in this textbook now, and we strongly encourage all readers and lecturers to utilize this work in class since it builds on many of the techniques introduced in the book and gives an excellent illustrative hands-on example.

Other additional efforts are more of an administrative nature, but we hope that these increase the usefulness of the book as well – above all, we have now named the JPEG images of the illustrations, which are found on the book's website at www.crcpress.com under supplementary materials in the folder "JPGs", in the same fashion as in the text. Lecturers may feel free to use these images in their presentations, and now it should be easier to assign these images to corresponding parts of the text.

Since a few more color images became necessary, we have also added a special folder "ColorImages" which holds these illustrations while they are still in grayscale in the book in order to keep the total cost of the volume to reasonable limits.

We were happy to see that the first edition of our textbook was well accepted, and we wish to thank you – the students and lecturers using this volume – for your support. We

---

[2]Available at the time of printing from http://rsbweb.nih.gov/ij/ for all major platforms.
[3]See http://www.slicer.org/.

hope that the second edition continues to serve the purpose of providing a basic introduction to the world of medical image processing.

Wolfgang Birkfellner, Michael Figl, and Johann Hummel

MATLAB® is registered trademark of The MathWorks, Inc. For product information, please contact:

The MathWorks, Inc.
3 Apple Hill Drive
Natick, MA 01760-2098 USA
Tel: 508 647 7000
Fax: 508-647-7001
E-mail: info@mathworks.com
Web: www.mathworks.com

User Guide

This is an introductory book for those who want to learn about the inner mechanics of medical image processing algorithms. Most likely, the course is not suitable for those who are interested in simply using available medical image processing software. An appropriate reference for this audience is given at the end of this section.

We have organized the course in such a manner that it gives an overview of the physics of medical imaging, which is followed by eight chapters that cover the most important aspects of medical image processing, from image file formats to reconstruction of volumetric images from projection data. Each chapter contains a rather short introduction of the basic concepts and several simple scripts for the Mathworks MATLAB® programming environment (`http://www.mathworks.com`). MATLAB is an interpreted environment for matrix computations, and does not require sophisticated programming skills.

All scripts provided on the accompanying CD were tested using MATLAB 7.7.0 (R2008b) under Microsoft Windows XP and Ubuntu 9.04 Linux. Furthermore, we made sure that all scripts also work with Octave, a freely available MATLAB clone that can be downloaded from `http://www.octave.org`. The scripts were therefore also tested using Octave 3.0.5 under various Linux brands and Microsoft Windows XP. A few tests were also successfully carried out with MATLAB under MacOS X. Some simple 2D image processing tasks are also demonstrated using the freely available GNU image manipulation program GIMP (`http://www.gimp.org`), although commercial programs such as Adobe Photoshop may be used as well. Furthermore, a number of image examples were made using the commercially available AnalyzeAVW software – however, AnalyzeAVW is not required to work with this volume. Public domain software – namely Octave and GIMP, which are both available for Microsoft Windows and Linux operation systems – is all you need. In a few examples, 3DSlicer and ImageJ, two more programs also available in the public domain, are used as well.

To a large extent, we have avoided the excessive use of mathematical formalisms, although a working knowledge of engineering mathematics, especially numerical mathematics and linear algebra, is inevitable. The other prerequisite is some knowledge of basic physics and a little bit of experience in programming, although the scripts are kept very simple. Furthermore, it is inevitable to have some knowledge about basic anatomy and medical terminology if one wants to start a career in medical imaging.

Furthermore, we have also abdicated the use of good MATLAB programming manners for the sake of simplicity, and we do only use very basic functionality of the MATLAB environment.[4] Above all, we do *not* use the *Image Processing Toolbox* of MATLAB. All algorithms are implemented from scratch. Good MATLAB programming would require the use of fast internal procedures and vector notations for optimum performance in such an interpreted environment. For instance, the use of multiple `for` loops, which you will encounter very often in this volume, is a classic example of bad MATLAB programming. Using such a structure in favor of the MATLAB specific vector notation tends to slow down the code. On the other hand, we wanted to keep our code as simple and readable as

---

[4] An exception is seen in Examples 9.9.5 and 9.9.6, where some functions from the Optimization Toolbox of MATLAB are used.

possible, and therefore we had to make a compromise here. The advantage of this approach lies in the fact that the resulting code is easy to understand, even for students not familiar with MATLAB. Basically speaking, it is more or less so-called *pseudo code*; for some arcane reason, this pseudo code works under MATLAB and Octave. If you are interested in proper MATLAB programming (which unfortunately is of limited use in medical imaging because of the sheer size of modern 3D datasets) you may resort to some of the references given below.

Since we have had the experience that experimenting with small code snippets is a more efficient approach to teaching the details of medical image processing compared to lengthy explanations, we have provided more than 70 MATLAB scripts illustrating the algorithms presented in a simple and straightforward manner. You can find those scripts, together with the associated images, in the `LessonData` folder on the accompanying CD. Working with those lectures and the associated additional tasks is a crucial part of studying this volume. Each script is well documented within the volume.

If the course is to be used in class, one may also use the illustrations from the book, which are provided separately on the CD in a folder `JPGs` – some of them in color, whereas they are printed in grayscale. We have to point out that the algorithms are provided for teaching purposes only. They are not suitable for clinical work; all datasets were completely anonymized, and while the illustrations are made by us, we have indicated the source of the image data in the text where applicable.

LITERATURE

S. Attaway: MATLAB: A Practical Introduction to Programming and Problem Solving, Butterworth-Heinemann, (2009)

G. Dougherty: Digital Image Processing for Medical Applications, Cambridge University Press, (2009)

E. Berry: A Practical Approach to Medical Image Processing, Taylor & Francis, (2007)

Acknowledgments

Many people have contributed to this volume; first of all, I have to thank my co-authors Michael Figl and Johann Hummel, not only for their contribution but also for their critical comments, their review work and for being colleagues for quite a while by now. In the preparatory phase, Leo Joskowicz, Terry Peters, Georg Langs, Julia Schnabel, Olivier Clatz and Stefan Vanderberghe gave very valuable input. Richard Robb provides us with Analyze AVW, which is an inevitable tool in our research work, and he kindly also wrote the foreword – for both, I am grateful. Franz Kainberger, Sonja Plischke, André Gahleitner, Stephan Gruber and Christian Herold (Department of Radiology, Medical University Vienna), Peter Schaffarich (Department of Nuclear Medicine, Medical University Vienna), Dietmar Georg, Markus Stock and Richard Pötter (Department of Radiotherapy, Medical University Vienna), Peter Homolka, Wolfgang Drexler and Helmar Bergmann (Center for Medical Physics and Biomedical Engineering, Medical University Vienna), Claudia Kuntner (AIT Seibersdorf, Austria) and Ziv Yaniv (ISIS Center, Department of Radiology, Georgetown University) provided some of the image data used, or gave their kind permission to do so.

Among those who took the great challenge of proofreading are Helmar Bergmann, Martin Meyerspeer, Peter Homolka, Stefan Witoszynskyi, Rene Donner, Michael Figl, Christelle Gendrin, Christoph Bloch, Daniella Fabri, Rudolf Pfeiffer, Christoph Weber, Supriyanto Ardjo Pawiro, Jakob Spoerk, Begoña Fuentes, Dieter Hönigmann and Ziv Yaniv. Thomas Fahrner deserves a special mentioning – he not only did the proofreading but also tested all scripts on two environments and two operating systems in a painstaking manner. Luna Han, Jill Jurgensen and David Fausel from Taylor & Francis provided all the support we needed from our publisher.

And I have to mention my colleagues at the Center for Medical Physics and Biomedical Engineering for all their support, as well as my students at the Medical University Vienna and the Universities of Applied Sciences Technikum Vienna and Wiener Neustadt for bearing the lectures that finally evolved in this volume. Finally, my university, the Medical University Vienna, gives me the possibility to work as a researcher and academic teacher in the exciting field of medical image processing. Many thanks to all of you, and to all of those that I may have forgotten unintentionally.

Wolfgang Birkfellner
Center for Medical Physics and Biomedical Engineering
Medical University Vienna

CHAPTER 1

A Few Basics of Medical Image Sources

Johann Hummel

CONTENTS

1.1	Radiology	2
1.2	The electromagnetic spectrum	2
1.3	Basic x-ray physics	3
	1.3.1 The x-ray tube	4
	1.3.2 X-ray detectors	6
1.4	Attenuation and imaging	7
1.5	Computed tomography	10
	1.5.1 Basics of CT and scanner generations	10
	1.5.2 Imaging geometries and CT technologies	12
	1.5.3 Image artifacts in CT	15
	1.5.4 Safety aspects	16
1.6	Magnetic resonance tomography	17
	1.6.1 Basic MRI physics	17
	1.6.1.1 Relaxation processes	20
	1.6.1.2 Spin-echo	22
	1.6.2 Tissue contrast	23
	1.6.3 Spatial localization	23
	1.6.3.1 Slice selection	24
	1.6.3.2 Frequency encoding	24
	1.6.3.3 Phase encoding	24
	1.6.4 Image artifacts in MR	25
	1.6.5 The elements of an MR system	27
	1.6.5.1 The main static magnetic field	27
	1.6.5.2 Gradient fields	27
	1.6.5.3 The RF system	27
	1.6.6 Safety aspects	27
1.7	Ultrasound	28
	1.7.1 Some physical properties of sound	28
	1.7.2 Basic principles	29
	1.7.3 Image artifacts in B-Mode US imaging	30
	1.7.4 Doppler effect	30
	1.7.5 3D imaging	31

	1.7.6	Safety aspects	32
1.8		Nuclear medicine and molecular imaging	33
	1.8.1	Scintigraphy	33
	1.8.2	The γ camera	34
	1.8.3	SPECT and PET	34
1.9		Other imaging techniques	36
1.10		Radiation protection and dosimetry	39
	1.10.1	Terminology of dosimetry	39
	1.10.2	Radiation effects on tissue and organs	40
	1.10.3	Natural and man-made radiation exposure	42
1.11		Summary and further references	43

1.1 RADIOLOGY

Medical imaging plays a crucial role in modern medicine and image data are found in a wide variety of clinical specialties. Planar x-ray and fluoroscopy data are acquired for routine diagnostics in chest imaging, for guidance and diagnosis in cardiac interventions, and for monitoring intraoperative progress during surgical procedures. Computed x-ray tomography and magnetic resonance imaging, both being 3D imaging modalities, are among the most important diagnostic tools in hospitals around the world. Ultrasound and endoscopy provide direct insight into the body in real-time, and nuclear medicine allows to monitor function and metabolism where pathological changes in anatomy are not yet visible. Besides the broad impact of radiological techniques in diagnosis and therapy, molecular imaging – an umbrella term for a number of imaging methods – has become a vital tool in basic biomedical research and drug development. This course introduces the basic techniques for handling those images. Some knowledge about the basic physics of the imaging modalities used is nevertheless inevitable. In this chapter, an overview of radiological imaging physics is given. You may use this chapter as a refresher, or as a starting point for more intense studies in medical imaging physics.

1.2 THE ELECTROMAGNETIC SPECTRUM

Most images encountered in clinical medicine are generated by recording the physical properties of tissue when being exposed to a certain type of electromagnetic radiation or – in the case of ultrasound – mechanical excitation. Electromagnetic radiation consists of quantum objects, so called *photons*. The energy of a photon is given by the following formula:

$$E = h\nu[\text{J}] \tag{1.1}$$

where h is *Planck's constant*, given as $6.626 * 10^{-34}$Js. The unit is *Joleseconds* – the product of energy and time, which is the physical quantity of *Action*. ν is the frequency of the photon – that is the number of oscillations of a wave per second, and its unit is *Hertz*. It is also equivalent to the reciprocal value of time: $1\text{Hz} = \frac{1}{\text{s}}$. The product of action and frequency is therefore an energy: $\frac{\text{Js}}{\text{s}} = \text{J}$. We can grossly classify different types of electromagnetic radiation by its frequencies:

$1 - 10^4$Hz: Alternating current (AC) is used only for *electrical impedance tomography*, a rather exotic medical imaging technique.

$10^4 - 10^8$Hz: Radiofrequency is used not only for broadcasting but also in *magnetic resonance imaging* (MRI), a widespread imaging technology for acquiring 3D volume data of excellent soft tissue contrast.

$10^8 - 10^{12}$Hz: Microwaves, well known by connoisseurs of unhealthy food, do not play a major role in medical imaging.

$10^{12} - 7 * 10^{14}$Hz: Infrared, invisible to the human eye but perceived as heat, is used in some medical applications like *near infrared imaging*.

$4.6 * 10^{14} - 6.6 * 10^{14}$Hz: The rather narrow spectrum of visible light, the one part of the electromagnetic spectrum most important to man. Used for *light microscopy* and *histological imaging*, *endoscopy*, and *optical coherence tomography* (OCT) in medical imaging.

$4 * 10^{14} - 10^{18}$Hz: Ultraviolet (UV) radiation plays a role in *fluorescence imaging*. Even more important is the fact that from this frequency domain onward, the photons have sufficient energy to *ionize* molecules. It is therefore possible to damage biological tissue by removing electrons from molecules, thus changing the chemical properties of matter. The energy per mass deployed by ionizing radiation is called a *dose*.

$10^{18} - 10^{20}$Hz: X-rays are possibly the most important type of radiation for medical imaging.

Beyond 10^{20}Hz: γ-radiation is usually a product of radioactive decay. Since γ radiation may penetrate tissue easily, it is widely used for diagnostic purposes in nuclear medicine (namely *scintigraphy*, *single photon emission computed tomography* – SPECT, and *positron emission tomography* – PET). These high energy photons are also used for therapeutic purposes in radiation therapy, where malignant tissue is destroyed by a focused deployment of high dose in the tumor. The treatment beam of this *linear accelerator* (LINAC) can also be used for imaging by means of so called *electronic portal imaging devices* (EPIDs).

As we can see, medical imaging devices use a large part of the electromagnetic spectrum; since the mechanisms of tissue interaction with electromagnetic radiation are different, these machines deliver different information which may be used for diagnostic and therapeutic purposes. The only widespread imaging modality that relies on a completely different principle is, as already mentioned, *ultrasound*. In the following chapter, we will briefly discuss the most important medical imaging technologies.

1.3 BASIC X-RAY PHYSICS

X-rays are generated when fast electrons interact with metal objects. The kinetic energy of an electron acquired during acceleration by a high voltage is partially transformed into electromagnetic energy. X-ray machines provide a large number of electrons focused on a small spot (called the *focal spot*) in a metallic material, the *anode*. As the kinetic energy of the electrons is increased, both the intensity (that is, the number of x-ray photons) and the energy (which is related to the ability of the x-ray to penetrate tissue and solid materials) of the radiation are increased as well. Generally, more than 99% of the kinetic energy of the electrons is converted to heat, leaving less than 1% available for the production of x-radiation. The x-ray spectrum consists of two types of radiation:

Characteristic x-radiation is generated when the incoming electron interacts with an electron of the target atom located at an inner orbital. If the kinetic energy is sufficient to ionize the target atom by removing the inner electron characteristic x-radiation may result.

If a fast electron interacts with the nucleus of a target atom, *Bremsstrahlung* is created. In this type of interaction, the kinetic energy of the electron is converted to electromagnetic energy. An electron that avoids the orbital electrons while passing an atom of the target material may come sufficiently close to the nucleus for interaction. As it passes the nucleus, it is slowed down and deviated from its course, leaving with reduced kinetic energy in a different direction. This loss in kinetic energy reappears as an x-ray photon. These types of x-rays are called Bremsstrahlung radiation, or Bremsstrahlung x-rays.[1] As opposed to characteristic radiation, its energy distribution is continuous. Figure 1.1 shows the general shape of an x-ray spectrum.

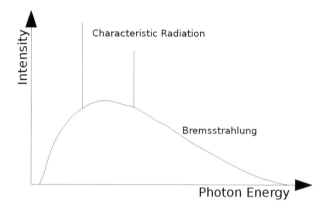

FIGURE 1.1: The shape of a typical x-ray spectrum. The lowest energy available is limited by self absorption of the anode and intentionally added metal filters. The upper end of the spectrum is reached if all the energy of one single electron is converted to a single x-ray photon. The sharp peaks correspond to the characteristic radiation; they are defined by the energy levels in the orbitals of the atom. The continuous part of the spectrum stems from the Bremsstrahlung.

1.3.1 The x-ray tube

Figure 1.2 shows the design principle of an x-ray tube. It consists of a vacuum tube, the cathode for electron creation and focusing, and the target anode. The cathode is composed of one or more electron emitting heated filaments and an auxiliary electrode, the so-called *Wehnelt electrode* or *focusing cup*. The task of the heated filament electrode is to generate free electrons. Electrons in metal can move freely between atomic cores in the lattice. If the

---

[1]Bremsstrahlung is the German word for "braking radiation"; Bremsstrahlung can be considered radiation resulting from the deceleration of fast electrons by the nucleus.

temperature in the metal exceeds a certain point, the electrons may gain enough energy to leave the compound of atomic cores. Besides the geometry and the material used for the heated filament, the number of emitted electrons depends on temperature. In operating mode a temperature of about 2700 K is necessary. At this temperature one may also observe evaporation of the cathode material. For this reason the cathode is heated only for the short exposure time of the x-ray image. The electrons released from the heated filament are accelerated towards the anode by high voltage called the *tube potential*. The focusing of this current of free electrons to a small focal spot at the anode is the task of the Wehnelt electrode. The area of the anode where the accelerated and focused electrons impact determines the structure and dimension of the electronic focal spot. Since the anode heats up in this process, most x-ray tubes have a rotating anode so that the thermal energy deployed at the focal spot is distributed.

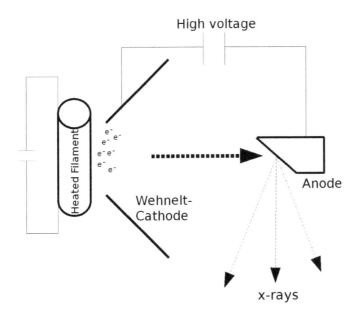

FIGURE 1.2: The principle of an x-ray tube. A high current heats up the hot cathode; electrons (marked as e⁻ in the sketch) gain enough energy to leave the lattice of the conductive material of the heated filament and are freely available within the evacuated x-ray tube. A second voltage supply accelerates the electrons away from the heated filament towards the anode, where the kinetic energy of the electrons is converted to electromagnetic radiation – the x-ray photons. The number of electrons available is controlled by the current supplied to the heated filament. The energy of the photons is governed by the voltage between the anode and the cathode.

As already mentioned in Figure 1.1, the shape of the x-ray spectrum is defined by the energy of the electrons and the anode material. The two quantities defining the quality and intensity of the radiation are the number of electrons from the heated filament and the *voltage* used for acceleration. These are usually given in units of milliampereseconds [mAs] and kilovolts [kV]. Since current is defined as the number of charge carriers per second, mAs simply give a measure of the electrons impinging on the anode. Each of those electrons is accelerated by the high voltage given in kV, which is directly proportional to the energy of this electron.

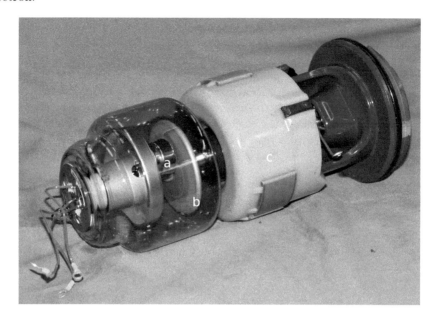

FIGURE 1.3: An x-ray tube. **a** marks the Wehnelt-electrode, which also contains the heated filament. **b** is the anode. The path of the focal spot on this rotating anode is clearly visible. **c** is the drive for the rotating anode. Image courtesy of P. Homolka and A. Taubeck, Center for Medical Physics and Biomedical Engineering, Medical University Vienna.

1.3.2 X-ray detectors

Detectors for x-rays can be classified as *direct* and *indirect* detectors or *analog* and *digital* detectors. Direct detectors measure the electrical charge that results from the ionization of the atoms in the detector. Indirect systems are scintillator based. The x-rays interact with luminescent materials; these emit light in or near the visible range when being hit by an x-ray photon. These converted light photons are then routed to a photodetector which records the pattern as an image. Analog detectors cover the "classical" way of imaging such as *radiographic film*, *intensifier screens* and *computed radiographic plates* (CR plates). Only the first of these three works as a direct system; the latter two are indirect systems.

Radiographic film consists of a polyester layer that is laminated on one or both sides with photographic emulsion. This emulsion contains light sensitive silver halides. Many types of film/developer combinations differing in contrast, density, noise and spectral sensitivity exist. The right choice depends on the particular application.

Intensifier screens consist of a luminescent layer that is coated on a polyester sublayer. The luminescent substance converts x-rays into light. Therefore, the film or CR plate – embedded between two intensifier screens – is also exposed by luminescence light. This concept was first invented by T. A. Edison in 1896 and reduces the necessary dose significantly.

Computed radiographic plates: The physical principle of CR plates is similar to intensifier screens. The main difference is based on the emission of light which does not only occur immediately after exposure with x-rays. Rather, the energy from the x-rays excites electrons to higher energy levels in the lattice of the CR plate where they are stored as a latent image. These levels are called *traps*. For readout of the latent image, the CR plate is excited linewise by a laser beam. The laser light frees the stored energy producing *stimulated luminescence*. The emitted light is detected by means of an electronic detector. In the following, the resultant signal is amplified and converted to digital numbers. The great advantage of this technology is the fact that CR plates can be reused. However, not all electrons are read out at once; therefore, the plates must be erased by intense light before they can be exposed again.

Indirect flat panels: These detectors are built up by a layer of *cesium iodide*, a *scintillator* which emits light when being hit by an x-ray photon.

Direct flat panels: Here, in contrast to conventional technologies, x-rays are not converted into visible light but directly into an electrical signal. Instead of a scintillator, *amorphous non-crystalline selenium* is used here. The surface of the selenium layer is charged before the exposure. Then x-rays release charge carriers in the layer which dissipate the surface charge and leave an image of the remaining charge pattern. Capacitors assigned to each pixel store the charge which is then read out by means of a *thin film transistor* (TFT) matrix. Therefore, the resolution of the image only depends on the assembly of the detector. The amount of stored charge per pixel is directly proportional to the incident radiation.

The characteristic measure giving the efficacy of a detector is its *detector quantum efficiency* (DQE); it is the ratio of photons imparted to the detector versus the number of photons counted by the detector.

1.4   ATTENUATION AND IMAGING

Attenuation of x-rays follows the *Beer – Lambert law*. It can be derived from the basic idea that the number of absorbed and scattered photons of a beam dI in a thin slice ds of matter is proportional to the intensity $I(s)$ of the beam in this particular slice. Mathematically, this reads as follows:

$$\frac{dI}{ds} = -\mu I(s) \tag{1.2}$$

This differential equation can easily be solved and results in

$$I(s) = I_0 * e^{-\mu s} \tag{1.3}$$

where I_0 is the initial number of photons, and s is the thickness of the absorber. μ is a material-specific quantity, the *linear attenuation coefficient*; it depends on the energy of the photons and the absorbing material.

Generally, there are three effects responsible for x-ray attenuation:

the *photoelectric effect*,

the *Compton effect* and the

pair production effect.

Therefore, μ can be written as $\mu = \mu_{\text{photo}} + \mu_{\text{Compton}} + \mu_{\text{pair}}$. In addition, elastic scatter of electrons may also contribute. The photoelectric effect causes attenuation of photon energy by emitting an electron from the electron shell of an atom where the energy of the photon is transformed into ionization and kinetic energy. Referring to the Compton effect, the photon only partly dispenses energy to the electron producing a scattered photon with slightly less energy. At energy levels higher than 1.022 MeV a photon can be converted near the nucleus to a pair of particles, namely an *electron* and a *positron* – the positron being an anti-particle of the electron with the same mass and positive elementary charge.[2] Figure 1.4 shows the principle of these three mechanisms.

The principle of x-ray imaging is based on the different attenuation in tissue. The attenuation is governed by the *atomic number of the material, tissue density, photon energy* and *material thickness*. A higher density of the tissue causes greater attenuation. According to Equation 1.3 this effect is not linear but exponential.

Since overlapping structures are merged to an image, the laws of *central projection* have to be considered for correct interpretation of the x-ray image. Regarding x-ray imaging, the most important consequence lies in the fact that structures with different distances to the focal spot are imaged with different magnifications. We will encounter central projection several times in this book (for instance in Chapters 7, 9 and 8). Depending on attenuation properties of the tissue to be imaged and detector energy response, tube voltage as well as spectrum quality have to be selected. Bones show high attenuation properties and are easy to distinguish from soft tissue. Therefore, in the early days of x-ray imaging, bone imaging was most common. It is much more difficult to visualize tissue or vessels. To emphasize small differences in attenuation one has to use low tube voltages and maybe also computer assisted contrast enhancement. Another possibility for contrast enhancement is the use of *contrast media*. These are substances applied to the patient with either high or very low attenuation properties.

Image quality is also affected by *scatter radiation, noise* and *blurring*. The first is mainly a problem when the object to be imaged is thick. Photon beams that pass the body are either attenuated or penetrate the body without any interactions. For a thorax exposure, the fraction of scattered radiation is more than 50% of the available imaging radiation, which results in a loss of image contrast due to scatter. *Anti-scatter grids* are positioned between patient and detector to reduce the effect of scatter radiation.

Noise is generated by various sources. The most important source is statistical fluctuations of the photons called *quantum noise*. The statistical model for stochastic events with very small probability is the *Poisson distribution*; this distribution is a model for all processes where there is only a small chance of an event (for example the incidence of a single photon on a large matrix of x-ray detector elements). The Poisson distribution is given as

$$P(x) \quad = \quad \frac{1}{x!}\bar{x}^x e^{-\bar{x}} \tag{1.4}$$

$$P(x) \quad \dots \quad \text{Probability for the occurrence of } x \text{ events}$$
$$\bar{x} \quad \dots \quad \text{Mean of } x$$

Perceptual image noise can be reduced by *increasing* the number of photons; however, this also increases the applied dose, and dose may cause detriment to tissue (see also Section 1.10.2). Other sources of noise are structural characteristics of the detector, electronic noise in the amplifiers and system noise in the whole signal processing chain. Image degradation caused by noise can be quantified by the *signal-to-noise ratio* (SNR), which will be introduced in Chapter 3.

---

[2]The inverse effect, *annihilation*, is used in *positron emission tomography* imaging.

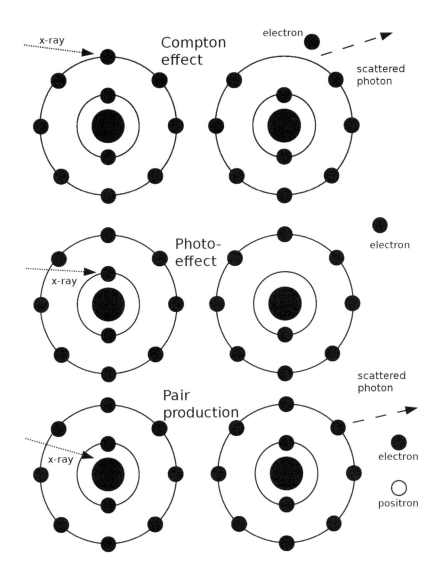

FIGURE 1.4: The three main attenuation effects using the example of neon. The first illustration (top row) shows the Compton effect, where an electron is removed from an outer orbital, leaving an ionized atom. The remaining energy from the incident high-energy photon is transported by a photon of lower energy. In the case of the photo-effect, all photon energy is absorbed. Finally, a high-energy photon from the γ radiation domain may produce a pair of matter and anti-matter – an electron and its positively charged counterpart, the positron.

Finally, image blurring arises from the finite size of the focal spot which is not point-shaped as supposed in geometrical imaging theory. The blurring effects depend on the physical size of the focal spot and the imaging geometry.

1.5 COMPUTED TOMOGRAPHY

1.5.1 Basics of CT and scanner generations

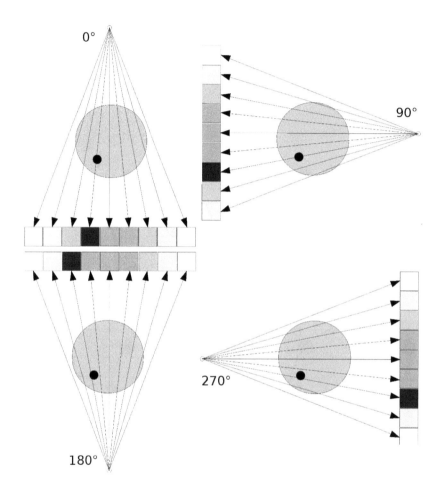

FIGURE 1.5: The principle of CT. An array of x-ray detectors opposing an x-ray tube rotates around the object to be imaged. The attenuation profile changes depending on the geometry of the object and the rotation angle. By means of a *reconstruction algorithm*, one can derive a planar slice image from these projections.

The principle of a *computed tomography* (CT) machine is shown in Figure 1.5. A collimated x-ray fan beam penetrates a slice of the patient. A detector on the other side measures the intensity of the residual beam, which is attenuated according to Equation 1.3. After a small rotation of the tube-detector assembly, the procedure is repeated. In this way, projections from many different directions are recorded and a two-dimensional integral of attenuation is obtained. Figure 1.6 illustrates this. J. Radon has already shown back in 1917 that it is possible to reconstruct a two-dimensional image from such a set of intensity profiles. The exact formalism is explained in Chapter 10. In CT, a gray value proportional to the attenuation is displayed. This voxel value is given in *Hounsfield units* (HU). In this scale air has a value of -1000 HU, water is equivalent to 0 HU, many metals exhibit more than 1000 HU and bony tissue can be found in a range between approximately 50 to more than 1000 HU.

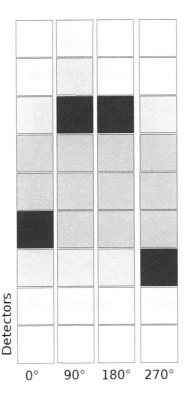

FIGURE 1.6: The four attenuation patterns from Figure 1.5, re-arranged as a function of the rotation angle of the x-ray tube and detectors. The heavily attenuated signal from the radioopaque black spot in our simple structure apparently wanders across the detectors. This diagram is called a *sinogram*.

Over the years several generations of CT devices have been developed. Devices of the *first generation* (see Figs. 1.7 and 1.8) employed just one detector. The motion was composed of translation and rotation. The sampling time was up to 5 minutes per slice which restricted the field of applications. Therefore the first CTs were only used for cranial applications. The next generation was improved by using a fan beam in combination with multiple detectors. Multiple profiles were recorded in one translation cycle and the number of angular steps was reduced. This allowed for better exploitation of radiation by simultaneously decreasing the scan time to 20 seconds per slice. Devices of the *third generation* are very efficient at exploiting the generated radiation. The imaged object is inside the fan of x-rays at any point in time. Translational movements are obsolete and the tube is rotating together with a curved detector array around the object. In the *fourth generation* the same configuration is used but radiation is detected by a fixed detector ring while the tube is rotating around the object. The detector elements are arranged in a full circle. Because the distance between two detector elements is crucial for the spatial resolution, a huge number of detector elements is necessary. For this reason newer machines use third generation technology.

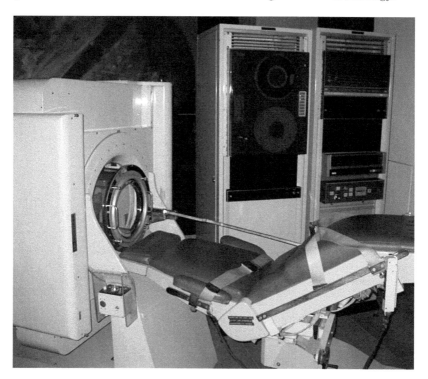

FIGURE 1.7: The EMI-scanner, developed by Sir Godfrey Hounsfield and introduced to the world of medical imaging in 1971. It is a first generation scanner, useful for brain imaging only. The photograph was taken in the Science Museum London, UK. Besides the computers in the background, the machine looks pretty modern and one would not guess that it is actually an early ancestor of modern tomographic medical imaging. For a comparison, one may take a look at Figure 1.9.

1.5.2 Imaging geometries and CT technologies

In contrast to contiguous "step and shoot" CT, *spiral* or *helical CT* is a volumetric recording technique. The x-ray tube and detector assembly are rotating around the patient while the radiographic table is translated continuously. Therefore, the focus of the system moves on a *helical path* around the patient and the data of the full volume can be acquired completely. Advantages include short examination times, which reduce artifacts due to patient movement, and gapless volumes, which avoid slice intersections. Due to the continuous motion, raw data from helical CT cannot be used directly for reconstruction. Therefore, the raw data from different helical segments are interpolated[3] to planar slices. The simplest method of interpolation uses the projections adjacent to the desired table position. The weight for

---

[3]In Section 7.2, we will learn more about interpolation.

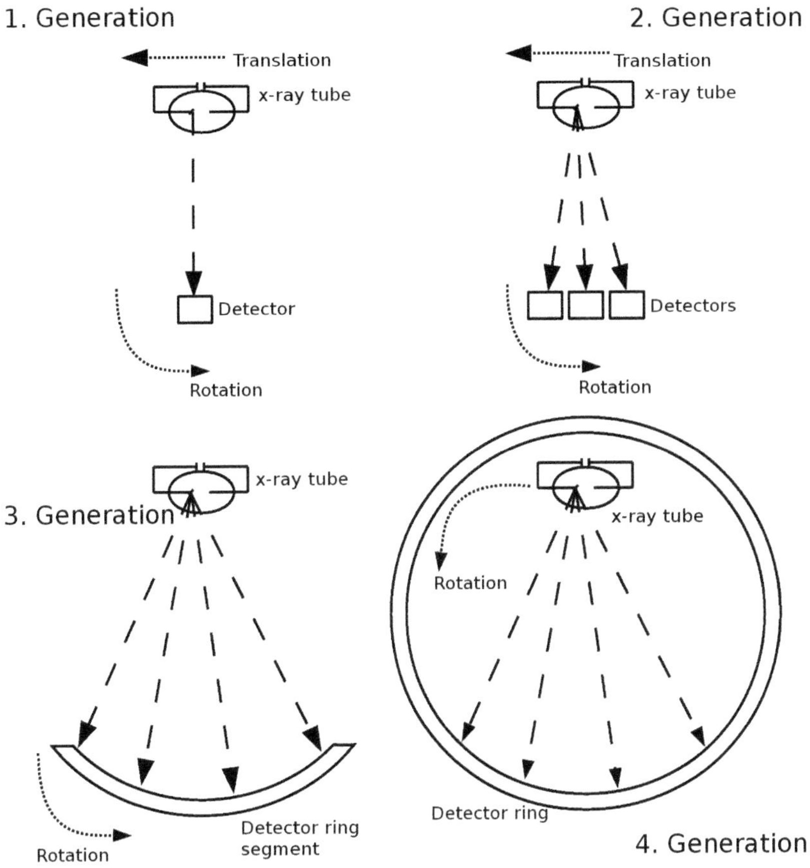

FIGURE 1.8: The four generations of CT. *First generation* scanners consisted of a single detector and a sharply collimated x-ray beam. The attenuation profile was recorded during a translation, which was followed by a rotation of both the detector and the x-ray tube. *Second generation* scanners acquired the data in the same manner, but utilized several detector elements and an x-ray fan beam with less collimation. A separate translational movement was still part of the acquisition process. In *third generation* scanners, only a rotation of the curved detector element together with the x-ray tube is carried out. A stationary detector ring with rotating x-ray tube is called a *fourth generation* system. The technological advantages such as a smaller form factor of the third generation geometry have, however, caused the fourth generation scanners to vanish.

linear interpolation coincides with the distance from measurement position to a given table position.

An important parameter for image quality in single slice spiral CT is the *pitch factor*, which is the ratio of table translation per gantry rotation (in mm) to the slice thickness in the final volume. Pitch factor 1 means that the table is moved the equivalent of one slice thickness during one rotation. Small pitch factors decrease pixel noise but increase the examination time and the dose.

Another advantage of spiral CT came with the implementation of the *slip ring* technology. Here, the power supply of the x-ray tube is provided by sliding contacts instead

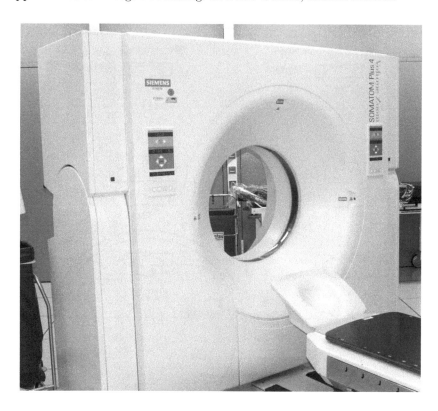

FIGURE 1.9: An early multislice CT (with four detector rows) used in clinical routine.

of cables; this enables continuous recording in contrast to the start-stop mode of older CT systems. In those old-fashioned wired setups, the rotation was started clockwise. After a full rotation, the x-ray tube stopped, the patient table feed was turned on, and the next slice was acquired during a counter-clockwise motion. Nowadays, modern systems also use the generator as a counterweight, and therefore the generator is rotating together with the detector and the x-ray tube.

To enlarge scanning range and achieve greater volume coverage in shorter time, *multi-detector spiral CT* was developed. These systems enable acquisition of up to 640 slices simultaneously at a rotation time of 0.2 s per rotation. The technical challenge, on the one hand, lies in the design of detectors capable of measuring several thousand channels at the same time. The greater difficulty is the development and design of suitable reconstruction algorithms; for this reason, early multislice systems featured only two or four slices. All multi-slice systems are built with rotating detectors in a third generation setup. The reconstruction algorithm, however, is different to single slice spiral CTs.

Cone beam CTs (CBCTs) are somewhat similar to multislice CTs but use two-dimensional detector arrays measuring the transmitted radiation. Although multislice detectors can be interpreted as two-dimensional arrays, the main difference lies in the fact that multi-slice CTs scan large volumes still sequentially and the detectors of cone beam CT are flat compared to the curved detectors used in multi-slice CT. Two-dimensional cone beam detectors collect data from a 3D volume during a single rotation; axial motion of the patient is usually unnecessary. On the other hand, multi-slice CT still requires a motion of the detector array on a helical path to create large volumetric data sets. The recon-

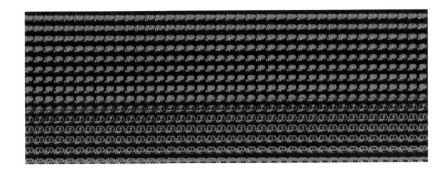

FIGURE 1.10: An illustration of the data volume produced by a modern multislice CT scanner. These are the 600 original slices produced by a single scan of a patient's torso with a slice spacing of 1 mm. Data acquisition took approximately 14 seconds. Image data courtesy of the Department of Radiology, Medical University Vienna.

struction algorithm for CBCT imaging, which allows for very compact small systems used in dentistry and intra-operative imaging, was already introduced in 1984.[4] However, the broad introduction of CBCT type devices in clinical routine is actually a phenomenon of the last decade. An image of a system for interventional CBCT, x-ray and EPID imaging in radiation oncology can be found in Figure 1.11. CBCT has also gained a huge interest in dental radiology, where it replaces classical x-ray and orthopantomographic devices (Figure 1.12).

1.5.3 Image artifacts in CT

Partial volume effects are caused by high contrast differences in an object and are displayed as blurring of sharp edges. Here, higher sampling rates are often helpful as well as the use of a finer pitch.

Ring artifacts occur when one or more channels of the detector fail. This effect will also show up if there are differences in sensitivity between two neighboring detector channels that are not corrected properly. Figure 1.24 shows a similar artifact in single photon emission computed tomography. A demonstration of how a ring artifact generates is also to be found in Chapter 10.

Noise artifacts. Noise causes grainy images and is the result of a low *signal-to-noise ratio*. As a remedy, the signal-to-noise ratio can be increased by higher tube current and tube voltage.

Motion artifacts are caused by movements of the patient during image acquisition. These appear as local blurs and streaks on the reconstructed image. Shorter acquisition times are the simplest and most effective way to avoid such artifacts although there are sophisticated algorithms available which can partially correct this effect.

Beam hardening artifacts result from high attenuation coefficients. This is corrected for radiologically water equivalent tissues. Nevertheless, especially bone will harden radiation, resulting in dark streaks in the image.

---

[4]The classic reference is Feldkamp LA, Davis LC, Kress JW: Practical conebeam algorithm, J Opt Soc Am A 1, 612-619, (1984). A simple implementation of this algorithm can be found in Example 10.6.5.

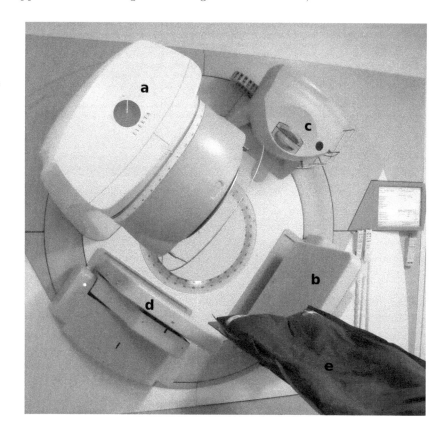

FIGURE 1.11: A linear accelerator (LINAC) for radiation therapy treatment of cancer at the Department of Radiotherapy, Medical University Vienna. Besides the LINAC itself (**a**), one can also see a direct flat panel detector for electronic portal imaging (**b**) – the acquisition of attenuation image data using the high-energy treatment beam – and for x-ray imaging (**d**). The x-ray source for planar radiographic imaging and CBCT is also visible (**c**). The patient is immobilized by a vacuum mattress (**e**).

Metal artifacts. If the attenuation is so large that the measured signal is dominated by electronic noise (as it is with metallic objects within the body) the image shows overall deterioration. Dark lines appear which radiate from sharp corners of the object – see Figure 1.13 and also Chapter 10.

1.5.4 Safety aspects

Both x-ray imaging and CT utilize ionizing radiation, which is potentially harmful; the effects of *dose* will be discussed in Chapter 1.10.

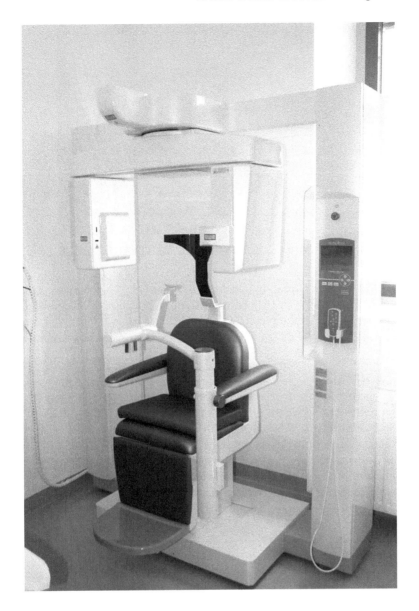

FIGURE 1.12: A small cone beam CT for dental radiology; these devices are also called digital volume tomography units.

1.6 MAGNETIC RESONANCE TOMOGRAPHY

1.6.1 Basic MRI physics

MR imaging was introduced to clinical diagnostics in the early 1980s. Since then, it has evolved into a routine diagnostic method. Due to its manifold possibilities to generate specific image contrasts, it has become the gold standard for diagnosis of many disorders. Standard MRI works on the basis of exciting the *magnetic moment* of hydrogen ^1H nuclei bound in tissue water and fat molecules. In a simple picture, electromagnetic radiation in

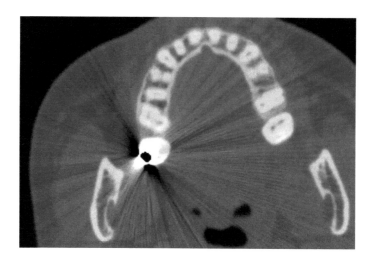

FIGURE 1.13: Metal artifacts, caused by a dental filling in CT. The complete absorption of x-ray quanta leads to a dark spot in the center of the filling since no information for image reconstruction is available. Star-like reconstruction artifacts emerge from the source of the artifact. Image courtesy of the Dept. of Radiology, Medical University Vienna.

the radiofrequency (RF) range is transmitted to the human body lying in a large magnet. The nuclei in the tissue respond to the excitation by emitting RF signals with the same frequency whose amplitude and phase information are used to form an image. The spatial information on slice location is obtained by superimposing spatial field gradients to the main magnetic field.

MR imaging is based on the physical phenomena of the *spin* of atomic nuclei – a property similar to the *angular momentum* in classical mechanics. Although the exact interpretation of this effect requires knowledge in quantum mechanics, a classical view can explain the main principle. Let's suppose a *proton* to be a spinning particle with a positive electrical charge. From the laws of electrodynamics it follows that this object must have a *magnetic moment*. This magnetic moment can be described as a vector with a given length and direction in analogy to the magnetic field caused by moving charges in a conductive loop.

From basic physics we already know a few things about matter. *Mass* is the one property of matter that is responsible for the interaction with a *gravity field*. *Charge* interacts with the *electric field*. The magnetic moment connected to the *spin* is responsible for the interaction of matter with a magnetic field. MR utilizes this property.

In addition, we have to add two quantum mechanical facts: *neutrons* (which do not carry an electrical charge) possess a magnetic moment as well since they are composed of three unequally distributed *quarks*. Also, the magnetic moment of bound protons and neutrons only appears in two different states named *up* and *down*. According to its composition from protons and neutrons, a nucleus may have a net spin. For instance, ^{1}H, ^{13}C, ^{19}F and ^{31}P possess a detectable residual magnetic momentum. In absence of an external magnetic field, these spins are distributed in arbitrary directions, therefore matter is non-magnetic.

Things are changing when we introduce a strong magnetic field. Here, we can measure a weak macroscopic magnetization in the direction of the applied magnetic field. As we know, each nucleus was already "spinning" around its own axis. With the influence of the magnetic field the nucleus starts a complex motion called *precession* around the direction

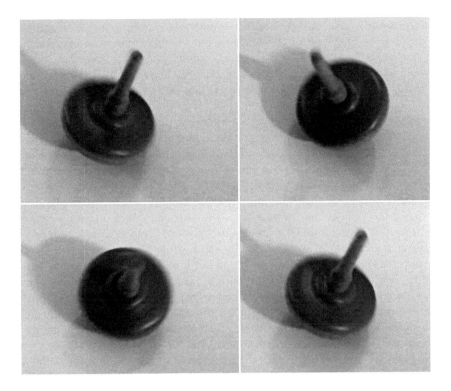

FIGURE 1.14: A spinning top, under the influence of gravity, starts to exhibit a phenomenon named *precession* – the axis of the top shows a circular motion. In this sequence of four photographs, one can easily see how the axis of the top points in different directions at different times. The spin, a property of elementary particles that exhibits an analogous mathematical behavior compared to the angular momentum, is responsible for the same behavior in the presence of an external magnetic field.

of the external field (see Figure 1.14). Due to the discrete nature of quantum mechanical phenomena, this precession can only appear in two states: *spin-up* and *spin-down*. Since the energetic level of spin-up is lower than the one of the spin-down, we will find a small abundance of spins in *up* state which is responsible for the macroscopic magnetization. This abundance is very small – typically lower than the thermal energy of the molecules, and the population of energy levels follows a thermal equilibrium. For example, in a magnetic field of 1.5 Tesla only 9.6 ppm (parts per millions) abundant spins can be found. Given the fact that one milliliter of water consists of $3 * 10^{22}$ protons, we get about $3 * 10^{17}$ abundant spins which result in the weak magnetization described above. Since there are now more spins in a lower energy state than before, the total energy of the ensemble has decreased. The missing energy is transported to the surrounding lattice. The abundance of spins-up increases with the *density of protons*, the *magnetic field* and *decreasing temperature*.

The rate of precession of a spin in an external magnetic field is called *Larmor frequency*. It is given as:

$$\omega_0 = \gamma B_0 \left[\frac{\text{rad}}{\text{s}} \right] \tag{1.5}$$

Here, ω_0 is the precession frequency in $\frac{\text{rad}}{\text{s}}$ while B_0 represents the external magnetic flux density in *Tesla* and γ is a constant called the *gyromagnetic ratio* in $\frac{rad}{sT}$. The magnitude of the latter depends on the type of the nucleus. For example the gyromagnetic ratio for the hydrogen nucleus is $\gamma = 2.67 * 10^8 \frac{rad}{sT}$, which equals $42.6 \frac{MHz}{T}$. Therefore, the Larmor frequency for such a nucleus in a magnetic field of 1 T is 42.6 MHz or $42.6 * 10^6$ Hz. According to Section 1.2, this corresponds to the radio frequency (RF) range of the electromagnetic spectrum.

All spins are precessing arbitrarily and have different phases – their components in the plane orthogonal to the direction of the magnetic field compensate each other and sum to zero. To simplify things, we may choose an arbitrary coordinate system where the magnetic field vector is aligned in z-direction. Then the orthogonal plane to this direction is the xy-plane and the components of the magnetization vector in xy-direction are zero. To excite the magnetization along $\vec{z}$ from its thermal equilibrium state and hence introduce a detectable in-phase net magnetization in the xy-plane, we have to *add* energy. Energy will only be absorbed by the system if it is applied at the same frequency that is in accordance with the *resonance frequency* of the nuclei to be excited – the Larmor frequency.

This absorption of energy at the resonant frequency is called *nuclear magnetic resonance*. The energy of the RF pulse is responsible for tipping the net magnetization vector toward the xy-plane. The more energy is applied, the higher the tilt angle after the RF pulse. At a certain energy the magnetization vector is tipped through 90° and leaves the z-component zero. This corresponds to an equal number of *up* and *down* spin states. Further energy supply tips the vector toward the negative z-direction until the tilt angle reaches 180° – more spins are in the spin-down state now. It is important to emphasize that, despite the name, nuclear magnetic resonance is a purely electromagnetic phenomenon. Neither radioactive decay nor ionizing radiation play a role in this process.

To supply the system with energy, additional RF coils are used that can transmit and receive pulsed electromagnetic waves with a frequency in the RF range. Let's suppose we applied an RF pulse so that the tilt angle of the spin vector is 90°. Then the magnetization in z-direction M_z is zero and the xy-magnetization M_{xy} is at its maximum. This state is called *saturation*. As we know from electrodynamics this changing magnetic field induces currents which can be received by appropriate receiver coils. After the RF pulse has ended, the xy-magnetization disappears due to the dephasing of initially coherent xy-magnetization. This process is called *Free Induction Decay (FID)*.

1.6.1.1 Relaxation processes

When an RF pulse is applied the spin ensemble is brought to a physical state of disequilibrium. After ending the pulse the system changes back to the equilibrium state, and energy is dissipated as RF radiation. Hereby, the magnetization in z-direction M_z recovers while the xy-magnetization M_{xy} decays. Each of these processes has typical time constants.

The recovery of M_z is called *longitudinal relaxation*. During this process the energy from the RF-pulse stored in the spin system is transferred from the excited nuclei to its surroundings, the lattice. For this reason the longitudinal relaxation is also called *spin-lattice relaxation*. The recovery of the M_z can be described by an exponential curve, similar to Equation 1.3. Its characteristic variable is the decay time T_1. It represents the time needed to recover approximately 63% of the final relaxed magnetization. After a period of five times T_1, the M_z magnetization is almost completely recovered. The T_1 time constant depends mainly on the size of the molecules in tissue and their bonding. Small, movable water molecules in a loose bonding in liquids are limited in interaction with their surrounding. Therefore, tissues such as brain fluid (CSF) show long relaxation times. In contrast, large fat molecules in dense atomic lattice bonding of a solid body recover quickly and have a short

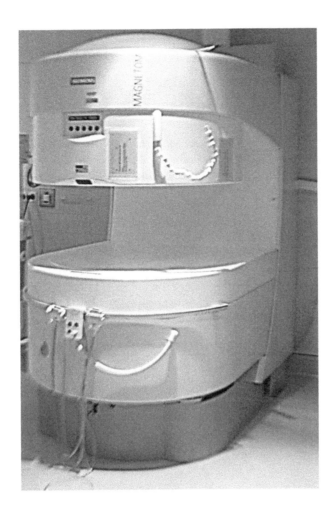

FIGURE 1.15: A low field open MR-machine. As opposed to conventional MR-machines, which generate the main static magnetic field by using a large coil – a so-called solenoid – this machine has the geometry of a horseshoe magnet. The field between the north and south pole of the horseshoe is not as homogeneous as in the case of a solenoid, resulting in image distortions such as shown in Figure 1.17. But the geometry allows for accessing the patient directly, therefore these machines are used in interventional radiology, brachyther-apy and surgery; another field of application is pediatric imaging since this scanner allows for soothing the patient during image acquisition. Another possible geometry for such an interventional MR is the use of two large, thin coils. In physics, such an arrangement is known as *Helmholtz coils*. The interventional MRI using such an arrangement was therefore nicknamed "double donut".

	T_1 [ms]	T_2 [ms]
Grey brain matter	813	101
White brain matter	683	92
Muscle	732	47
Liver	423	43
Fat tissue	241	84

TABLE 1.1: T_1 and T_2 constants in ms for various tissues for B=1 Tesla. Data from W.R. Hendee: Medical Imaging Physics, Wiley, 2002.

T_1. The variation of T_1 values for different tissues is the important property for imaging and image contrast. Table 1.1 shows some values for T_1 and T_2 constants for different tissues.

In contrast to the longitudinal relaxation, the *transverse relaxation* is not induced by energy transfer but by interaction between the magnetic moments of neighboring nuclei. The signal decays because the precession of the spins running out of phase and the phase coherence between the nuclei is lost. Therefore, the transverse relaxation is also called *spin-spin relaxation*. The loss of coherence is based on the slightly different chemical environment of each nucleon which results in slightly different magnetic fields for different nuclei. This spin-spin interaction is much stronger than the spin-lattice interaction and leads to significantly smaller time constants T_2. In solid bodies with strong atomic bonding, the local fluctuations of the magnetic fields are extensive and T_2 is accordingly short. In liquids, the nuclei can move in relatively loose bonding and we can experience longer T_2 relaxation times.

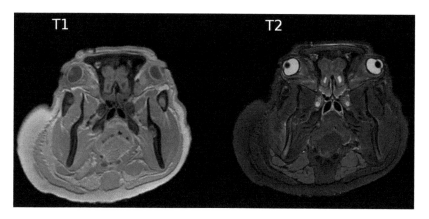

FIGURE 1.16: The effects of T_1 and T_2 weighted MR image acquisition – we will encounter the subject of this scan, a pig, many more times in this text. The considerable differences in T_1 and T_2-constants given in Table 1.1 produce the obvious differences in image contrast.

1.6.1.2 Spin-echo

The lifetime of the FID given as relaxation times is only valid for a perfectly homogeneous magnetic field B_0. Inhomogeneities in the magnetic field cause additional de-phasing of the spins and lead to an effective time constant T_2^* that is shorter than T_2. But since these inhomogeneities are constant in space and time, there is the possibility to reverse their effect. The idea is to apply a second $180°$ pulse after a specific time period τ, which tilts the net magnetization by 180°. Now the effect of the inhomogeneity also reverses and after another time period τ, the spins have recovered and we can measure a new signal called *spin-echo*. However, this signal is smaller in amplitude than the original FID signal because the de-phasing caused by the spin-spin interaction is irreversible. The time period 2τ is called *echo time*. Longer echo times decrease the amplitude of the spin-echo.

1.6.2   Tissue contrast

The high sensitivity of MR imaging is based on the varying time constants for different tissue types. To create a contrast between different types of tissue, both time constants T_1 and T_2 can be used. Additionally, contrasts based on different time constants can be enhanced by varying the temporal sequence of the RF signals. Images where the contrast is based on T_1 differences are called T_1 *weighted images* while in T_2 *weighted images* contrast is based on different T_2 values.

Let's examine two different tissues A and B with corresponding time constants $T_{1,A}$ and $T_{1,B} < T_{1,A}$; a sequence of 90° pulses is applied with a frequency f. After a time period (the *repetition time*, T_R) the 90° pulse is repeated. As we already know a 90° pulse leads to the state of saturation where M_z is zero and the net magnetization vector is tipped into the xy plane. Then M_z recovers partially before the next 90° pulse is applied after the repetition time T_R. The magnitude of the resulting FID signals measured after a certain time (the *echo time*, time between the application of the RF pulse and the measurement of the signal T_E) depends on the time constant T_1. Short T_1 means that M_z recovers faster and therefore the FID signal from the tissue characterized by T_1 will be greater than the FID signal with longer T_1. For short T_R, both longitudinal magnetization cannot build up significantly and the difference in magnitude in transversal magnetization after the 90° pulse is small. If T_R is too long, both M_z are almost totally recovered and the magnitudes of the resulting FID signals are almost the same. The greatest difference in magnitude appears when T_R lies between $T_{1,A}$ and $T_{1,B}$, e.g., $T_{1,B} < T_R < T_{1,A}$. This 90°-90° pulse sequence is called *progressive saturation*.

It is easier to measure a spin-echo than the fast declining FID signal. The *spin echo sequence* is designed to minimize the effect of magnetic field inhomogeneities. When the first 90° pulse is followed by a 180° pulse after a time period τ we can measure a spin-echo after an echo time of $T_E = 2\tau$. For T_1-weighted images, T_R should be of the magnitude of the mean T_1. T_E should be as short as possible because the difference between the transversal magnetization decreases with T_E in this case.

The influence of the longitudinal magnetization can be decreased using long repetition times T_R. This is desirable when the time constants T_2 of the tissues differ more than the T_1 constants. In this case we have to choose long echo times T_E to benefit from the varying decay of M_{xy} to get T_2-weighted images.

1.6.3   Spatial localization

When an RF pulse is applied, we can measure a FID or a spin-echo signal. But this signal represents only the sum of all spin-signal responses of the whole tissue compound and has no spatial information. For the spatial decoding of the MR signals *three additional field gradients* are necessary. According to this hardware requirement the following description is separated into three steps. First, we define an (arbitrary) coordinate system for better clarity and easier understanding. In accordance with most introductions to MRI, the z-axis lies in caudal/cranial direction, the patient is lying supine, parallel to the direction of the static main field, which runs also in z-direction. Then slices parallel to the xy-plane are transversal slices. The x-axis runs across the body from left to right and consequently, the y-direction is defined from posterior to anterior. The three gradient fields are switched on at certain points in time in the image sequence.

1.6.3.1 Slice selection

To select a transverse slice, an additional magnetic gradient field in z-direction is added. This means that the magnetic field is no longer constant but varies in z-direction. This additional magnetic field (as well as the others described below) is much smaller in size than the static field and is zero at the center, with a positive value at one extreme and a negative value at the other. As a result, the Larmor frequency for the proton also differs, depending on the location in the magnet. Therefore, it is possible to determine from which transversal slice of the body a signal was emitted by excitation. For example, let the static field be 1 T and the gradient field in a distance of 1 m -0.001 T. Then the RF frequency in the center is 42.6 MHz while the Larmor frequency at a caudal slice is 42.2 MHz.

The slice selection gradient is switched on **before** the RF pulse is applied. Only spins in the affected transversal slices are excited. In practice the applied RF pulse contains a range of frequencies (called *transmitted bandwidth*). A single frequency would only select a physically impossible slice of "zero thickness". Therefore, the transmitted bandwidth has a crucial impact on the slice thickness – the broader the bandwidth, the thicker the selected slice. The slice thickness also depends on the strength of the gradient field; a steeper gradient leads to thinner slices.

1.6.3.2 Frequency encoding

For frequency encoding we use a second gradient field which has to be perpendicular to the slice selection field. In our example we choose (arbitrarily) the x-direction for this purpose although the y-direction would fulfill our requirement as well. Then, we can determine the position of the signal in x-direction corresponding to columns in the image.

In contrast to the slice selection gradient, the frequency encoding gradient is switched on **before** the measurement of the spin-echo. This gradient leads to the effect that the spins along the x-gradient are precessing with different frequencies across the selected slice. Each of these signals has a frequency associated with its x-location and has an amplitude that is summed by all signals along the same x-location, e.g., x-coordinate. When we record this signal we can use the *Fourier transform* to reconstruct the amplitude for each x-location (see also Chapter 5). This *receiver bandwidth* also defines size of the *field of view* (FOV).

As we will learn in Chapter 10, we could apply the frequency gradient from different angles through 360°, as done in CT, and the reconstruction problem can be solved by *filtered backprojection*. This technique was indeed used in early MR research but was too slow and too sensitive to inhomogeneities in the main field and in the gradients. Furthermore, it only allowed small FOVs.

1.6.3.3 Phase encoding

The phase encoding gradient is switched on **between** the RF pulse and the time of measuring the spin-echo signal. The field gradient is applied along the y-direction. Although this direction is arbitrary, it has to be aligned perpendicular to the slice secretion field and the frequency encoding gradient. Again, there is a variation in frequency when the gradient is switched on. That introduces phase differences between the different y-locations. These differences still remain when the gradient has already been switched off. After the application of the phase gradient, all spins are again precessing with the same frequency, but the phase shifts remain for the measurement step of frequency encoding. Each y-position is now represented by a unique phase and each x-position is represented by a unique frequency. This results in a unique combination of frequency and phase for each pixel in the selected slice. But it is not possible to encode the phases by means of Fourier analysis as for frequency encoding because at each measurement only one signal can be acquired. Therefore, the phase gradient has to be applied as often as the number of rows in the image is required. Each time the phase gradient is applied, the phase shift must increase by an amount that is the same size at every phase encoding step. Then each separated step can be identified with a row of pixels and the Fourier analysis distinguishes the amplitude of the different x-locations. Finally, a change in the static magnetic field does not influence the phase-shift but does influence the encoding frequency.

1.6.4 Image artifacts in MR

Aliasing artifacts occur when the field of view is smaller than the object being imaged. Anatomical structures outside the FOV are mapped to the opposite side of the image. Therefore, the simplest way to compensate for aliasing is to enlarge the FOV to encompass the entire anatomical dimension of the object. Another possible approach is to use digital filters to cut off frequencies greater than the *Nyquist frequency*. Image artifacts due to nonrandom inhomogeneities are removed by the use of 180° RF pulses for refocusing. This artifact is also called *wraparound artifact* – see Figure 5.17 – and will be discussed in Chapter 5.

Chemical shift artifacts occur in the frequency encoding direction when signals from tissues with slightly different resonance frequency compared to water (for instance, fat) are mistaken as signals from water molecules. This frequency difference is then interpreted as spatial translation in the gradient direction. The frequency difference is due to different electron environments of the protons of water and, for example, fat.

Motion artifacts occur due to motion along the phase encoding gradient because of wrong phase accumulation. While object motions are generally slower than the time used for the frequency encoding step, these kind of artifacts are common due to the long time that elapses between phase encoding steps. Here, both periodic movements (such as cardiac motions or bold flow) and random motion (such as breathing or coughing) cause artifacts of this kind. Motion artifacts in MR will be discussed in Chapter 5. An example can be found in Figure 5.18.

Edge artifacts can be seen in areas of boundaries between tissues with strongly different signals.

Field inhomogeneity: A poor field homogeneity, especially at the borders of the field-of-view, may distort the image, just as small non-ferromagnetic conductive objects. If the conductive objects such as implants made of non-ferromagnetic alloys are larger, a complete extinction of the image in the surrounding of the implant may be the consequence. Figures 1.17 and 1.18 show the effects of field inhomogeneity in different MR machines.

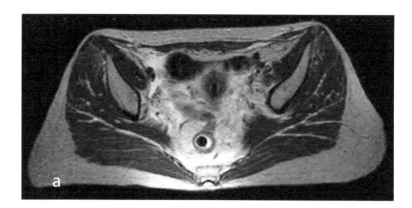

FIGURE 1.17: An MR image from an open low-field MR scanner. The field homogeneity at the edges of the volume is poor in this type of scanner. **a** points out an area where the image is distorted due to these inhomogeneities of the main static magnetic field. Image courtesy of the Dept. of Radiology, Medical University Vienna.

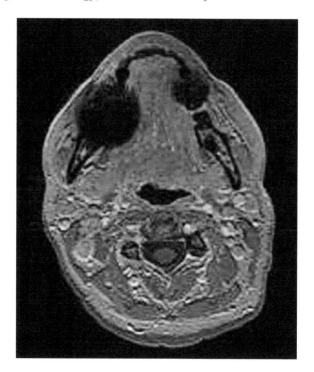

FIGURE 1.18: Large metal fillings in this patient's teeth caused massive local field inhomgenieties. As a result, two large void areas are found in this case since no signal was received by the MR machine. Compare this artifact also to the CT-artifact found in Figure 1.13. Image courtesy of the Dept. of Radiology, Medical University Vienna.

1.6.5 The elements of an MR system

1.6.5.1 The main static magnetic field

This part of the system is the most important element of a modern MR system as well as its most expensive one. We can distinguish between two types. The field of *superconducting magnets* is built up by a large coil made of an niobium-titanium or niobium-tin alloy cooled by liquid helium to extremely low temperatures of approximately 4 K. The process of superconduction implies that the magnet shows no resistance, thus allowing for very high currents. Once loaded to the desired field magnitude no further energy supply is necessary to maintain the field. Magnetic fields between 1.0 and 7.0 Tesla can be found in clinical use. There are also up to 9 T magnets for scientific purposes. *Permanent magnets* are built out of large blocks of ferromagnetic alloys (for instance steel alloys containing rare earth elements such as neodymium) and do not need any energy supply. The disadvantage of these types of magnets lies in their enormous weight and their bulkiness although they are cheaper and provide better homogeneity.

Generally, inhomogeneities in the static field lead to image distortions and dislocations. To avoid this effect, the magnets are adjusted or *shimmed*. For this purpose, small *shim coils* are added to create small magnetic fields which compensate for the inhomogeneities. In the case of permanent magnets, small iron plates are pasted onto the magnet to compensate for distortions. The process of shimming prior to each image acquisition is a bare necessity for good image quality.

1.6.5.2 Gradient fields

The gradient fields are generated by coils arranged in couples. These are driven by currents of the same strength but inverted polarity. Therefore, the one resulting electromagnetic field increases the static magnetic field, while the other coil on the opposite side decreases the static field. In the middle of the gradient field both coil fields annihilate each other – the static field remains the same. The change along the axis of the gradient is always linear.

1.6.5.3 The RF system

The RF transmission system consists of an RF synthesizer, power amplifier and transmission coils, while the receivers include the coil, pre-amplifier and a signal processing system. Because the RF signals are in the range of radio waves, effective shielding is compulsory – the magnets and coils are installed in a Faraday cage. Another challenge arises from the desired low signal-to-noise ratio (SNR). The main source of noise is Brownian motion inside the body. The SNR is better with small coils, which also reduces the imaged volume on the other side. Another way of improving the degree of efficiency is to increase the space factor, the ratio of sensitive volume to the total volume of the core. Therefore, the receiver coils are adapted in shape and size to different relevant human anatomies such as head, thorax or extremities.

1.6.6 Safety aspects

There is no proof that the electromagnetic fields used in MRI damage tissue. However, the very strong magnetic field may cause the displacement of cardiac pacemakers, which may result in a loss of electric contact to the cardiac muscle. Ferromagnetic materials in the body such as hemorrhage clips made from surgeon's steel can be torn off, and ferromagnetic structures such as wheelchairs and oxygen flasks can be drawn into the magnet at high speed.

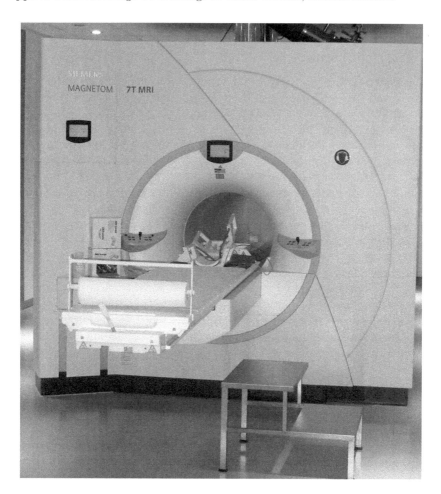

FIGURE 1.19: A modern 7 Tesla high-field MR machine at the MR Center of Excellence at the Medical University Vienna. The machine features a long coil for maintaining the main static field; due to the very high field strength of this machine, all ferromagnetic material is kept at maximum distance and the impressive tomograph stands rather solitary and solemn in an otherwise empty room.

1.7 ULTRASOUND

1.7.1 Some physical properties of sound

Sound is a longitudinal pressure wave based on compression and decompression of the carrier medium. So the speed of sound c depends on the compressibility and density of the carrier medium and equals the product of *wave length* λ and *frequency* ν ($c = \lambda\nu \left[\frac{m}{s}\right]$). The average speed of sound in tissue is approximately $1540\frac{m}{s}$. An exception from this rule is bone, which features a very high speed of sound, and air.

While passing the body, the acoustic signal may undergo *reflection* on tissue boundaries; furthermore, there is also *refraction* and *scattering*. Refraction only occurs on border structures that are large compared to the wavelength of the acoustic signal. On structures with sizes comparable to the wavelength of sound, ultrasound (US) is scattered, with small structures of different density acting as centers of scatter. Scatter is never directed but isotropic. The appearance of refraction can lead to misinterpretation in position and extension of the structures under exam (see also Section 1.7.3). The intensity of transmitted, reflected and scattered pulses depends on the ratio of the acoustic impedance of the structures and also on the angle of incidence.

The depth of penetration by the acoustic signal is limited by *attenuation*. The intensity of the wave decreases exponentially with the depth, and the attenuation coefficient depends on the material – a similar behavior we have already encountered in Equation 1.3 and in the case of the relaxation time in MR. The energy of the wave is converted to heat. An important property of attenuation with respect to ultrasound imaging is that it depends heavily on the frequency of the wave – the higher the frequency the larger the attenuation and the lower the penetration depth.

1.7.2 Basic principles

US imaging is based on the reflection of acoustic signals; high frequency signals are generated by the *piezo effect*. The *direct piezo effect* describes the phenomenon that voltage can be measured in certain solids under deformation – for instance, certain lighters use this for ignition, and some musical instruments feature piezo-electric pickups. Inversely, the application of a voltage to these solids causes deformations, which is known as the *inverse piezo effect*.

This inverse effect is used for the generation of ultrasound signals in US imaging. A piezo-electric US transducer transforms an electrical pulse into an acoustic signal which penetrates the object and is reflected on internal structures. These reflected pulses – the echos – are detected by the US transducer, which utilizes the direct piezo effect, and converts back to electronic signals. This kind of imaging represents the simplest way of ultrasound imaging and is called *amplitude modulation* or *A-mode ultrasound imaging*. The percentage of reflected US waves is determined by the difference in acoustic impedance of the tissue involved. Because this difference is generally relatively small the main part of the sound energy passes such boundary surfaces and makes possible localization of diverse organs lying behind each other by exploiting the temporal distance between the echoes. The distance z of a boundary surface is easily calculated as

$$z = \frac{ct}{2} \left[\frac{m}{s} \right], \tag{1.6}$$

where t indicates the return time of the echo signal in seconds and c describes the velocity of sound in the tissue in $\frac{m}{s}$.

Due to absorption of ultrasound in tissue, echos with longer run time are weaker and produce smaller electrical signals in the US transducer compared to echoes coming from closer surfaces. Therefore amplification has to be increased with increasing run-time. Since the A-mode technique only provides one-dimensional information, other imaging methods were developed. *B-Mode* or *brightness modulation* is the most widespread of these techniques. Here, the echo amplitudes are converted to gray values in a 2D image. In the beginning of ultrasound imaging the transducer was manually moved over the body surface. This technique was known as *compound scan*. Nowadays, an *ultrasound scan head* consists of a row of US transducers forming a one-dimensional (or – in the case of 3D ultrasound imaging – a two-dimensional) array; the elements of the scanhead are switched on and off one after the other.

Different shapes of transducer configuration exist: linear configuration can be found in *linear scan heads* while *convex scan heads* form a curve (see also Figure 1.20). With *sector scan heads* the single transducers are operated in a sequential manner. The group width can vary from 8 to 128 elements.

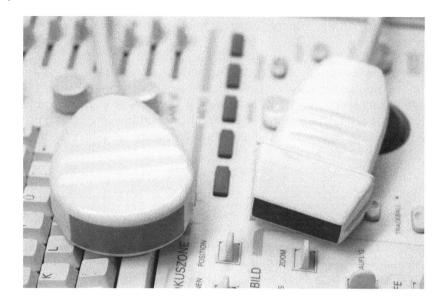

FIGURE 1.20: A linear and a convex B-mode transducer lying on the keyboard of a modern medical US-machine.

1.7.3 Image artifacts in B-Mode US imaging

Noise: One of the most obvious ultrasound artifacts is *speckle*. It is a consequence of the reflection of sound waves on microscopic tissue inhomogeneities. The reflected waves always emerge at random phase. When these random phases align, high intensity echoes may occur. With a small change in frequency or in location of the imaging transducer, the precise relationship will change and a complete change in the speckle pattern can be observed. Figure 1.21 illustrates this.

Shadowing: Objects with strong echos reflect sound waves in a way that produces a shadow behind the reflecting object while the object is displayed with greater brightness. Another similar but inverse effect can be observed on objects with little absorption. Here, an *amplified signal* behind the object is the result.

Multiple reflections between two strong reflectors are displayed as multiple echos where the distance between each of the echo artifacts correlates to the distance between the two reflectors.

Mirroring: If an object is placed between the transducer and a strongly reflecting layer, the object is *mirrored*.

1.7.4 Doppler effect

The *Doppler effect* is used in US imaging to display flow velocities of blood and other liquids. This effect, discovered by Christian Doppler in 1842, can be described as follows: when a

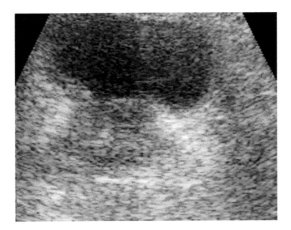

FIGURE 1.21: An illustration of speckle in an ultrasound image of the prostate. The anatomical structures – namely the bladder at the top of the image, and the prostate below the bladder – are somewhat hard to identify. Image speckle, however, is obvious.

source of acoustic waves is moving towards an observer, the waves undergo a shift towards a shorter wavelength. When the source is moving away from the observer, the wave is shifted towards longer wavelength. A well-known example is the shift in audible frequency when an ambulance car approaches with a siren. In US Doppler imaging red blood cells inside the vessels can be seen as a source of ultrasound waves when they reflect US signals. The frequency shift of the measured reflected wave depends on the velocity v and direction of the blood flow. The measured frequency difference $\Delta \nu$ is given as

$$\Delta \nu = 2\nu \left(\pm \frac{v}{c} \right) \text{[Hz]} \qquad (1.7)$$

where ν is the emitted frequency in Hertz and c the velocity of ultrasound given as $\left[\frac{m}{s} \right]$.

The echoes from within the vessels are much weaker than the original signal by a factor of 10^2 to 10^3. Therefore, this imaging technique is much more sensitive to artifacts, namely shadowing, compared to normal B-mode imaging. The echo also gives information about the direction of the flow where velocities towards the transducer are usually displayed on the positive axis in the spectral curve and encoded red while flow velocities away from the transducer are displayed in blue color.

The Doppler signals are obtained by *demodulation*. When a Doppler signal hits an object in motion, a low-frequency kHz signal is superimposed on the high-frequency MHz carrier signal. *Continuous wave (CW) Doppler* demodulates the resulting signal continuously. The transducer elements are divided into two parts, where one emits continuously while the other one receives the incoming signal. Here, it is not possible to determine the origin of the signal. *Color Doppler* is a technique that enables a spatial 2D distribution of velocities. This is accomplished by converting the time between transmitted and received pulses into distances. *Color flow mapping* (CFM) combines color Doppler and B-Mode imaging. Grayvalues are used to describe anatomy while color-values characterize the blood flow.

1.7.5 3D imaging

3D US imaging has been around for more than a decade. There are three different approaches. *Wobblers* use conventional curved array transducers with attached small motors

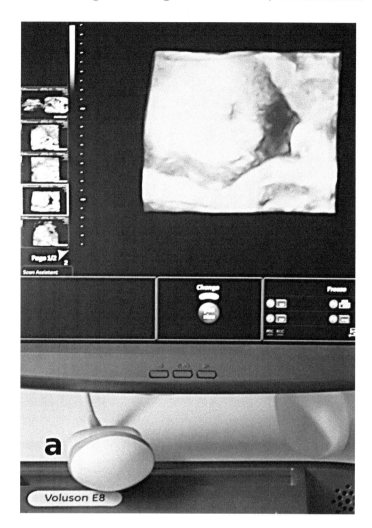

FIGURE 1.22: A modern 3D transducer (**a**), and the display showing a 3D rendering of a fetus. This type of transducer consists of a moving linear array, acquiring a fan of single slices. Therefore it is somewhat more clumsy compared to the 2D transducers from Figure 1.20. Figure 1.21 was acquired with this machine.

that wobble the transducer up and down to scan the missing dimension. They are often applied for obstetric imaging. Because of their simple additional technical requirements they are supported by many conventional systems that render the three-dimensional data on the two dimensional screens. Furthermore, 2D transducer arrays are feasible, and one may also determine the spatial location of the scanhead by means of a *tracking system*. Tracking systems are introduced in Section 7.5.

1.7.6 Safety aspects

One of the greatest advantages of ultrasound imaging compared to modalities using ionizing radiation stems from its innocuousness to tissue as long as sound pressure and sound intensity do not exceed certain thresholds. These are not defined sharply but lie somewhere in the range of 100 $\frac{mW}{cm^2}$ for unlimited examination time. There are two major effects of damaging: *cavitation* effects and *temperature* effects, which are both independent from each other.

Cavitation occurs in a low-pressure phase when cavities are formed inside the biological tissue. This effect can be amplified by already existing micro bubbles or cavitation seeds. In the diagnostic range of ultrasound of 2 to 20 MHz the negative pressure necessary for this effect has to exceed at least 15 MPa to create cavitation in pure water while the maximum negative pressure appearing with US is about 1.5 MPa. Therefore, tissue damage by cavitation can be excluded for medical US diagnostics.

Temperature effects emerge from the conversion of sound wave energy to thermal heat through absorption. The absorption coefficient increases proportionally with frequency. With B-mode imaging, the absorbed energy is dispersed to a relatively large body volume and each single pulse is as short as possible ($< 1\,\mu s$) at a frequency of about 5 kHz. Therefore, the power delivered from US is very small (about 1 to 10 mW). Considering the large irradiated volume, this power is not sufficient to cause a measurable increase in temperature. In contrast, for Doppler examinations the irradiated volume is much smaller, and for frequencies of up to 30 kHz, overheating is possible.

1.8 NUCLEAR MEDICINE AND MOLECULAR IMAGING

Imaging in *nuclear medicine* is similar to x-ray imaging. The fundamental difference is that in nuclear medicine, the patient emits ionizing radiation, whereas in x-ray diagnostics, the radiation is applied from the outside. In order to visualize metabolic activity in organs, the *tracer method* is commonly used. Here, the radio nuclide is bound to a chemical complex that is taken up by the organ like any metabolic substance. In most clinical applications technetium ^{99m}Tc is established as tracer. It emits γ-quanta of an energy of 140 keV due to the transition from an excited *metastable state* to a basic state.

In diagnostic nuclear medicine a small quantity of radioactive tracer is injected into the patient; the tracer is preferentially stored in a target organ due to its biochemical properties. The γ-quanta from inside the body, emitted due to the decay of the nuclide, are then detected and displayed as image intensities. The distribution of the activity allows visualization of the metabolism of the particular organ. Therefore, these methods primarily show the physiological function of the system, not the anatomic structure. This information can be fused with images from other modalities such as CT or MR to give more anatomical information – some of the methods to combine images from different modalities will be introduced in Chapter 9. A classical example of a substance used in nuclear medicine is iodine-123 (^{123}I), which is taken up by the thyroid like non-radioactive iodine. An iodine-123 scan visualizes the metabolic activity of the thyroid gland.

1.8.1 Scintigraphy

Scintigraphy is the common term for imaging the distribution of radioactivity by detecting photons emitted from inside the body. Although there are remarkable advantages in the field of semi-conductor detectors the classical *scintillation detector* is the physical base of nuclear imaging. The detector is a transparent scintillator crystal that converts the incident γ-ray into visible light photons. The most common crystal for this purpose is sodium iodide (NaI) contaminated with a small amount of thallium (NaI(Tl)) because of its high light efficiency. The next step in the detection chain is a *photomultiplier* which first converts the photons to electrons using the well-known photoelectric effect. Then the so-called *dynode* system of the photomultiplier tube multiplies the electrons and a preamplifier finally processes the current from the photomultiplier to an electrical signal.

1.8.2   The γ camera

The detector of a γ camera (or Anger camera, after its inventor H. O. Anger) is a large area scintillation crystal made of NaI(Tl). In front of the crystal, a parallel *collimator* is placed. Only quanta impacting perpendicular to the plane of the crystal are able to pass the collimator, while oblique quanta causes are absorbed by the collimator walls, the so-called *septa* – see also Figure 1.23.

The design of the collimator crucially impacts the sensitivity and spatial resolution. The collimator holes are rotationally symmetric. Larger holes and smaller length of septa increases the detector sensitivity while spatial resolution deteriorates. There are a large number of different collimators available, depending on the energy of the γ and the clinical applications.

Another important feature of γ-cameras is the technique of localizing a single event. The *internal* or *inherent* resolution of the camera is given by the electronic accuracy to determine the position of an interaction in the detector. The camera's detector assembly can be seen as a two-dimensional configuration of *photo multipliers* (PM) in a hexagonal form mounted on a thin rectangular NaI-crystal. The number of PMs in a typical modern Anger camera amounts from 60 to 100; the diagonal of a camera head is in the range of 550 mm. An incident photon on the crystal releases a two-dimensional distribution of light photons on the exit side of the crystal that is more or less rotationally symmetric. The generated light photons create a pattern of signals at the exit of the involved PMs which is characteristic for the event location (see also Figure 1.23). The exact location is calculated as the center of gravity of the light distribution as measured by the surrounding photomultipliers. However, the homogeneity and linearity of the camera images have to be improved by applying several corrections.

1.8.3   SPECT and PET

Single Photon Emission Computed Tomography (SPECT) uses rotating γ-cameras; it is the technique in nuclear medicine analogous to x-ray computed tomography. Projections of the activity distribution are recorded at discrete angles during the rotation, and from these projection data a 3D volume is reconstructed. The detector head allows for gathering projections of several slices simultaneously. For image reconstruction, filtered back projection is used as in x-ray CT (see Chapter 10).

Positron emission tomography (PET) uses *positron* (β^+) emitters as tracers. These tracers are nuclides with an excess number of protons compared to the number of neutrons. Therefore, these isotopes are unstable and decay by converting a proton p into a positron e^+, a neutron n and a neutrino ν:

$$p \mapsto e^+ + \nu + n, \tag{1.8}$$

which is also known as β^+ *decay*.

The positrons cannot be detected directly because their *mean free path* before annihilation – which is the inverse effect of pair production – with an electron is limited to several tenths of a millimeter. But there is an effect that produces detectable gamma quanta: the positron, being the anti-particle of an electron – annihilates when interacting with an elec-

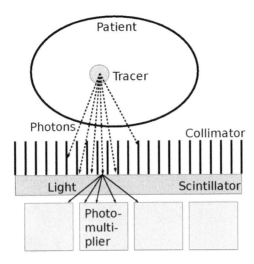

FIGURE 1.23: The principle of a γ-camera. A tracer substance emits γ radiation. The rays are "focused" by the septa of the collimator, which block incoming radiation with an oblique angle of incidence. The γ photons that pass the collimator hit the scintillator, where the photon produces a scintillation consisting of an avalanche of low-energy photons. Several photomultipliers are hit by the photons; the centroid of the signal intensities from the photomultipliers allows for a localization of the original scintillation event with an accuracy in the range of $2-3$ mm.

tron e^- by converting both masses to γ quanta:

$$e^+ + e^- \mapsto 2\gamma \tag{1.9}$$

The two resulting γ-quanta are emitted in exactly opposite directions with an energy of 511 keV each – the formula for this amount of energy E is well known and given by:

$$E = mc^2 [\mathrm{J}] \tag{1.10}$$

m is $1.8218764 * 10^{-30}$ kg, twice the mass of a single electron, and c is the velocity of light in vacuum, $299792458 \frac{\mathrm{m}}{\mathrm{s}}$.

Some of the medically important positron emitters are ^{11}C (half-life 20.4 min), ^{13}N (9.9 min) and ^{18}F (110 min), which is mainly used for labeling PET tracers. In more than 90% of all PET imaging procedures FDG (2-[^{18}F]fluoro-2-deoxy-D-glucose) is employed as the biologically active molecule. This analog of glucose is the tracer of choice in oncology since most tumors have a high glucose metabolism due to the rapid growth of the malignant tissue. It is also used in cardiology and neurology.

To distinguish the annihilation γ-quanta from quanta resulting from other effects, *coincidence detection* is used. Only events where two quanta are detected simultaneously by opposing detectors are counted. For fast detectors, the coincidence window is on the order of about 5 ns. This principle of event detection requires ring detectors. While early PET scanners had a single ring and allowed for reconstruction of single transverse planes only, modern scanners feature multiple detector rings.

If the two quanta are not scattered along their path to the detectors, the event is called *true coincidence*. Here, the origin of the detected event is localized along a straight line called

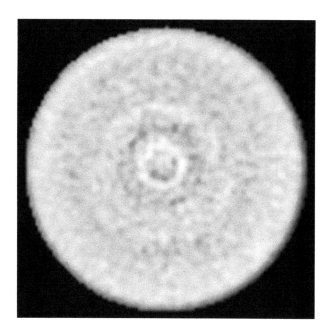

FIGURE 1.24: A ring artifact in SPECT reconstruction. The brighter areas in the homogeneous phantom are a consequence of local irregularities in detector sensitivity. A similar artifact is also known in CT and will be simulated in Chapter 10.

line of response (LOR). For scattered quanta, the event is referred to as *scatter event*. These events are only measured if the energy of each quanta falls into a predefined *energy window*.

Another requirement for image reconstruction is *attenuation correction*. Since the photons traverse tissue of different thickness, they are attenuated in a different manner according to Equation 1.3. This can be corrected for by additional measurements of external sources. A transmission scan measures the local distribution of the attenuation coefficient in the patient. Then, an attenuation map for each LOR can be calculated. A transmission scan can also be obtained by creating a CT scan of the patient, for example with PET-CT scanners (see also Figures 1.25, 1.26 and 9.1).

Image reconstruction is similar to the reconstruction of CT, but with PET the raw data set is of lesser quality. Each event represents a line in space which connects the two simultaneously recorded photons. Modern systems providing a high time resolution can even measure the time between the detection of the two photons and therefore allow to determine the position of the event on the LOR to some extent. This technique is called *time of flight PET*.

1.9 OTHER IMAGING TECHNIQUES

Optical coherence tomography (OCT) allows for acquisition of 3D images with microscopic resolution in tissue. Usually, light in the near-infrared range is used; the scattering of quanta with a short coherence length allows for acquiring high-resolution images of tissue with a penetration depth of several millimeters. An important clinical application is diagnostics of retinal disease in ophthalmology on a micrometer scale. Figure 1.27 shows an example of an image rendered from OCT image data.

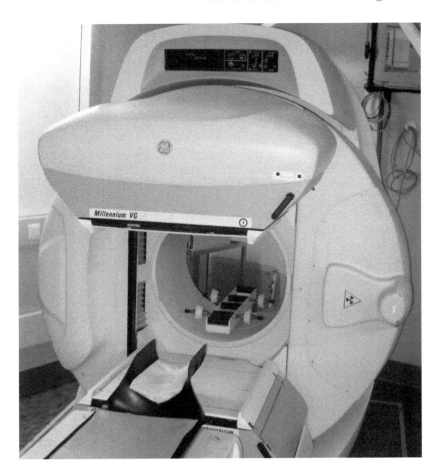

FIGURE 1.25: A very interesting γ-camera. This dual head camera allows for acquisition of planar images and SPECT. Beyond that, it can also acquire CT-data using a small x-ray unit mounted perpendicular to the two detectors, and it can detect the specific radiation from β^+ annihilation in coincidence mode – therefore, it also allows for PET imaging. Machines of this type were the first clinically available systems for PET-CT. A modern PET-CT machine can be found in Figure 1.26.

Electron beam CT (EBCT) allows to rotate the focal spot of an x-ray tube electronically on an anode ring, resulting in very fast image acquisition. Electrons are emitted by an electron gun and the electron beam is magnetically deflected towards the circular anode surrounding the patient. No mechanical parts are involved. Therefore, a sweep can be accomplished within 50 ms. By comparison, an average CT x-ray tube requires more than 200 ms for one sweep. These devices are primarily used for heart imaging in real time. Disadvantages of this technology are related to the large amount of scatter radiation, a bad signal-to-noise ratio, a bad ratio between production volume to size of the device and finally its high costs. It is now replaced by multislice CT.

Near infrared imaging (NIR) is another optical imaging technique. Similar to the tracer method in nuclear medicine, an optical dye is bound to a metabolically active

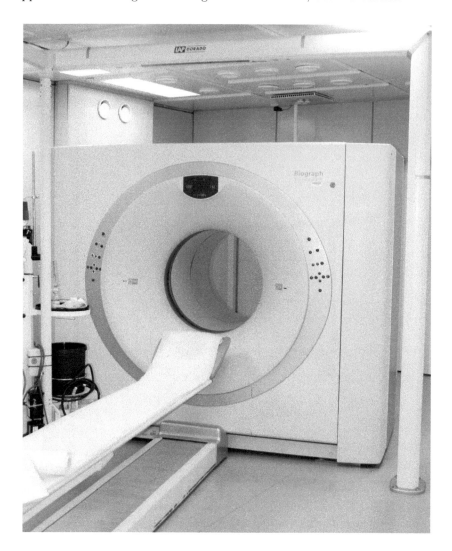

FIGURE 1.26: A modern state-of-the-art PET-CT machine. Here, a modern PET scanner is integrated with a 64-slice multislice CT. One can see that the machine is quite thick since the detector ring of the PET and the CT are combined in one housing. Machines like that give images such as Figure 9.1. Its main clinical application is oncology, where cancer metabolism and metastases are visualized in the context of the patient's anatomy.

substance. Fluorescence phenomena, preferably in the near-infrared domain, show the localization of the substance to be tracked. The method is widely used in small animal imaging.

Histology: By using a *microtome*, it is possible to produce very thin slices of tissue which can be inspected under a microscope in transmitted light. Images taken from these samples can also be reconstructed as 3D volumes.

Endoscopy: An endoscope is a device that allows for acquisition of optical images, histology samples, and simple interventions inside the body. It consists of a rigid or

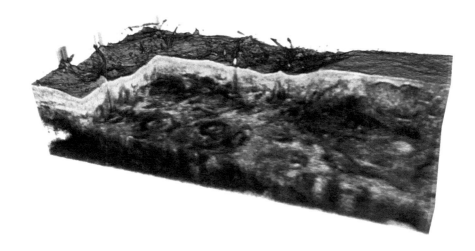

FIGURE 1.27: A 3D rendering of OCT image data of layers of the epidemis, also showing a basalioma. The volume covers an area of 6 x 3.5 mm. Image data courtesy of W. Drexler and B. Hermann, Center for Medical Physics and Biomedical Engineering, Medical University Vienna.

flexible tube with an end-effector that can be controlled from the outside. Usually small videocameras acquire the image data.

1.10 RADIATION PROTECTION AND DOSIMETRY

1.10.1 Terminology of dosimetry

The definition of *absorbed dose* or *energy dose* D is the quotient of energy (dE) from *ionizing* radiation absorbed in a mass element dm:

$$D = \frac{dE}{dm} [\text{Gy}] \tag{1.11}$$

The *SI unit* is *Gray* (Gy); it replaces the old unit *rad* (radiation absorbed dose). One Gray is defined as

$$1\,\text{Gy} = 1\frac{\text{J}}{\text{kg}} = 100\,\text{rad} \tag{1.12}$$

The quantity *Kerma* (kinetic energy released in matter) describes the energy dE_{tr} which is transferred to material in the first step of interaction. dE_{tr} is the sum of the initial kinetic energy of all electrons excited by the uncharged photons, ρ is the density of matter, m is the mass, and V is volume.

$$K = \frac{dE_{\text{tr}}}{dm} = \frac{1}{\rho}\frac{dE_{\text{tr}}}{dV} \left[\frac{\text{J}}{\text{kg}}\right] \tag{1.13}$$

From the definition, it is clear that this quantity depends on the material in which the interaction takes place and therefore has to be indicated (air Kerma, water Kerma, ...). The Kerma is directly proportional to the photon energy fluency $\psi = \frac{E_{ph}dN}{dA}$, where dN

Radiation type	α	neutrons	γ-rays	β
q-factor	20	5–20	1	1

TABLE 1.2: Quality factors of different radiation types in regard to radiation protection. The factors are due to interpret in the way that 1 Gy of α-radiation equals 20 Gy of γ-radiation with respect to its biological effects.

is the number of photons and dA the area. Kerma is always maximal at the surface and decreases with depth while the dose builds to a maximum value (dose maximum) and then decreases at the same rate as Kerma.

A very important term with respect to radiation protection is the *equivalent dose H*. It refers to the fact that with the same energy dose different types of radiation show different impact in biological tissue. It is defined as

$$H = Dq \left[\frac{J}{kg} \right] \tag{1.14}$$

q is a dimensionless factor; it defines equivalent dose that causes the same biological damage to tissue. Although the quality factor q is dimensionless and the SI unit for the equivalent dose is the same as for the energy dose $\frac{J}{kg}$, there is a special unit *Sievert (Sv)* to distinguish between the two terms. Table 1.2 shows the quality factor q for the most important types of radiation.

1.10.2 Radiation effects on tissue and organs

The major impact of ionizing radiation with a low linear energy transfer such as photons and electrons to cells is the generation of free radicals. These are mainly created when cellular water molecules are cracked into OH- and H- radicals, which are very reactive due to their unpaired electrons. The most fatal effects are caused when DNA molecules get damaged. Here, we distinguish between single- and double-strand cracks and base defects. Damage to a DNA molecule does not necessarily lead to cell death. Most DNA damages can be fixed by special cell repair mechanisms. Exposure with 1 Sv causes about $4000 - 5000$ DNA damages with approximately 3000 base breaks, 1000 single strand cracks and 40 double strand cracks per cell. Most of the damage can be repaired and $20 - 30\%$ of the exposed cells are destroyed – the cell loses its functional capability and is dissolved. Cell types showing high radiation sensibility are for example the ovule, spermatogonial, mucosal tissue cells or lymphocytes, while muscle cells, neurocytes or liver cells are less sensitive to radiation damage.

For the description of the impact on living organisms, two different types of tissue damages can be distinguished. *Deterministic damages* occur above a certain exposure threshold. If the threshold is exceeded, the number of killed cells influences cell proliferation and tissues and organs are harmed. The severity of the effects increases with the energy dose. Table 1.3 shows the effect of three different equivalent doses to case of exposure to the whole body.

Stochastic radiation effects are not associated with a minimal dose. In the dose range relevant for radiation protection purposes, inheritable damages, cancer and leukemia are indicated as stochastic effects. The probability of damage differs crucially for the irradiated organs or tissues. The International Commission on Radiological Protection estimates a probability of developing cancer of 5.5% per Sievert at low effective dose rates.

For estimation of the risk to develop cancer at low dose data from epidemiological analysis are used. These data come mainly from survivors of Hiroshima and Nagasaki, job

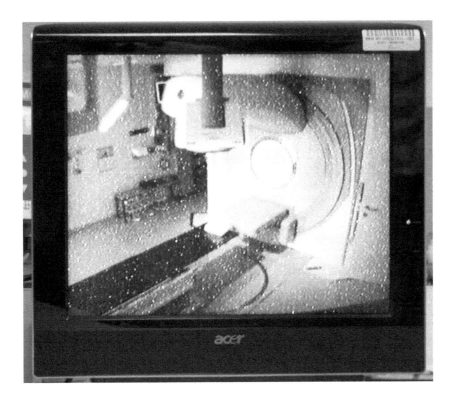

FIGURE 1.28: Ionizing radiation does not only have effects on living tissue; it also changes the properties of materials like semiconductors. This is an image of a surveillance monitor used in a radiation therapy treatment station. In radiotherapy, a highly focused dose is applied in several treatment sessions to the cancer tissue, with the purpose of destroying every single cancer cell in the target area. As a side effect, a considerable amount of scatter radiation (see also Section 1.4) is produced, which can amount up to 0.1 Gy. Therefore, the treatment room is heavily shielded and no personnel must be inside during treatment. The video camera is necessary to observe the course of treatment. However, over time, the image detector of the video camera is destroyed by radiation. What you see here is a standard LINAC (similar to the machine shown in Figure 1.11), and the image noise is not caused by transmission noise or a faulty monitor, but by dead pixels on the detector. Usually, these cameras have to be replaced within a few months.

related radiation exposures and from radiotherapy patients – the statistical significance and accuracy of these data is, however, under discussion.

Sporadically, effects of *hormesis* can be observed. Generally spoken, hormesis means that low doses of toxic substances can show beneficial effects. It seems that a low dose challenge may induce body repair effects that not only neutralize the destructive effect of radiation but even repair other defects not caused by irradiation. However, this effect was only proved to enhance growth of plants when the seeds were irradiated, and benefits for the human body are still questionable.

Time after exposure	Sub-lethal dose 1 Sv	Critical dose 4 Sv	Lethal dose 7 Sv
1st week	reduction of lymphocytes	reduction of lymphocytes	symptoms after 3 days: bloody diarrhea, emesis, fever
2nd week	no symptoms	no symptoms	
3rd week	hair loss, diarrhea, indisposition	same as sublethal internal bleeding	
4th week	recovery likely	50 % fatality	100% fatality

TABLE 1.3: Symptoms from deterministic damage after whole body exposure with photons (q-factor 1).

Exposition	Dose [mSv]
North atlantic flight (round trip)	0.1
Chernobyl incident (accumulated to 50 years)	0.55
Side-effects of nuclear weapon tests (accumulated to 50 years)	1.5
Cosmic background	1
Terrestrial background	1
Average annual exposure (natural and human-caused)	3.6
Radiotherapy treatment in oncology in target volume	40000 – 80000
Sterilization dose for medical instruments	30000

TABLE 1.4: Some examples of radiation exposures.

1.10.3 Natural and man-made radiation exposure

Natural radiation exposure has two main sources. Primary *cosmic radiation* consists of an high energy galactic component and a solar component. It is built up by 86% protons, 12% α-particles, 1% electrons and 1% heavy particles. This primary radiation undergoes a strong shift in components when it comes in contact with the magnetic field of the earth. Spallation and neutron capture create so-called cosmic radionuclides (for example ^{3}H, ^{22}Na, ^{7}Be). Some of these nuclides reach the food chain and are partly responsible for *internal radiation exposition. Terrestrial sources* are radioactive elements such as *uranium, thorium, radium* and *radon*. The latter can be found in high concentration in many areas of the world although it is, generally speaking, a scarce element. It diffuses from soil, water and construction materials and can be found in the air at ground level. The annual average dose from natural background radiation amounts to approximately 2.2 – 2.4 mSv, with local peaks much higher. In Kerala India, for example the average annual dose can sum up to 32 mSv due to monazite sand which can be found on the coast. In Table 1.4 one can find some selected examples of average radiation exposures from natural and artificial sources. A typical average natural radiation exposure is 2 mSv/year.

Radiation caused by humans is not distributed uniformly as it is for natural background radiation. *Radiography* is the major component, with an average exposure dose of 1.5 mSv per person and year. In this context, the effective dose depends crucially on the part of the body under examination. Table 1.5 shows the absorbed equivalent dose for different examinations. Another source of irradiation that stems from medicine stems from the use

Exposition	Dose [mSv]
Thorax CT	20
Skull CT	3
Mammography	2
Chest x-ray	0.1
Dental x-ray	0.01

TABLE 1.5: Some examples of x-ray exposures.

of radionuclides in nuclear medicine. Here, the average dose is approximately a tenth of the x-ray exposure (approximately 0.15 mSv per person and year).

1.11 SUMMARY AND FURTHER REFERENCES

This chapter is a very short synopsis of the physics associated with most common medical imaging techniques. For someone working in medical image processing, it is important to understand the intrinsic properties of the various imaging methods. One of the differences of medical image processing compared to conventional image processing is the fact that the images are usually not recorded in the domain of visible or infrared light, thus requiring different methods to retrieve images from the data recorded. Furthermore, everyone working in medical image processing should have a clear understanding of the dose concept and related issues of radiation protection.

Literature

J. T. Bushberg, J. A. Seibert, E. M. Leidholdt Jr: The Essential Physics of Medical Imaging, Lippincott Williams & Wilkins, (2001)

W. R. Hendee, E. R. Ritenour: Medical Imaging Physics, Wiley, (2002)

P. P. Dendy, B. Heaton: Physics for Diagnostic Radiology, Taylor & Francis, (1999)

W. A. Kalender: Computed Tomography: Fundamentals, System Technology, Image Quality, Applications, Wiley VCH, (2006)

D. Weishaupt, V. D. Köchli, B. Marincek: How does MRI work?: An Introduction to the Physics and Function of Magnetic Resonance Imaging, Springer, (2006)

E. Berry, A. Bulpitt: Fundamentals of MRI – An interactive learning approach, CRC Press, (2009).

A. Oppelt (Ed.): Imaging Systems for Medical Diagnostics: Fundamentals, Technical Solutions and Applications for Systems Applying Ionizing Radiation, Nuclear Magnetic Resonance and Ultrasound, Wiley VCH, (2006)

S. R. Cherry, J. Sorenson, M. Phelps: Physics in Nuclear Medicine, Saunders, (2003)

CHAPTER 2

Image Processing in Clinical Practice

Wolfgang Birkfellner

CONTENTS

2.1	Application examples	45
2.2	Image databases	45
2.3	Intensity operations	46
2.4	Filter operations	47
2.5	Segmentation	48
2.6	Spatial transforms	49
2.7	Rendering and surface models	51
2.8	Registration	54
2.9	CT reconstruction	56
2.10	Summary	56

2.1 APPLICATION EXAMPLES

In order to provide you with some insight on the possibilities and the potential of medical image processing, we have gathered a few examples of what is being done in hospitals right now using the image processing methods presented in this book. Reference to the algorithms as presented in the volume are given where appropriate. This compilation does not claim to be complete; rather, it is an effort towards linking the concepts you will learn with clinical reality.

2.2 IMAGE DATABASES

As you may have already learned from the previous chapter, medical image data can be of quite enormous size, and they are quite often three-dimensional. The organization of such huge data volumes, which have to be linked to other data such as laboratory exams, histology and data on treatment methods is of course a major challenge. In radiology and affiliated disciplines, the common standard for handling, storing and administrating image data is called *Digital Imaging and Communications in Medicine – DICOM*, and it will be introduced in Chapter 3. Figure 2.1 shows a screenshot of a browser window for a DICOM database. This image must not be confused with the similar looking listings of DICOM header data, which can, for instance be found in Figure 3.8. Here, we only see the dialog of a clinical dose planning system where a number of patients currently under treatment can be selected.

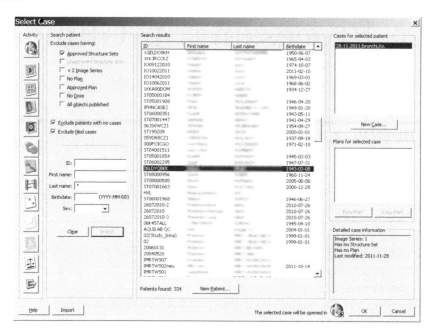

FIGURE 2.1: A screenshot from a radiotherapy planning system – Oncentra Masterplan by Nucletron/The Netherlands showing a selection of patients currently under treatment. The patient names were blurred for the sake of anonymity. DICOM datasets contain a lot of information on the patient, and the DICOM standard also manages the storage and administration of patient data. By selecting one of the patient names, the physician or radiographer can retrieve the image data, together with dose plans for tumor irradiation and other information relevant for patient treatment.

2.3 INTENSITY OPERATIONS

Medical image data are – technically speaking – mathematical functions of measured values. For instance in CT, measurements of absorption coefficients are translated to gray values. These measured values are stored with the greatest accuracy reasonably achievable, and therefore, there are many possible shades of gray between black (= no signal) and white (= the maximum signal). In the case of CT, absorption values are measured by means of 4096 Hounsfield units, and in principle, measurement values from MR can take 65536 values. The same holds true for measurements from nuclear medicine devices.

The eye cannot resolve such subtle detail in gray levels; therefore, all kinds of operations that manipulate the display of gray levels are widely used. These *intensity operations* are discussed in Chapter 4. Figure 2.2 shows the effect of the most important of these operations known as *windowing*. By choosing a gray level range that corresponds to the typical absorption coefficients of a specific type of tissue, contrast is selectively enhanced for that type of tissue. Windowing is performed on virtually every tomographic image data set. The fact that medical images are stored with greater depth (or, to put it simply, higher precision) than "normal" image data renders this visualization method much more powerful compared to a simple adaptation of brightness and contrast, which is well known from conventional image processing applications.

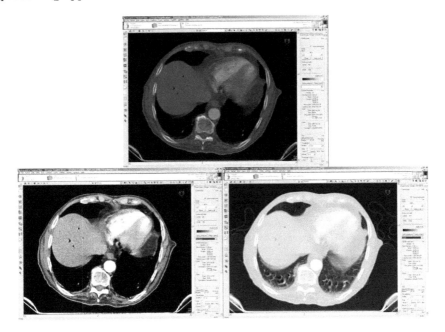

FIGURE 2.2: Here, we see *windowing*, the most widespread visualization technique in diagnostic radiology, in action. As we know from Chapter 1, absorption coefficients in computed tomography are stored in Hounsfield-units (HU), ranging from -1024 to 3072. Humans can only perceive approximately 100 shades of gray. Windowing allows for selectively enhancing the contrast of certain tissue types. The upper screenshot shows the original screenshot from Oncentra Masterplan, displaying the upper abdomen of a radiotherapy patient. The lower left image shows the same image data, but its intensities are displayed in a soft tissue window; it corresponds to the absorption of parenchyma such as the liver. The lower right images shows the same slice in a lung window, where the subtleties of the lung are shown with optimum contrast.

2.4   FILTER OPERATIONS

Chapter 5 will deal with local operations to modify images, and with image transforms. Filters (sometimes referred to as pointwise operations) modify an image; they can be used to reduce noise by local averaging of gray values, and can also be used to sharpen images, which is for instance being done automatically in reconstruction of CT images (see also Chapter 10 and Figure 5.5). Figure 2.3 shows the use of another filtering application, namely edge detection, for the assessment of image fusion results.

In Chapter 5, we will also encounter some *image transforms*, mainly the *Fourier-transform*, which is of great relevance for all kinds of signal processing. In medical imaging, it is of special importance for the reconstruction of tomographic MR-images, and for the convolution of complex filter kernels with images.

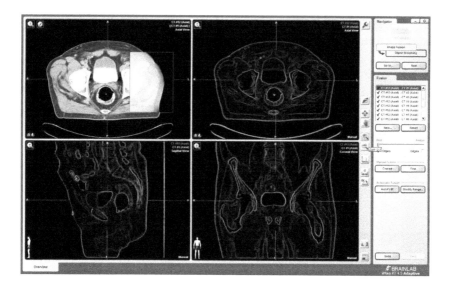

FIGURE 2.3: An edge-detection filter used for assessment of image fusion results. This screenshot of the iPlan software suite (BrainLAB AG, Germany) shows an application of an edge detection filter. Two image datasets of the same patient, one from conventional CT (upper left quadrant of the screenshot), the other from CBCT (which is partially displayed in the rectangle inserted into the conventional CT), were merged by means of *image registration* – see also Chapter 9. In order to assess the success of this fusion, the images undergo a filtering operation with a so-called *Sobel-kernel*, which will be introduced in Chapter 5. A Sobel filter is an edge-detection method which determines sudden changes in image brightness by means of computing a gradient. Overlap of edges in the CT and CBCT images are used for registration validation in this application.

2.5 SEGMENTATION

The identification of certain regions in an image is usually referred to as *segmentation*, and it will be introduced in Chapter 6. Segmentation is a field with a plethora of applications, including physiological measurements in a defined region of interest, measurement of area and volume in medical image datasets, definition of geometrical models from medical image data (see also Figure 6.8) and definition of target areas and organs-at-risk in radiotherapy. Unfortunately, the definition of a given region of interest (which is often simply an organ) is a difficult and ill-posed problem. Figure 2.4 shows a straightforward effort towards identifying anatomical structures by assigning a certain intensity range. This technique is called *intensity thresholding*. It is based on the simple assumption that image areas above a certain gray level belong to a particular type of tissue. However, this is not always true. Figures 6.2 and 6.30 give an idea of the limitations of this method.

Therefore, numerous other techniques such as *region growing, snakes, statistical shape models, level-set techniques* and others were developed. An example of *atlas-based* segmentation, where an approximate statistical shape model of certain structures is adopted to the patient specific anatomy, can be found in Figure 2.5.

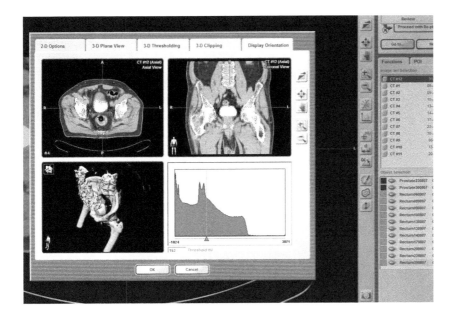

FIGURE 2.4: An application example of simple segmentation by means of intensity thresholding. In the lower right of the screenshot you see a distribution of intensity values in the given image, a so called *histogram*. In this histogram, a threshold is identified. All image elements above that gray value are considered to belong to a specific class of tissue – in this case, bone. The areas whose gray values are higher than the threshold are identified as white areas. In the color version of this screenshot, which may be found on the accompanying CD, these areas are shown in red.

2.6   SPATIAL TRANSFORMS

Spatial transforms, which will be introduced in Chapter 7, are another important class of image manipulations, which do not deal with the gray values assigned to a picture element, but are connected to the manipulation of image element positions. Two common spatial transforms are *interpolation*, the redistribution of gray values in a new discrete mesh of image elements, and *reformatting*, the computation of new 2D slices from 3D tomographic data.

Figure 2.6 illustrates the effect of changing the resolution of an image on a CT-slice that shows a magnified part of the pelvis, the pubic arch. In the original resolution (upper part of the image), single picture elements (so-called *pixels*, which will be introduced in more detail in Chapter 3) are clearly visible. A similar illustration can also be found in Figure 3.1. After defining a grid with more pixels, the gray values are redistributed in a specific manner, which gives a smoother appearance (lower part of Figure 2.6). Details on interpolation techniques in 2D and 3D are given in Section 7.2.

Many times in this book, you will encounter the statement that tomographic medical images are not "stacks of slices" – a simple collection of 3D images. Instead, they are true 3D images with three dimensional picture elements, so-called *voxels*. Voxels will be discussed in more detail in Chapter 3. A major difference to "conventional" image processing therefore lies in the fact that we have to deal with spatial transforms (namely rotations and translations) in three dimensions. The main difference here lies in the fact that we do not

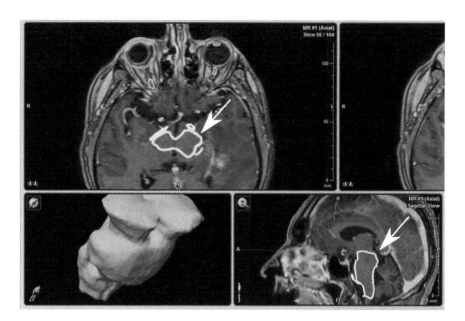

FIGURE 2.5: An application example of a more sophisticated segmentation method compared to intensity thresholding. In this case, we see an *atlas-based* segmentation method at work on a MR-image of the brain. Again, radiotherapists tried to delineate an *organ-at-risk* – a sensitive anatomical structure in the proximity of a tumor that must not be irradiated. A statistical shape model of the brain stem is adopted to the anatomy of the patient. The arrows in the upper left axial slice and in the lower right sagittal slice point at the contours of the brain stem. Based on these contours, a 3D model of the brain stem is derived. This model is visualized by means of *surface rendering* – see also Chapter 8. In the color version of this screenshot, which can be found on the accompanying CD, other structures such as the eye balls, the optical nerve and the cornea are also clearly visible as colored organs-at-risk. The screenshot shows the iPlan software suite, BrainLAB AG, Germany.

have to deal with three degrees of freedom (one angle of rotation and a shift in the direction of the two coordinate axes of a Cartesian coordinate system), but we are facing six degrees of freedom. The handling of this more complex formalism will also be discussed in detail in Chapters 7, 8 and 9.

A simple and very common application of such a 3D transform is *reformatting*, another very widespread visualization technique for 3D image data. Here, a new imaging plane is positioned in the 3D volume image, and those voxels of the volume that intersect with the pixels of the imaging plane determine the gray value in the pixels of the new image. A very simple geometric example for this process can be found in Section 7.6.4; in this case, the well-known curves derived from cone sections – the circle, the ellipsoid, the parabola and the hyperbola – are generated by reformatting. Figure 2.7 shows a clinical example. In this illustration, three views are generated from a clinical CT volume of the abdomen. Given its imaging geometry, CT can only take axial slices of the patient; still, one has to keep in mind that modern CT machines do not acquire single slices. This is also a major difference from MR machines, which can take the original image data at arbitrary orientations. However, once the volume is stored, reformatting allows for computation of new slices in all directions.

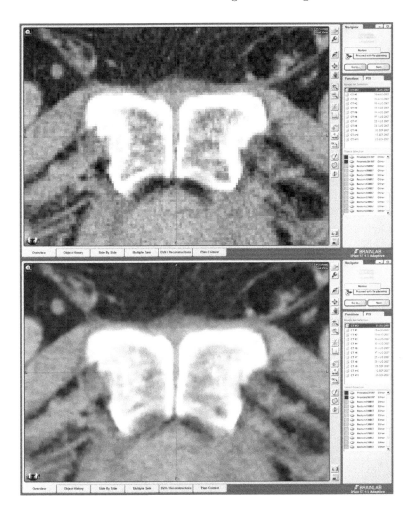

FIGURE 2.6: Interpolation of gray value distributions in a refined mesh of picture elements. In this CT-slice, we see a part of the pelvis – the symphysis of the os pubis, or the pubic arch – in the original resolution of the CT volume (upper screenshot). After *interpolation*, a smoother high-resolution version of the same image is seen (lower screenshot). Interpolation does not add image information, but improves visualization and simplifies mathematical handling of image data. The screenshot shows the iPlan software suite, BrainLAB AG, Germany.

2.7 RENDERING AND SURFACE MODELS

A direct application of 3D spatial transforms is the visualization of 3D datasets; Figure 1.10 gave an impression of the amount of data produced by a modern CT machine. *Volume* and *surface rendering* provide methods to visualize these large amounts of data in a comprehensive manner. Technically speaking, we utilize physical models and spatial transforms to produce images such as Figures 2.8, 2.9 and 8.5. In Chapter 8, we will learn about the basics of generating such images.

Figure 2.8 shows a clinical application of *volume rendering*. Here, a virtual x-ray (a so-called *simulator image* or *digitally rendered radiograph (DRR)* is generated from CT data.

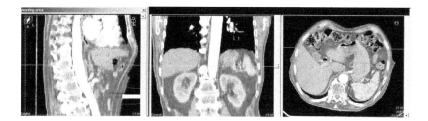

FIGURE 2.7: A clinical example of orthogonal reformatting. The rightmost image shows the original slice of a patient's abdomen, taken with a CT scanner. The slice orientation is given in an axial direction – the body stem of the patient is normal to the imaging plane. By placing a new "virtual" imaging plane in the 3D volume dataset, other images can be derived. The leftmost image shows a sagittal view of the same dataset; in the middle, we find the coronal view. The screenshot shows the Oncentra Masterplan software, Nucletron/The Netherlands.

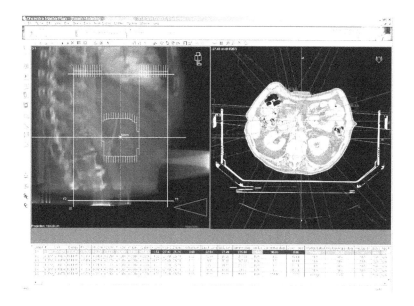

FIGURE 2.8: An application of volume rendering, used for target area verification in radiotherapy dose planning. The right part of the image shows the treatment plan developed by the radiotherapist. Radiation with various angles of incidence is used to destroy the tumor cells in the target area. In order to verify this plan, a virtual x-ray – called a simulator image or digitally rendered radiograph – is generated from the CT-data by means of rendering. This rendering can be seen on the left-hand side of the image. The shape of the collimator (a device used to shape the treatment beam) is also overlaid as a graphical structure. The screenshot shows the Oncentra Masterplan software, Nucletron/The Netherlands.

The dose application for a radiotherapy treatment is planned on a CT volume dataset. In order to visualize the *beam's eye view* – the anatomy of the patient as it is "seen" by the linear accelerator – this DRR is superimposed with the target area and the shape of the collimator (a structure made of lead plates that acts as a stop for the γ-radiation).

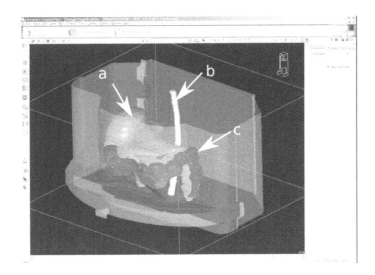

FIGURE 2.9: Another example from radiotherapy; this time, organs-at-risk were *segmented* and are visualized as opaque, colored surfaces; a.) shows the diaphragm, which tightly covers the liver, b.) is the spinal cord and c.) is the ileum. These structures have to be spared during irradiation. A few more anatomical structures are also shown in this image; the target volume in this case is the pancreas, which is also delineated. The patient is fixated in a rigid perspex structure, which deforms the body surface. The screenshot shows the Oncentra Masterplan software, Nucletron/The Netherlands.

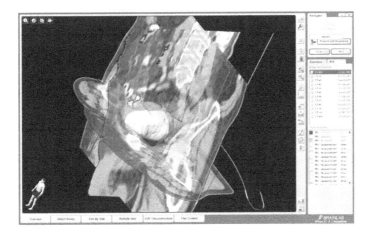

FIGURE 2.10: An example of 3D visualization of reformatted slices – shown in their actual spatial position within the volume – and surface rendering of segmented structures. Here, mainly the bladder which was segmented as an organ-at-risk is visible. Screenshot taken from the iPlan software suite, BrainLAB AG, Germany.

Figure 2.9 is an example of *surface rendering* in clinical practice. Several anatomical structures were *segmented* (see also Figure 2.5). These are the organs-at-risk and the planned target volume for tumor irradiation. The contour information was used to generate surface models, whose optical properties such as reflection and absorption were simulated, giving a 3D impression of the structure. Another example for surface rendering can be found in Figure 2.5. In Figure 6.2, surface rendering is also used to visualize the shortcomings of segmentation using simple intensity thresholding.

Connected to surface rendering is the generation of *surface models*, which consist of small geometric primitives. Such models can be generated from tomographic volume data; in a subsequent step, it is possible to use these structures in computer-aided design or stereolithography. Figure 6.8 shows the result of such a process, where a model of the left ventricle of the heart was segmented, and a surface model was generated and printed using a 3D stereolithography printer. If done properly, surface rendering might generate impressive views, but it is usually also connected to a loss in diagnostic image information.

Finally, Figure 2.10 shows another application of 3D visualization and surface rendering. In this screenshot, three reformatted slices are visualized in a 3D model at their actual location within the volume, together with a surface rendering. In Example 8.5.7 using *3DSlicer*, we will generate such a view.

2.8 REGISTRATION

In Section 1.8.3, we heard about combined modalities such as PET-CT, and other machines that allow for multimodal imaging such as PET-MR which are currently introduced in clinical practice. But sometimes, combined imaging is not available or unfeasible, while datasets which contain information from different sources are desirable. PET-CT images that display both morphologic information on the patient's anatomy and functional information on metabolism are only one example for such an application of multimodal imaging, and an example for such an image can be found in Figure 9.1.

The basic problem of *registration* or *image fusion* is the fact that all data from an imaging system are reported in a coordinate system that is related to the imaging machine, not to the patient. In other words, if we want to merge image information, we need a common frame of reference, and the physical entity that defines that frame of reference is the patient. Registration algorithms are used to find such a common frame of reference. This can be achieved either by identifying well-defined landmarks which are present in all different coordinate systems (or image data sets), by optimizing statistical measures, or by merging image edges which can be identified by methods similar to the filter example shown in Figure 2.3. In Chapter 9, we will learn about these registration techniques, which are not only useful for fusion of images, but also for defining a common frame of reference with the real world. Such a registration of image space to a physical coordinate system is, for instance, inevitable in *image-guided therapy* and medical robotics. Figure 2.11 shows the registration of a diagnostic conventional CT dataset to a CBCT dataset acquired prior to treatment with a LINAC. A LINAC capable of producing such CBCTs can also be found in Figure 1.11.

If we are only interested in compensating different coordinate systems, a spatial transform defined by six degrees of freedom is sufficient. Every image element undergoes the same transform, and therefore we call this type of transformation a *rigid registration*. Human beings are, however, not rigid. It is therefore sometimes necessary to compensate for additional deformation of soft tissue after the rigid alignment of coordinate systems. This expansion of the registration problem is called *deformable registration*. The result of a deformable registration algorithm is, aside from a spatial transform, a deformation field that deforms one of the volume datasets to compensate for soft tissue motion. Figure 2.12 shows a clinical application, again with a diagnostic CT scan and a CBCT scan taken prior to

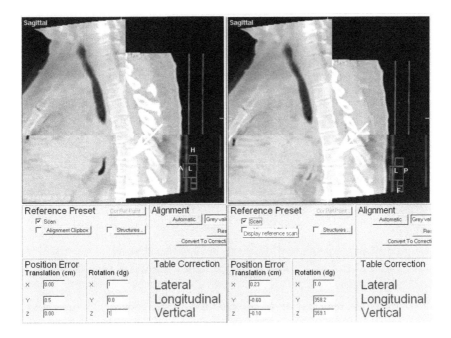

FIGURE 2.11: Two screen parts of the control software of a LINAC capable of CBCT-imaging. The left part of this image shows a fused visualization (usually referred to as *checkerboard visualization*) of a diagnostic CT taken prior to treatment and a CBCT-scan taken immediately before a therapy session. The diagnostic CT dataset is used for treatment planning, and the CBCT dataset is used for position verification of the patient with respect to the LINAC. The two datasets are not very well aligned, which is, for instance, visible from the mismatch of the intervertebral disk spaced denoted by the white arrow. The right screen shows the result of *rigid registration*, where six degrees of freedom were optimized to give an optimum match. Again, the arrow points at an intervertebral disk space, but this time, the two images match. In the lower part, one can also see that under the heading "Position Error", the translation and rotation of the coordinate systems was changed. By changing the position of the patient, misalignment prior to irradiation can be minimized. The screenshot shows the XVI software suite, Elekta AB, Sweden.

prostate irradiation. Here, the deformation of the target region – in this case, the prostate – due to different filling of the bladder and the rectum is being compensated for by deformable registration of the diagnostic CT scan (again taken prior to the the start of treatment) to a more recent CBCT scan. The deformation is visualized by means of a grid that reflects the displacement of areas in the volume dataset.

Finally, it is also possible to register modalities that deliver image data of different dimensionality. In Figure 2.13, we have an example of *2D/3D registration*. Volume rendering is used to produce a DRR from a volume data set. The DRR does exhibit the same characteristics concerning perspective, field-of-view and other image parameters as an x-ray taken with known relative orientation. By iterative comparison of a sequence of DRRs with changing rigid-body parameters, one can determine the position of the patient in 3D in relation to the x-ray device. Applications include *image-guided surgery* and *image-guided radiotherapy*.

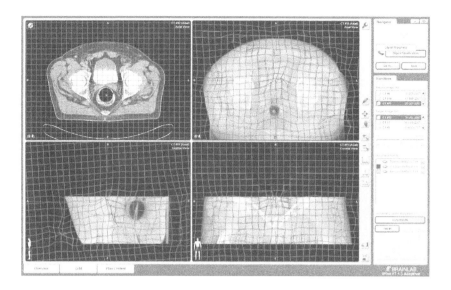

FIGURE 2.12: Deformable registration of pre-therapeutic diagnostic CT data and CBCT data taken immediately before radiation therapy treatment of the prostate. Here, additional degrees of freedom are introduced besides rotation and translation of coordinate systems. The relative change in the patient's anatomy is being compensated by displacing smaller regions in the volume data. This displacement is visualized by means of a grid in this case. The treatment plan is deformed in accordance to the result of the deformable registration process. The screenshot shows the iPlan software suite, BrainLAB AG, Germany.

2.9 CT RECONSTRUCTION

Finally, in Chapter 10, we will learn about the basics of tomographic medical imaging. *Tomographic reconstruction* is the art of retrieving 3D image data from projections, and it is possibly the earliest application of computers for medical image processing which has facilitated a whole new field of diagnosis and treatment. In short, reconstruction deals with the computation of 3D volume datasets from projective data such as the sinograms shown in a simplified sketch in Figure 1.6. All tomographic example data from CT or nuclear medicine (but not necessarily from MR, where image reconstruction usually takes place by a *Fourier transform*, discussed in detail in Chapter 5) you encounter in this book are the product of reconstruction algorithms, and while the topic is too often neglected in standard textbooks on image processing, we felt that it makes a good conclusion for this textbook on medical image processing.

2.10 SUMMARY

Following a chapter that dealt with the basic physics of medical imaging – or, in other words, the machines that produce our subject of interest – this chapter is more of a pictorial essay on selected applications. However, it may provide the motivation to deal with the methods to be introduced in the following chapters. It may also help to put the algorithmic details of some methods into a wider context.

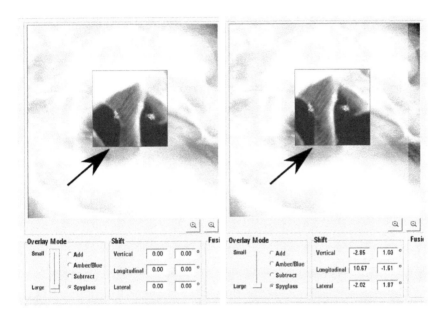

FIGURE 2.13: An example of 2D/3D registration. By iterative comparison of volume renderings and real projective x-ray data, the position of the patient in 3D can be determined. This image shows two views of the same screen – on the left, the patient is not registered. Since this is an x-ray of the pelvis region taken at an oblique angle, anatomical details are hard to figure. The arrow denotes an anatomical detail – the foramen obturatum – which is displaced prior to registration (left screenshot) and where alignment can be seen after registration (right screenshot). Below the heading "Shift", the parameters in terms of translation and rotation are also displayed. Screenshot shows the iPlan software suite, BrainLAB AG, Germany.

CHAPTER 3

Image Representation

Wolfgang Birkfellner

CONTENTS

3.1	Pixels and voxels	59
	3.1.1 Algebraic image operations	63
3.2	Gray scale and color representation	63
	3.2.1 Depth	63
	3.2.2 Color and look up tables	64
3.3	Image file formats	66
3.4	DICOM	71
3.5	Other formats – Analyze 7.5, NifTI and Interfile	73
3.6	Image quality and the signal-to-noise ratio	74
3.7	Practical lessons	75
	3.7.1 Image subtraction	75
	3.7.2 Opening and decoding a single DICOM file in MATLAB	75
	3.7.3 Opening a DICOM file using *ImageJ* and *3DSlicer*	81
	3.7.3.1 A single slice in ImageJ	81
	3.7.3.2 A CT-volume in 3DSlicer	82
	3.7.4 Converting a color image to gray scale	84
	3.7.4.1 A note on good MATLAB programming habits ...	85
	3.7.5 Computing the SNR of x-ray images as a function of dose	86
3.8	Summary and further references	89

3.1 PIXELS AND VOXELS

In digital image processing, every image is represented by numerical values associated with positions in a regular grid. A single position is usually referenced as *picture element*, or *pixel*, and the associated numerical value usually gives a gray value or a color. In medical image processing, we often deal with three-dimensional image elements. Here, the aforementioned numerical value is associated with a point in 3D space, and these positions are called volume elements or *voxels*. Therefore, an image can be regarded as a discrete mathematical function mapping a position in two- or three dimensional space to a number. Formally speaking, the image is represented as

$$I(x,y) = \rho \qquad (3.1)$$

for 2D images, and

$$I(x, y, z) = \rho \tag{3.2}$$

for 3D volume images, where x, y, and z are spatial coordinates, and ρ is the gray value.[1] The special case of color images will be discussed soon in Section 3.2. In short, one can imagine the 2D image something similar to a map, where the altitude of a mountain range is translated to different colors or shades of gray. Figure 3.1 shows a single CT slice of the lower abdomen with an enlarged area – the single pixels can be clearly identified.

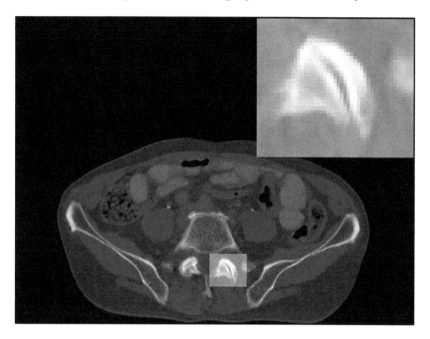

FIGURE 3.1: A CT-slice of the lower abdomen with parts of the pelvis and a pedicle. The area of one facet joint in the lumbar spine is highlighted and enlarged. In the enlarged image, single pixels are clearly identifiable. The brightness corresponds to the numerical value ρ, whereas the area of the pixel is given by its size and position in Cartesian coordinates. Image data courtesy of the Department of Radiology, Medical University Vienna.

By itself, this mathematical way of interpreting images is of little help; no assumptions on special mathematical properties like continuity and so on can be made. However, digital image processing is applied discrete mathematics, and in the next chapters, the concept of an image as a discrete mathematical function will be encountered numerous times. Figure 3.2 illustrates this concept.

An important property of medical images is, however, the fact that the grid of coordinate positions in medical images is not isotropic by nature. A frame of reference in image processing is usually defined by

its origin – that is the location of the first image element,

the orientation of its axes,

---

[1]ρ will be used by default as the dependent variable of an image. Whenever you encounter the character ρ, it refers to a shade of gray or a color.

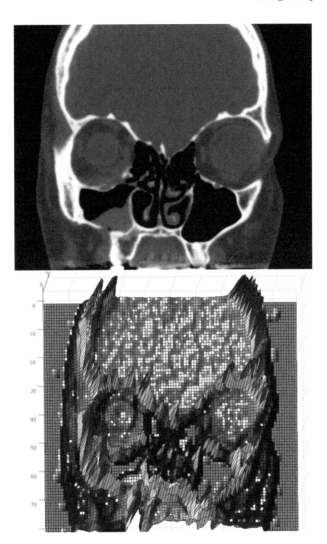

FIGURE 3.2: Images – no matter whether they are defined on a 2D or 3D domain – are mathematical functions that map a gray value to a coordinate. The upper part of the image shows a coronal CT view of a human skull. One can identify the calvaria, the orbitae, the paranasal sinuses, and the maxilla. By using MATLAB's `surf` function, the same image can be rendered as a 3D surface plot. Image data courtesy of the Department of Radiology, Medical University Vienna.

and the dimension of the image elements.

The latter two points are of considerable importance in the case of medical images. The handedness of a frame of reference for an image volume is not always defined, therefore it may be necessary to flip one or more image axes before further processing is possible. Most imaging modalities do also not provide isotropic voxels – the distance between slices, defining the depth of a voxel, is usually different from the other dimensions of the voxel, which are given by the image matrix of the imaging device. Figure 3.3 illustrates this common problem. *Flipping* of image axes and *scaling* by *interpolation* is therefore a common procedure before standard image processing algorithms can be applied to a dataset. In Chapter 7, operations like interpolation and scaling will be discussed.

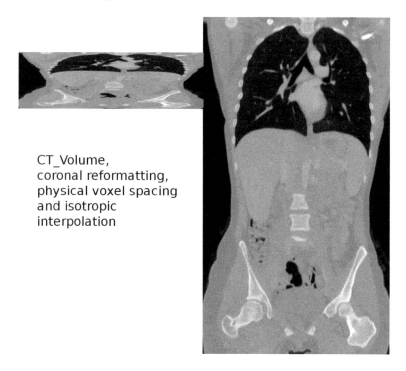

CT_Volume,
coronal reformatting,
physical voxel spacing
and isotropic
interpolation

FIGURE 3.3: An illustration of physical and isotropic voxel spacing in a CT–volume dataset of a human torso. The original resolution of the dataset is $0.5{\times}0.5{\times}3\,\mathrm{mm}^3$. In CT, images are acquired slicewise in an axial orientation. If an alternative slice is derived from the volume dataset by *reformatting* – a visualization technique that will be introduced in Chapter 7 – to a coronal orientation, the image appears compressed in the direction of the body stem. On the right side of the image, *interpolation* of the volume to an isotropic volume of $0.5\,\mathrm{mm}^3$ results in an image of correct proportions. Image data courtesy of the Department of Radiology, Medical University Vienna.

Another way of looking at an image is the interpretation of an image as matrix; a matrix is an array of numbers for which certain mathematical operations are defined. In general, a matrix of dimension $m \times n$ looks like this:

$$
I = \begin{pmatrix}
\rho_{11} & \rho_{12} & \cdots & \rho_{1n} \\
\rho_{21} & \rho_{22} & \cdots & \rho_{2n} \\
\multicolumn{4}{c}{\dotfill} \\
\rho_{m1} & \rho_{m2} & \cdots & \rho_{mn}
\end{pmatrix}
\tag{3.3}
$$

For each pixel, a numerical value ρ_{ij} is assigned to the matrix position given by the indices i and j. The matrix elements correspond to the pixels or, more generally, to the image elements. Since all practical lessons in this book are given in MATLAB,[2] a programming

---

[2]Throughout this book, the term "MATLAB" refers to both the MATLAB and its public domain counterpart Octave. All examples are compatible with both environments, and in fact, many of the examples were developed using Octave (`http:\\www.octave.org`).

environment for dealing with matrix computations, this way of image representation will also become pretty familiar.

Throughout this book, we will deal with two- as well as three dimensional image data sets. A tomographic three dimensional data set can be viewed as a cube that consists of single slices with a defined spacing and order. The pixels of those slices, together with the slice spacing, define the voxels of a volume data set. The matrix definition of a volume image is therefore only an augmentation by means of a further index, which is related to the relative position of the slice the pixel originates from. Spoken figuratively, the voxel is generated by raising the pixel to the third dimension until a new pixel is encountered in the next slice image.

3.1.1   Algebraic image operations

An important consequence from the fact that images are discrete mathematical functions is the possibility to use mathematical operations on images. The most important one is, as we will see from the examples in this chapter as well as Chapter 4, scalar multiplication. In this case, the gray value ρ for every single image pixel is multiplied with the same number. Therefore, scalar multiplication is an inevitable necessity for manipulating the gray scale representation of images, which will be introduced in Section 3.2. Beyond multiplication, it is also possible to add or subtract a number to the value ρ of each pixel, which is also necessary to manipulate ρ in such a manner that the range of gray values ρ matches the chosen datatype. In this book, mathematical formulations are used only if necessary; however, in the language of Section 3.1, a scalar multiplication of an image $I(x, y, z)$ and a scalar s would read $I'(x, y, z) = s * I(x, y, z)$, and a scalar addition is $I'(x, y, z) = s + I(x, y, z)$, where a constant value s is added to every single image element.

Beyond scalar operations, it is also possible to add or subtract whole images. The matrix representation as introduced in Eq. 3.3 is especially helpful for this purpose. Addition of two images I and I' takes place by simply adding each matrix element ρ_{ij} and ρ'_{ij} for images of the same width and height. Subtraction of two images can be very helpful to see if two images are identical, although a scalar intensity transform is usually necessary afterwards to make sure that one stays within the required data range of the resulting difference images. Adding images of the same subject, for instance, can be helpful to average images. By doing this, one can get rid of *image noise*, which may have a number of causes (see also Chapter 1).

More complex operations such as unsharp masking will be introduced in Chapter 5. Blending two images is usually also a simple image addition. Finally, it is sometimes also necessary to perform an elementwise multiplication of images. Elementwise or component-wise multiplication is performed by multiplying each matrix element with its counterpart: $\rho_{ij} * \rho'_{ij}$ is the new gray value at pixel position ij of the resulting image. Denote that elementwise multiplication is *not* matrix multiplication, which will be discussed in Chapter 7. Still it is a helpful operation, for instance when removing image content of a gray scale image by means of a binary region-of-interest (ROI) mask derived by segmentation, which will be introduced in Chapter 6.

3.2   GRAY SCALE AND COLOR REPRESENTATION

3.2.1   Depth

So far, we have seen that an image can be represented as a discrete mathematical function, or as an array of numerical values. The interesting thing here now is the nature of the scalar value ρ, which represents the gray scale value in a non-color image. In principle, the value ρ can be any number. For instance, in x-ray imaging ρ corresponds to the absorption of the high-energy electromagnetic radiation from the x-ray tube in the patient. However, a display device such as a computer monitor needs a defined protocol to translate those numbers in different shades of gray. In general, the number of shades is defined by the data type used for image representation.

It is generally known that a number in binary format is stored as a combination of the digits zero and one; one can convert an arbitrary number – let's say 0101 – given in binary format to the decadic system as follows:

$$\underbrace{0}_{\text{Multiples of } 2^3} \quad \overbrace{1}^{\text{Multiples of } 2^2} \quad \underbrace{0}_{\text{Multiples of } 2^1} \quad \overbrace{1}^{\text{Multiples of } 2^0} =$$

$$0 * 2^3 + 1 * 2^2 + 0 * 2^1 + 1 * 2^0 = 4 + 1 = 5 \tag{3.4}$$

The position of the single digit in the number governs its value – the number 5 in the decadic system requires at least three digits in the binary system. The number of digits available governs the maximal value to be represented. In the case of Eq. 3.4, a four bit number is given, and the maximal decadic value to be represented is 15 ($= 1111$ in binary format). This maximum possible value is – in the case of images – referred to as image depth. An image with four bit image depth can therefore contain a maximum of 16 shades of gray – $I(x, y) = \rho$, $\rho \in \{0, \ldots, 15\}$.

The human eye can approximately distinguish 100 shades of gray; for all practical purposes, a gray scale image is therefore sufficiently represented using 8 bit depth, which allows for $2^8 = 256$ shades of gray. Usually, the value $\rho = 0$ represents black, and $\rho = 255$ is white. In CT, ρ is stored in values between −1000 and 3000. The unit associated with the amount of absorption of x-ray energy is the Hounsfield unit [HU] which was introduced in Section 1.5. It is therefore handy to use an image depth of 12 bit, which allows to represent values ranging from 0 to $2^{12} - 1 = 4095$. Typical depths for gray scale images are 8 bit ($=$ `'char'` in MATLAB) and 16 bit ($=$ `'short'` in MATLAB). If a number can also take negative values, the first bit is a sign bit (which takes the values - and +). A signed 8 bit number can therefore, for example, take values from -127 to 127.

3.2.2   Color and look up tables

So far, we have only considered gray scale images. A value ρ is stored as a binary number of given depth, and this value is displayed as a shade of gray. So what about color?

The easiest way to introduce color is to provide a *look up table (LUT)*, which assigns each numerical value ρ a color. The choice of colors is, of course, arbitrary. Look up tables are sometimes used to emphasize subtle details in an image's gray scale content – this is related to the fact that the human eye can distinguish color better than shades of gray. An example from medical imaging is shown in Example 3.7.4. This is a single slice from PET; high concentrations of the radio tracer are marked as bright pixels. Introducing a LUT allows for better image interpretation, but does not provide any additional diagnostic information.

While a LUT is, in principle, a nice thing to have, it does nevertheless have severe drawbacks. Among those is the fact that the LUT always has to be stored with the image since it is an arbitrary selection. The other problem lies in the fact that for an image with lots of fine color detail, the LUT would become pretty big. Therefore it is easier to encode a color value ρ in an unambiguous manner. This can be achieved by mixing the color image from a basic color system such as red (R), green (G) and blue (B). An interesting example of such an RGB-encoded photograph can be found in Figure 3.4. The photograph shows an image of Austrian prisoners of war in a Russian camp during World War I in 1915. The Russian photographer Sergey Prokudin-Gorskii exposed three black-and-white plates through color filters. Projecting those weighted gray scale images resulted in color photographs before the introduction of the color film by Eastman-Kodak in 1935. An example demonstrationg the composition of color images from gray scale images can be found in Example 4.5.2.

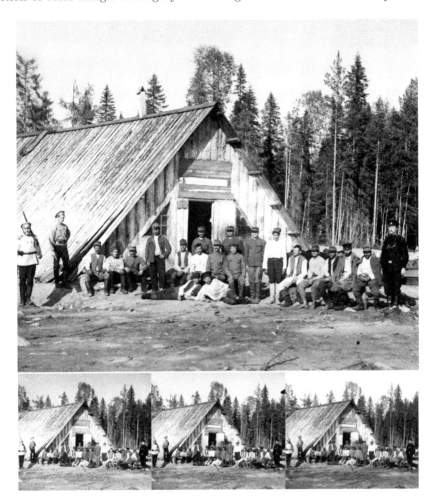

FIGURE 3.4: A photograph showing a prisoner of war camp in 1915. Color film was at that time not available, therefore Russian photographer Sergey Prokudin-Gorskii took three plates through red, green, and blue filters. Displaying an overlay with a slide projector resulted in these images, which can be found on the accompanying CD in color. The red, green, and blue components – which were produced using an image processing program and are not the original plates – can be seen in the lower part of the illustration. Image data are public domain.

It is therefore evident that a color image can be produced from three single gray scale images, which contain three color components. The decomposition in color space can follow many schemes – RGB for additive color mixing being just one of them. It is therefore straightforward to encode the three color values for a single pixel into one numerical value. This usually happens by assigning each pixel a 32 bit number; the first numerical value, the gray value ρ_{C1} for the first color component, occupies the first 8 bits in the number, followed by the 8 bits of ρ_{C2} and ρ_{C3}. The last 8 bits can be used for a fourth component, the alpha-channel, which is used to handle the transparency of a pixel. Therefore, a color image is simply a function that maps a spatial location to a 32-bit value, which is usually a floating point number. Retrieving the three components ρ_{C_i} is, however, necessary before an image can be displayed.

It has to be stated color images play only a little role in most medical imaging applications. The small color range used for color-encoding of low contrast detail, which is common in nuclear medicine or Doppler ultrasound, can also be handled using a LUT. An exception is the processing of histological image stacks acquired using light microscopy and the video sequences from endoscopic exams.

3.3 IMAGE FILE FORMATS

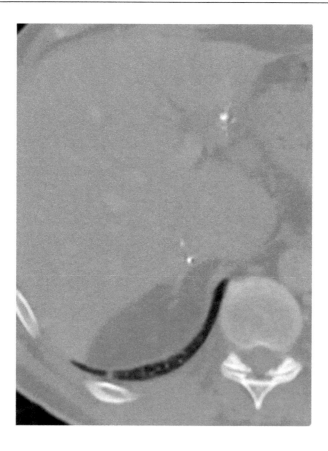

FIGURE 3.5: Part of a CT-slice, again showing the liver, some ribs, and a pedicle. The image was saved in PGM, which is an example of a very simple uncompressed file format. Image data courtesy of the Department of Radiology, Medical University Vienna.

The most straightforward method to store image data is certainly the so-called RAW data format – in this case, the numerical values ρ are stored one after another in a single file. All one needs to know is the depth of the image, and its dimensions in terms of width and height. With this information, it is easy to reassemble the image information in a matrix of dimension *image width * image height*; after this, each pixel position I_{ij} has a value ρ assigned, and the image can be displayed using the appropriate routines in an arbitrary computer program. Such simple file formats do exist. Two examples are PGM (Portable Gray Map) and BMP (BitMaP). The CT slice of Figure 3.5 was saved as ASCII-encoded PGM, and the first lines of the corresponding image file are as follows:

```
P2
# CREATOR: GIMP PNM Filter Version 1.1
472 632
255
4 4 4 2 1 1 0 0 0 0 2 6 12 22 34 48 62 79 92 104
109 112 113 112 110 107 105 102 102 101 101 102
102 102 103 101 102 102 103 103 103 102 101 100
...
```

P2 indicates that we are dealing with an ASCII-encoded PGM file – a binary encoded file, where the actual gray values ρ are not saved as literal numbers but as binary values, would start with P5.

The next line is a comment, which always starts with a # in the PGM-format.

The next two characters give the dimension of the image – it is 472 pixels wide and 632 pixels high.

Finally, the value 255, the highest gray value of the image, is stored in the next line.

What follows are the actual gray values for the subsequent pixels. While the first few are black (with values between 0 and 6), values rapidly increase to gray values as high as 113. This is the soft tissue visible in the upper left of the image.

As the name already indicates, PGM is a format for gray scale images. BMP also allows for storing color images by storing three values subsequently for the single color-channels in RGB format. Throughout this book, MATLAB is used as a tool for demonstrating low-level image processing routines; however, as an example of the storage of a gray scale image in BMP, a C++-example is given. If you are not familiar with C++, you may skip this paragraph.

```cpp
int myImageClass::saveToBitmap(const char* path) {
int retVal = 0;
int i, j, k;
FILE* BMP = fopen(path,'wb');
unsigned char Buff[54];
unsigned char tmpBmp[3 * PLAIN_SIZE_512x512];
unsigned char matrixImg[512][512];
unsigned char flippedImg[PLAIN_SIZE_512x512];

for(i = 0; i < PLAIN_SIZE_512x512; i++) {
        j = i/512;
        k = i% 512;
        matrixImg[j][k] = image8bit[i];
}
i = 0;
for (j = 511; j >= 0; j--) {
```

```
        for (k = 0; k < 512; k++) {
                flippedImg[i]=matrixImg[j][k];
                i++;
        }
}
for(i = 0; i < PLAIN_SIZE_512x512; i++) {
        tmpBmp[3 * i] = flippedImg[i];
        tmpBmp[3 * i + 1] = flippedImg[i];
        tmpBmp[3 * i + 2] = flippedImg[i];
}
memset(Buff, 0, 54);
Buff[0] = 'B';
Buff[1] = 'M';
Buff[10] = 54;
Buff[14] = 40;
Buff[18] = 0x00;
Buff[19] = 0x02;
Buff[22] = 0x00;
Buff[23] = 0x02;
Buff[26] = 0x01;
Buff[28] = 0x18;
fwrite(Buff, 1, 54, BMP);
fwrite(tmpBmp, 3, PLAIN_SIZE_512x512, BMP);
fclose(BMP);
return retVal;
}
```

PLAIN_SIZE_512x512 is a macro with the value 262144, which is actually 512×512 – the product of image width and image height. The first three for loops serve only one purpose – the image is flipped around the horizontal central line. It is pretty common that images appear mirrored, inverted or something similar after the first attempt to save the image matrix to a file. We will also encounter this problem in the examples, where we have to transpose the images usually. Here, it is necessary to flip the image horizontally to make it appear in the same orientation as on screen. The interesting part is the fourth for loop. The array tmpBmp is big enough to host three images of 512×512 of 8 bit depth, as can be seen from the definition of the variable. Obviously, the pixel value of the image flippedImg is copied three times to the array tmpBmp. This is simply because BMP can store color, but our image here is a gray scale image, as usual in most medical imaging applications. Therefore, all three color channels get the same weight. Finally, a BMP-compliant header is defined, and each pixel is written to the file. The result can be viewed with any common image processing program. Formats like PGM and BMP are uneconomic since they tend to consume considerable disk space, but they are a great aid in a quick visualization in debugging programs. Displaying an image in a graphical user interface (GUI) follows a similar fashion. GUI toolkits usually offer classes that hold pix maps and also provide methods for displaying them on-screen. You will find an example in the epilogue of this book.

More sophisticated formats usually employ compression techniques to save disk space and bandwidth. The easiest way to achieve compression is the implementation of techniques like run length encoding (RLE). RLE is the simplest compression algorithm – it replaces repetitions of byte patterns with the number of repetitions and the pattern itself. A simple example is a pattern of characters like AAAAAAAABAAAA; each character occupies one byte, which results in a total memory requirement of 13 bytes. Run length encoding this sequence would result in 8AB4A, which is only five bytes long. In practice, things are not that simple actually (one has, for instance, to manage the occurrence of numbers in the string to be encoded), but basically, this is the principle of RLE. If additional compression steps are taken, algorithms like the well known-compression methods for programs like ZIP may result. Numerous image formats have this type of built-in compression, PNG (Portable Network Graphics) and TIFF (Tagged Image File Format) being among the most popular ones. In general, RLE-type compression methods are lossless; one has to decode the compressed file to convert it into a raw image matrix, but the compression does not affect the information contained in the image. It is, however, also evident that the compression rates achievable are not extremely effective. Lossless compression is essential for program code and all kinds of binary documents – for images, it is not necessary, although the use of lossy compression methods is considered problematic in medical imaging.

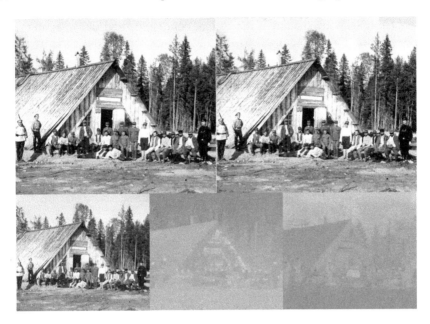

FIGURE 3.6: The photograph from Figure 3.4, encoded in good JPG-quality (upper left, file size 1477 KB) and in very low quality (upper right, file size 43.5 KB). The lower row images shows the luma, chroma blue, and chroma red from left to right (a color version of this image can be found on the accompanying CD). Image data are public domain.

The most famous example for a lossy compression method is the well-known JPEG (Joint Photographic Experts Group) recommendation, which serves as the basis of most imaging applications nowadays. It is noteworthy that the term JPEG summarizes a number of compression algorithms and is not a file format by itself, although an image compressed accordingly to the definition of the JPEG is usually referred to as .JPEG or .JPG file. Image size can be considerably reduced by lossy compression since small changes in pixel intensity do not necessarily affect image information. Two things about JPEG are remarkable – first, it does not use the conventional RGB color space but a YCbCr (Luma – Chroma Blue – Chroma Red) decomposition, an alternative representation of color space which already allows for reducing data size by definition; the other thing is the method of compression. The image is tiled in arrays of 8×8 pixels, which undergo a *discrete cosine transform* (which is related to the *discrete Fourier transform* to be introduced in Chapter 5) for reducing redundancy in images, and a so-called entropy encoding step. The result is a compression rate that usually cannot be achieved using RLE-types of compression at the cost of losing image quality. Figure 3.6 shows the image of Figure 3.4 compressed with different qualities together with the YCbCr – channels. If a JPEG-encoded image is to be processed in a program, it has to be decoded and stored in the computer's memory in the old way by assigning single positions a gray value ρ_{C_i}.

Other image file formats include the already mentioned TIFF, GIF, PNG and a variety of program specific formats like Photoshop Document (PSD) and Experimental Computing Facility (XCF), the native format of the GNU Image Manipulation Program GIMP. The Encapsulated Postscript (EPS) format deserves further special mentioning since it is a special case of a file format designed for printing graphics. Postscript by Adobe Systems is a programming language for printers rather than a simple image format; therefore, the contents of a Postscript file are usually a mixture of commands and image content. Again, all these formats require a decoding step to store its image contents in computer memory before processing them. What follows is the beginning of Figure 3.5, stored as an EPS-file using GIMP. The comments starting with %% are ignored by the Postscript-interpreter but give an overview of things like the title of the image file; image geometry and image depth are also stored (472 632 8), and the RLE encoded image data (stored as `unsigned char` 8 bit characters) finally follows the header of the Postscript file.

```
%!PS-Adobe-3.0 EPSF-3.0
%%Creator: GIMP PostScript file plugin V 1,17
%%Title: PGMLiver.eps
%%CreationDate: Fri Jul 18 13:03:57 2008
%%DocumentData: Clean7Bit
%%LanguageLevel: 2
%%Pages: 1
%%BoundingBox: 14 14 487 647
%%EndComments
%%BeginProlog
% Use own dictionary to avoid conflicts
10 dict begin
%%EndProlog
%%Page: 1 1
% Translate for offset
14.173228346456694 14.173228346456694 translate
% Translate to begin of first scanline
0 631.99578273054851 translate
471.99685039370075 -631.99578273054851 scale
% Image geometry
472 632 8
% Transformation matrix
472 0 0 632 0 0
currentfile /ASCII85Decode filter /RunLengthDecode filter
%%BeginData: 348998 ASCII Bytes
image
rWE9(!<N-!'ESII(*YFr:L%RME,fi7CM@BmAS ...
```

Finally, the class of formats for storing surface model data deserves mentioning. File formats such as STL (Surface Tessellation Language) or IGES (Initial Graphics Exchange Specification) are used to store 3D surface models which are constructed out of triangles or other graphics primitives. This representation of 3D models is very common in the world of *computer-aided design* (CAD); in diagnostic imaging, these formats are not suitable for storing radiological information. But some applications for visualization and further processing of radiological information do exist and will be discussed in Chapter 8.

3.4 DICOM

As said before, many medical imaging modalities produce three-dimensional volume image data sets. So far, we have only discussed 2D images, and unfortunately, most of the image processing literature is also pretty much restricted to two dimensions. The short presentation of file formats in Section 3.3 also only presents formats for storing 2D image data. It would be easy to expand such a format to 3D, but in real life, something else happened. Since many tomographic volume images are acquired on a slice-by-slice basis, it is a natural thing to store these single slices, and to fuse them to a volume. The standard that handles not only storage and the coherence of the slices but also communications between imaging hardware systems is called *Digital Imaging and Communications in Medicine* (DI-COM). It was defined by the American College of Radiology (ACR) and the US National Electrical Manufacturers Association (NEMA) and can be accessed via the NEMA website `http://medical.nema.org/dicom/`. DICOM also serves as the standard used for most *Picture Archiving and Communications* (PACS) systems, the infrastructure for acquiring, storing, retrieving, viewing and printing radiological images.

A short look at the standard reveals the considerable complexity of a DICOM-file set. One would expect that a single volume scan such as the data from a CT exam to be neatly packed in a directory with subsequent numbering and so on. This is, however, not the case. Rather than that, all single images are stored on one level of the file system and appear completely unorganized at first sight. The metadata, which introduce some kind of order into this apparently chaotic heap of single files, are contained in a single so-called DICOMDIR–file. The DICOMDIR–file organizes the image data hierarchically according to the logical structure *Patient – Study – Series – Image*. A single *patient* undergoes an exam (which results in a *study*) that may consist of several *series* of *images*. As an example, a patient receiving an MR exam (the *study*) leaves the radiology department with several volume data sets (the *series*), which were acquired for instance with different MR sequences and T_1 or T_2 weightings. All these volume data sets consist of several *images*. The DICOMDIR file itself does not contain any image information, but it references and organizes the files that belong together. If a DICOM–study is stored on a media such as a CD, it is mandatory to store the DICOMDIR alongside the image data despite the fact that all information regarding patient, study and series is stored in every single DICOM file as well.

The single DICOM files, on the other hand, are again organized just like standard image files and usually consist of a header and subsequently stored image data. The format of the image data is not strictly defined; rather than that, a number of compression methods like JPEG or RLE encoding are available but scarcely used. What is certainly special is the format of the DICOM-header, which contains a plethora of information not only related to the image itself but also for managing the patient data in a large relational database. The entries in the header (which is of arbitrary length) can be categorized as *mandatory*, *conditional*, or *user defined*. The mandatory entries are required in any case, whereas the conditional entries are dependent on an earlier entry; finally, users may define entries of their own, which has led to sub-formats such as DICOM-RT, where additional planning data for tumor irradiation planning are included as well. In general, a DICOM file starts with 128 bytes that are usually ignored; these 128 bytes are followed by the four characters DICM; the header entries themselves are marked by so-called data tags. The tags are defined in the DICOM standard and take the form of two four-digit hexadecimal number followed by the *value representation*, an optional entry on the length of the following data entry, and the data entry itself. One example is the tag (16,16), which actually is the tag for the entry *Patient Name*. Figure 3.7 shows the header of a DICOM image file in the Bless Hex-Editor of Fedora Linux. This is a CT-scan of a plastic skull phantom, and the technician named the phantom `Test^Maxi` – denote the space at the end, which is a padding character so that an even number of characters is achieved.

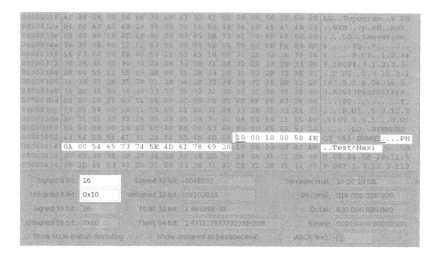

FIGURE 3.7: The header of a single DICOM file of a plastic head phantom viewed with a Hex-editor; right here, we are looking for the patient name entry, which starts with the tag (0x10,0x10). The prefix `0x` indicates that we are dealing with hexadecimal numbers. The corresponding entry is highlighted in this screen shot. Since the image is stored in *Little Endian* mode – which refers to the byte ordering in the representation – we find this doublet of number as `0x1000 0x1000`. What follows is two unsigned 8 bit numbers – `0x50 0x4E`. Transforming these two hexadecimal number to decimal numbers gives the values 80 and 78. These are the ASCII-codes for the characters P and N, obviously an abbreviation for *Patient Name*. The following value `0x000A` represents the length of the following entry. In a decimal base `0x000A` represents the number 10. This is the length of the following entry; the name of the phantom is `Test^Maxi` , which is a string 10 characters long when taking into account the space at the end.

From this example it is obvious that thorough parsing of a DICOMDIR and the associated files is a necessity if the volume is to be stored properly in the computer's memory. Furthermore, the plethora of possible header entries makes the header length a highly variable quantity. Usually, libraries and tool kits are available to decode DICOM files. When opening the file of the phantom scan, whose header is displayed in Figure 3.8 in AnalyzeAVW (Biomedical Imaging Resource, Mayo Clinic, Rochester/MN), the information stored in the header appears in a much more organized manner.

As said before, DICOM is a very wide standard, and the possibilities of misusing the header of DICOM files are endless. This has led to the unfortunate fact that DICOM files of different manufacturers are not always compatible. For all practical purposes, it is recommendable to use a standard tool kit for decoding DICOM data sets, or to use a viewer that allows for saving the image data. A large number of such applications exists. Furthermore, one must not forget that a complete DICOM data set always consists of the image data and the corresponding DICOMDIR file.

```
0008|0060="CT"
0008|0070="SIEMENS"
0008|0080="AKH - Wien"
0008|0081="Waehringer Guertel /678C90/Wien Waehring Austria"
0008|1010="ct28077"
0008|1030="Head^@EGN Plg. 1mm"
0008|103e="EGN 1/1  1.0 H31s"
0008|1050="GEN"
0008|1070="AHK"
0008|1090="Sensation 4"
0009|0010="SIEMENS CT VA1 DUMMY"
0010|0010="Test^Maxi"
0010|0020="08.04.08-18:11:59-DST-1.3.12.2.1107.5.1.4.24026"
0010|0030="20060808"
0010|0040="M"
0010|1010="020M"
0018|0015="HEAD"
0018|0050="1"
0018|0060="120"
0018|1020="VA47C"
0018|1030="@EGN Plg. 1mm"
0018|1100="238"
0018|1110="1040"
```

FIGURE 3.8: The beginning of the header of the image from Figure 3.7 as decoded by AnalyzeAVW. Tag (0x0008,0x0060) refers to the imaging modality (CT), (0x0008,0x0070) is the manufacturer (Siemens), (0x0008,0x0080) is the name of the Institution (AKH – Vienna General Hospital) and (0x0008,0x0081) is the postal address. The well-known tag (0x0010,0x0010) introduced in Figure 3.7 can also be found.

3.5 OTHER FORMATS – ANALYZE 7.5, NIFTI AND INTERFILE

Within the focus of this book, we consider DICOM simply a file format; it is, however, more than that. The DICOM standard contains all the formalisms to administrate the storage and display of medical image data in a large PACS. For simple image processing tasks, this type of format is overkill. A special nuisance of DICOM is the fact that 3D volume data are usually stored as single files containing one slice at a time. In order to complicate things further, the spatial structure of the volume is not reflected in the file names, but it is contained in the DICOMDIR and the header of the single files. All of this may be helpful in organizing image data in a large database, but for us, it is simply annoying since we usually end up with a plethora of unordered image files belonging to multiple studies. It would be preferable to have a file format like PGM, where all the information necessary is stored in a header, followed by the numerical value assigned to each voxel position. Such a format that became some sort of standard, although it is formally not as well defined by an official consortium like DICOM, is *Analyze 7.5*. It is the file format used by earlier releases of the Analyze software, which you will encounter many times throughout this book, and was developed by the Biomedical Imaging Resource (BIR) at Mayo Clinic, Rochester/MN.

In the Analyze 7.5 format, a medical image is stored in two files named ....hdr and ....img. The .hdr file contains the additional image information such as voxel dimensions in binary format, and the .img file contains the numerical image information. In Figure 3.9, we see a screenshot of an Analyze 7.5 header file as seen in a hex editor. Newer releases of Analyze called AnalyzeAVW[3] use a modified format called *AVW*; here, the header and image information is stored in one file. Nevertheless, Analyze 7.5 is still widely used and

---

[3]An older report on the principles behind Analyze can be found in R. A. Robb, D. P. Hanson, R. A. Karwoski, A. G. Larson, E. L. Workman, M. C. Stacy: Analyze: a comprehensive, operator-interactive software package for multidimensional medical image display and analysis, Comput Med Imaging Graph 13(6):433-54, (1989).

has become some sort of standard file format. The image processing toolbox of MATLAB also provides a function `analyze75read`.

Analyze 7.5 is also the basis for a file format called *NifTI*, an enhanced version of this format that mainly aims at storage of MRI image data for neuroscience. In nuclear medicine, another file format named *Interfile* is also widespread. It is interesting to note that only very few image formats support the storage of gray values ρ with more than 16 bit. Besides the mentioned medical formats like DICOM, a 16 bit variant of TIFF also exists but is not supported by all common image processing programs. And in astronomy, another field of science where subtle details in image content are apparently important, a specialized format named FITS (*Flexible Image Transport System*) which even supports 3D data, exists.

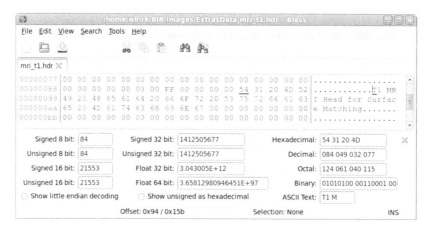

FIGURE 3.9: A header file from the Analyze 7.5 format, viewed using the Bless hex editor. Since this is a binary file, most of the information is not easily read. Some ASCII information can, however, be retrieved – see the right hand side of the dialog.

3.6 IMAGE QUALITY AND THE SIGNAL-TO-NOISE RATIO

In Chapter 1, we have already encountered some examples of imaging artifacts which stem from the particular properties of imaging systems. These artifacts can, of course, reduce diagnostic information content of images and are to be avoided. However, another source of reduced image quality is noise. The term *noise* describes all types of stochastic signals which are not related to image content. In x-ray imaging, noise is usually introduced by a lack of dose; in photography, images tend to get noisy if the ambient lighting is insufficient. The reason in both cases is simple – since image noise is a stochastic signal, its amplitude is independent of the usable signal. If the imaging signal itself is of small amplitude, the noise becomes more visible. A measure to quantify the noisiness of images is the *signal-to-noise-ratio* (SNR). One possible definition is given as:

$$\mathrm{SNR} \quad = \quad \frac{\bar{\rho}}{\sigma\left(\rho_{\mathrm{Uniform\ Area}}\right)} \tag{3.5}$$

$\bar{\rho}$ ... average pixel gray value

$\sigma\left(\rho_{\mathrm{Uniform\ Area}}\right)$ ... standard deviation in a signal-free area of the image

From Eq. 3.5, it is obvious why an underexposed image becomes grainy. The energy impacted (in terms of visible light or dose) is proportional to the gray value ρ, whereas the noise remains the same. The reason lies in the fact that the image noise, which can have numerous origins, is not necessarily connected to the original signal. While SNR is an important measure of detector efficiency and image quality, it does not give an idea of the ability of an imaging system to resolve fine detail, and it does not necessarily give a figure of the information content of an image. This is characterized by two more important measures, the point spread function (PSF) and the modulation transfer function (MTF), which will be introduced in Chapter 5. Lesson 3.7.5 gives an idea how the SNR can be computed from an image in dependence of the dose applied. However, since the average signal is not always a useful measure, one can also define the *contrast-to-noise-ratio* (CNR). Here, the average gray value is replaced by the absolute value of the difference between the maximal and minimal signal:

$$\text{CNR} = \frac{|\rho_{\max} - \rho_{\min}|}{\sigma\left(\rho_{\text{Uniform Area}}\right)} \tag{3.6}$$

$$\rho_{\max}, \rho_{\min} = \text{maximal and minimal gray value}$$

$$\sigma\left(\rho_{\text{Uniform Area}}\right) = \text{standard deviation in a signal-free area of the image}$$

3.7 PRACTICAL LESSONS

3.7.1 Image subtraction

In the script `dsa_3.m`, we see an example of image subtraction; two x-ray images of the pelvis, one before and one after injection of a contrast agent named `DSA1.jpg` and `DSA2.jpg` are provided in the **Lesson Data** folder. Figure 3.10 shows these two images.

If we subtract the two images, we will get an image that only shows the part of the image that has changed. In clinical routine, this method of visualizing vessels after application of a contrast agent is called *digital subtraction angiography* (DSA). As opposed to reading the images byte wise, we may use a MATLAB® function named `imread` for loading image data. This is definitely more handy than the verbose way of loading an image as shown in Example 3.7.2. For storing an image, a function `imwrite` also exists. If an 8 bit representation of our images is sufficient, we may therefore use `imread`. Two matrices `img1` and `img2` are filled with data from the x-ray images stored as JPG files using `imread`:

```
1:> img1=imread('DSA1.jpg');
2:> img2=imread('DSA2.jpg');
```

Next, we carry out the subtraction of the images, which have the same dimension; the result is displayed using `image` and can be found in Figure 3.11. The method is a little bit crude since we do not care about the proper image depth, or about subtle display details; these are about to come later:

```
3:> resimg=(img1-img2);
4:> colormap(gray);
5:> image(resimg)
```

3.7.2 Opening and decoding a single DICOM file in MATLAB

In this lesson, a single DICOM file will be opened and displayed using MATLAB or Octave; for this purpose, we provide a single slice of a T_2 weighted MR of a pig. The slice shows the

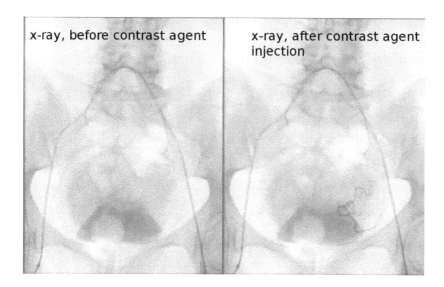

FIGURE 3.10: The images `DSA1.jpg` and `DSA2.jpg`, two x-ray images of a pelvis taken before and after injection used in Example 3.7.1. Subtraction of the two images yields an image that only shows the change between the two exposures – in this case, a vessel flooded by contrast agent. In clinical routine, this method is called digital subtraction angiography (DSA). Image data courtesy of Z. Yaniv, ISIS Center, Department of Radiology, Georgetown University.

remarkablly small brain and the huge temporomandibular joint of this species. The file is named `PIG_MR`. The image is uncompressed, has a matrix of $512 * 512$ pixels, and a depth of 16 bit. The machine used to acquire the volume was a 3T Philips Achieva MR. The script for this lesson is called `OpenDICOM_3.m` and can be found in the `LessonData` folder.

The single steps to be taken are as follows:

Determine the length of the header.

Open the image file in MATLAB using the `fopen(...)` function, and skip the header using `fseek`.

Assign a matrix of dimension $512 * 512$, and fill it with the values from the image file using `fread`.

Display the image using the `image` command

First of all, the header dimension has to be determined; under LINUX or other UNIX-variants, this can be accomplished by typing the `du -b` – command:

```
wbirk@vela: $ du -b PIG_MR
532734 PIG_MR
```

This is the size of the image file – 532734 bytes; under Windows-type operating systems, the size of the image can be determined using the `Properties`-dialog, where both the file size and the occupied disk space are presented. Figure 3.12 shows such a dialog from a GNOME-based Linux flavor.

Sometimes, two sizes for a file are given under some operating systems – the true file

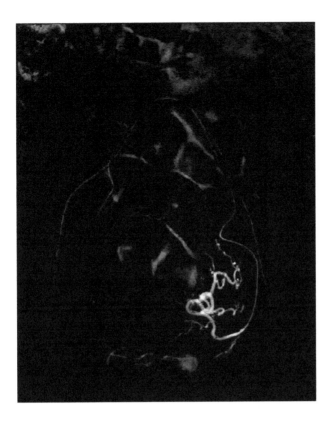

FIGURE 3.11: The result of `dsa_3.m`; only the vessel which shows up in the second x-ray `DSA2.jpg` is clearly visible after image subtraction. Image data courtesy of Z. Yaniv, ISIS Center, Department of Radiology, Georgetown University.

size, and the disk space occupied. We are only interested in the smaller number of the two, the file size. The image size of `PIG_MR` is also known, and it can be computed as $512*512*2$. The first two numbers are the matrix size of the image, and the last one is the image depth – the number of bytes per pixel (16 bit = 2 byte). This results in an image size of 524288 bytes; computing the difference between the file size and the image size results in the header size, which is 8446 bytes. The first step now is to open the file in MATLAB, and to skip the header so that the relevant image information can be read. For this purpose, a file pointer – a variable that holds the actual information as read from the file – is to be assigned using the command `fopen(...)`. The working directory (the directory accessed by MATLAB/Octave unless specified otherwise) is to be assigned using the `cd` command, or in the menu bar of MATLAB (see also Figure 3.13). If `fopen('...')` is successful, a value different to -1 is returned by the interpreter. The first 8446 bytes – the header – are to be skipped. This is achieved using the `fseek(...)` command, which positions the file pointer.

```
1:> fpointer=fopen('PIG_MR','r');
2:> fseek(fpointer,8446,'bof');
```

By now, the working directory is set to the location of the DICOM file, a file pointer with read-only access (specified by the `'r'` character in `fopen(...)`) is successfully assigned, and this file pointer is shifted for 8445 bytes starting from the *beginning of the file* (thus the

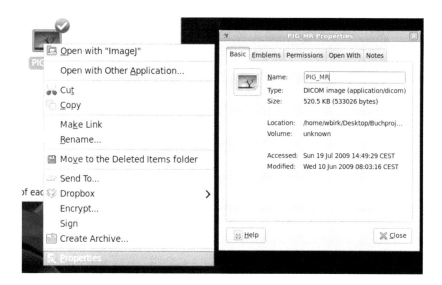

FIGURE 3.12: The size of the PIG_MR DICOM file as displayed by clicking the Properties ... button on a GNOME-Desktop (left hand side of the image). We are interested in the filesize. Based on this information, we can determine the size of the DICOM-header.

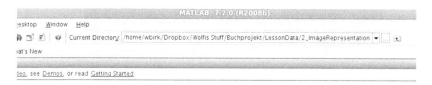

FIGURE 3.13: A screenshot of the MATLAB main menu; the working directory – the directory where all scripts and images are found – has to be set in this text entry-widget. Alternatively, one can also type in the cd command, followed by the path to the LessonData folder provided with this book.

'bof' qualifier in line 2). The operation is successful, therefore the interpreter delivers a non-negative number for the file pointer. However, output is suppressed here by using the ; character at the end of each line.

The next step is to assign a $512*512$ matrix that holds all the gray values ρ; this matrix is initially filled with zeros using the zeros(512,512) command. The trailing ; is of great importance here since it suppresses the output.

```
3:> img = zeros(512,512);
```

The next step is to read the following $512*512 = 262144$ values of ρ, represented as numbers of two bytes length. This is accomplished by assigning each position in the matrix to a value of data type 'short' using the command fread:

```
4:> img(:)=fread(fpointer,(512*512),'short');
```

The suffix (:) prompts the interpreter to read the values in the order of 512 numbers per row of the matrix. This notation is referred to as colon notation in MATLAB, and it is pretty useful to speed up matrix operations – see also Example 3.7.4.1. Again, the semicolon suppresses output of the full matrix. `'short'` is the datatype of the image, in this case 16 bit. Finally, the matrix can be displayed graphically. For this purpose, the command `image` is used. The result depends on the actual version of MATLAB or Octave used; my Octave version spawns *gnuplot* as an external viewer, but this may vary and we witnessed problems with Octave sometimes; if such problems occur, it may be necessary to install another viewer application for Octave. In MATLAB, an internal viewer is started. It has to be noted that `image` is a method to show general geometrical features of a matrix, and it is not a genuine tool for viewing images. Therefore, a rather colorful image is the result since a standard-LUT is applied. The LUT can, however, be changed by calling the command `colormap(gray)`. Finally, it is obvious that rows and columns are interchanged, therefore the matrix has to be transposed. This is achieved by using the command `transpose(img);`. Denote that the `image` command does usually not care about the proper ratio of width and height for an image – this has to be adjusted manually.

```
5:> img=transpose(img);
6:> colormap(gray)
7:> image(img)
```

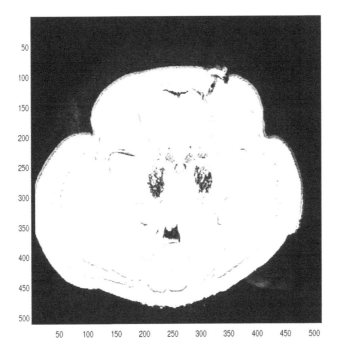

FIGURE 3.14: The outcome of calling the `image` command; the range of gray values ρ is not optimized, therefore the image is too bright. Optimizing the intensity range of images will be introduced shortly in Chapter 4.

It is of course also possible to store the results of our efforts using the PGM format;

according to the example given in Section 3.3, the header of an ASCII-encoded PGM file consists of three lines containing the format prefix P2, the image format ($512 * 512$ pixels in this case), and the maximum data value. The maximum value of a matrix is computed in MATLAB by applying the operator `max(max(...))`. Calling the function `max` for a matrix returns a vector with the maximum element for each column of the matrix; calling `max` the second time returns the biggest value from this vector, which is the maximum value for the array.

All we have to do now is open another file pointer for *write* access – that is the `'w'` character in `fopen(...)`; all values to be saved have to be converted to strings, which is done by using the function `sprintf`. `sprintf` – well known to C-programmers – assigns a series of characters to a single string `str`, whereas `fprintf` writes this string to a file specified by the file pointer `pgmfp`. The character `\n` is a non printable *newline* character that causes a line feed. The `%d` specifier tells `sprintf` that an integer number – `maximumValue` in our case here – is to be inserted.

```
8:> pgmfp = fopen('PIG_MR.pgm','w');
9:> str=sprintf('P2\n');
10:> fprintf(pgmfp,str);
11:> str=sprintf('512 512\n');
12:> fprintf(pgmfp,str);
13:> maximumValue=max(max(img))
14:> str=sprintf('%d\n',maximumValue);
15:> fprintf(pgmfp,str);
```

By now, we have made a perfectly fine header for an ASCII-encoded PGM-file that contains an image of $512 * 512$ pixels and a maximum gray value of 892; now, the single gray values ρ have to be saved, separated by spaces. In the following `for`-loop, the semicolon-suffixes for suppressing output are especially important.

```
16:> for i=1:512
17:> for j=1:512
18:> str=sprintf('%d ',img(i,j));
19:> fprintf(pgmfp,str);
20:> end
21:> end
22:> fclose(pgmfp);
23:> fclose(fpointer);
```

By now, a PGM-file readable by any graphics program that supports this format should appear in your working directory. The final call to the function `fclose` is especially important for forcing all data to be written to the hard disk. Figure 3.15 shows the looks of `PIG_MR.pgm` in GIMP.

Those who have the Image Processing Toolbox of MATLAB available may also use the command `dicomread`. Throughout this book, however, MATLAB is used as a teaching vehicle, and we therefore abstain from using ready made solutions for decoding image data when possible.

Additional Tasks

Repeat the same procedure with the data set `PIG_CT`, which is a 512×512 image of 16 bit depth. Saving the image as PGM is, however, problematic due to to the fact

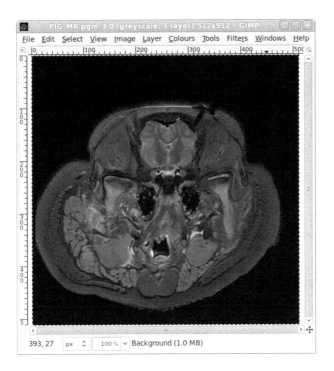

FIGURE 3.15: The `PIG_MR.pgm` file as generated by the `OpenDICOM_3.m` script, opened in GIMP. The gray values are now represented properly, and we can identify several anatomical structures such as the temporomandibular joint, the brain, and huge amounts of muscles and fatty tissue.

that the minimum value is negative, not zero. If you cannot figure out a way to deal with this range of image intensities, you may read Chapter 4 first.

3.7.3   Opening a DICOM file using ImageJ and 3DSlicer

3.7.3.1   A single slice in ImageJ

Usually, one does not have to write a program to inspect the contents of a DICOM-file. There is of course a plethora of programs available to do that. Two of them, which are available in the public domain, are *ImageJ*[4] and *3DSlicer*.[5] Both programs are available for all major computer platforms. Let us take a look at ImageJ first.

Figure 3.16 shows us how to select a DICOM file in ImageJ – which is pretty standard and does not need further explanation. Once you have located the `PIG_CT` DICOM file in your `LessonData` folder (actually, it is contained in the subfolder `3_ImageRepresentation`), the image will be loaded and the result is shown in Figure 3.17. As one can see, the intensities are already scaled properly, and as additional information, the image dimension in millimeters and the image depth (16 bit) is given. By using the item "Show Info..." in the "Image" menu of ImageJ, you can also retrieve the information of the DICOM header.

While ImageJ is a great tool, it also has disadvantages; the main problem lies in the

---

[4]ImageJ can be found, for instance, in `http://rsbweb.nih.gov/ij/`.
[5]The official 3DSlicer website is `http://www.slicer.org`.

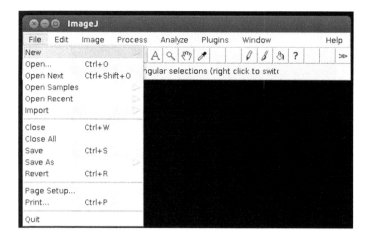

FIGURE 3.16: The toolbar of ImageJ; opening a DICOM file is simply done by choosing the "Open..." item in the "File" menu.

fact that, while one can load volume data as a "stack of slices", it is not a genuine 3D image processing program. We already know that our medical images are not a sequence of 2D images but a mathematical function that maps from three spatial coordinates to a physically measured quantity, as implied at the beginning of this chapter. 3DSlicer, as the name already implies, does take this into account.

3.7.3.2 A CT-volume in 3DSlicer

Once 3DSlicer is installed, the initial screen should look similar to Figure 3.18. The original CT scan of our porcine specimen already known from Section 3.7.2 is provided in the Lesson Data folder on the accompanying CD. It is stored in a folder named PigCT and features the DICOMDIR file as well as the original data. In order to load this dataset, we have to press the "Load DICOM Data" button, which can be found in the left panel of the main screen of 3DSlicer (see also Figure 3.18). As newer releases of 3DSlicer become available, there might of course be changes in this setup.

After releasing the "Load DICOM Data" button, 3DSlicer prompts you to import the data on the selected dataset into its local database. In Figure 3.19, the button for importing a DICOM-dataset can be found in the upper left of the screenshot. You may also be prompted to provide a location for the database file. The image data of the CT scan are found in the subfolder S102160 of the PigCT folder. Import those image data – this may take some time. Once you were successful, the name of the patient ("001" in the case of the provided dataset appears in the list of patients that are stored in the local database. Select this patient and press the "Load Selected Patient to Slicer" button.

The result of these efforts is shown in Figure 3.20. 3DSlicer offers three views of the volume. One can display the original slices by moving little sliders atop each panel. Since 3DSlicer is a true 3D program, it also computes different views, so-called reformatted slices. Therefore, not only the original (axial) slices are shown, but we also see two more orthogonal views. These slices were not acquired by the CT – they were computed from the volume data file. More on this process called reformatting can be found in Chapter 7. 3DSlicer is also aware of the fact that voxels are not necessarily isotropic – it interpolates the volume also to proper scaling. We will also encounter interpolation in Chapter 7 again.

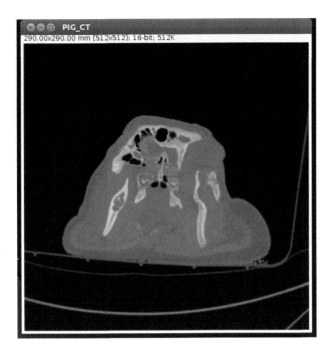

FIGURE 3.17: One of the sample DICOM files, PIG_CT, as displayed by ImageJ. Information such as the scale of the image in millimeters (290 × 290 mm) and the depth (16 bit) are given directly. Additional information from the DICOM header can also be retrieved and displayed separately by ImageJ.

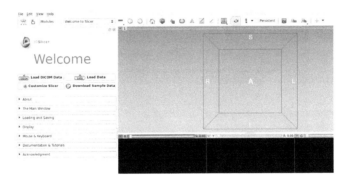

FIGURE 3.18: After startup, 3DSlicer presents itself in this screenshot. The right part of the screen is reserved for display of images. While the functionality of 3DSlicer is huge, we are right now only interested in loading a DICOM volume. For this purpose, the "Load DICOM Data" button in the upper left has to pressed.

Additional Tasks

At least in the release 4.0.1 of 3DSlicer, which was used when this book was written, there is a possibility to download sample data – see also Figure 3.18, where the appropriate button is found close to the "Load DICOM Data" button. Try to download a few of them and take a look at them.

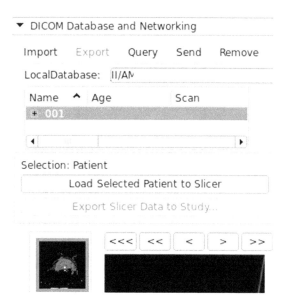

FIGURE 3.19: 3DSlicer does not simply load DICOM data – rather than that, it analyzes a directory and retrieves relevant information on the internal organization of the volume dataset and the patient from the DICOM headers. This information is stored in an internal database.

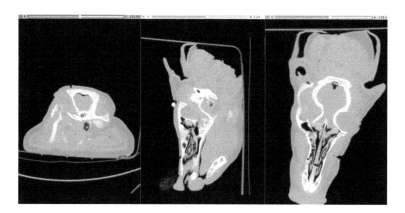

FIGURE 3.20: Three views of the imported DICOM dataset `PigCT` after loading the volume to 3DSlicer. These are the three panels shown on the lower right hand of Figure 3.18. The left panel shows the original slices as taken by the CT machine. The little sliders atop each panel allow you to browse the volume. The other views were generated by reformatting, a technique that generates slices at an arbitrary orientation from the volume data (see also Chapter 7).

3.7.4 Converting a color image to gray scale

In the case of a color image, `imread` returns three 3D-arrays of numbers containing the three color channels. This information can be fused to a gray scale image by computing the luminance of the single colors as perceived by the eye. Therefore, a gray scale image (as seen, for instance, by a color blind person) is computed from the RGB-images as $\rho = 0.3\rho_R + 0.59\rho_G + 0.11\rho_B$. The factors stem from the spectral sensitivity of the eye in daylight, which is highest at a wavelength of approximately 550 nm – which is actually green. First of all, the working directory has to be determined, and the color PET-image is loaded; the script for this example is called `ConvertColorImage_3.m`:

```
1:> colorimg = imread('PET_image.jpg');
```

We can determine the size of `colorimg` by calling the function `size`, which returns the actual dimensions of an array.

```
2:> size(colorimg)
```

The script returns the following line: `ans = 652 1417 3`. Apparently, three images, each of size 652×1417 pixels were loaded. MATLAB has to decode the JPG-type file first into a raw data format. The color components are therefore also converted from the JPG-type color space Y-Cr-Cb, and the three images in the array `colorimg` contain the R-G-B components. The only thing left to do is to allocate memory for the gray scale image and to compute the gray value ρ from the three components. Finally, the result of our efforts is scaled to 64 gray values ranging from 0 to 64 and displayed. The result should look similar to Figure 3.21.

```
3:> grayimg=zeros(652,1417);
4:> for i=1:652
5:> for j=1:1417
6:> grayimg(i,j) = 0.3*colorimg(i,j,1) + ...
0.59*colorimg(i,j,2) + 0.11*colorimg(i,j,3);
7:> end
8:> end
9:> imin=min(min(grayimg));
10:> grayimg=grayimg-imin;
11:> imax=max(max(grayimg));
12:> grayimg= floor(grayimg/imax*64);
13:> image(grayimg)
14:> colormap(gray)
```

`floor` generates an integer value by cutting off the numbers behind the decimal point – it is a crude operation that always rounds off.

3.7.4.1 A note on good MATLAB programming habits

As already pointed out in the introduction, we have tried to keep the code as simple and as straightforward as possible, at the cost of performance. In this example it is, however, easily possible to demonstrate the strengths of MATLAB's vector notation style for avoiding `for` loops. Lines 4 to 8 in `ConvertColorImage_3.m` can be replaced by a single line that shows the same effect:

```
4:> grayimg(:)=0.3*colorimg(:,:,1) +
0.59*colorimg(:,:,2) + 0.11*colorimg(:,:,3);
```

By utilizing the vector notation (:), the double `for` loop becomes obsolete. In the `LessonData` folder, you find this modified example under `BetterConvertColorImage_3.m`.

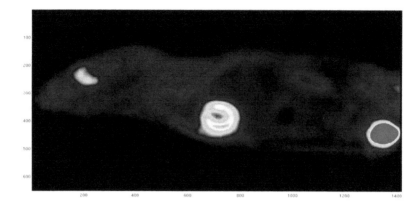

FIGURE 3.21: Result of converting a color PET image to a gray scale image using the weighted addition of red, green and blue channels according to the photopic sensitivity of the eye. Image data courtesy of C. Kuntner, AIT Seibersdorf, Austria.

With larger datasets, the result of this programming technique is a considerable improvement in performance. One cannot replace all statements which access single matrix elements, but if you run into performance problems with one of the scripts provided, you may try to apply the vector notation instead of nested loops.

3.7.5 Computing the SNR of x-ray images as a function of dose

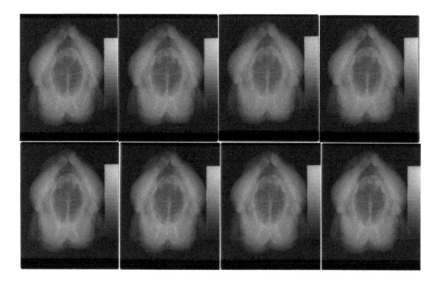

FIGURE 3.22: The eight x-ray images of a chicken, stored in original resolution as DICOM-files acquired from a CR plate reader. All images were acquired with different dose; while the overall appearance is similar due to the large tolerance of CR plates to under- and overexposure, the SNR varies considerably. Image data courtesy of P. Homolka, Center for Medical Physics and Biomedical Engineering, Medical University of Vienna.

Next, a set of eight x-ray images of a dead chicken is provided; the images were exposed using 1/8, 1/4, 1/2, 1, 2, 4, 8, and 16 times the dose required. We will compute the SNR of these images and take a look at the SNR-values in dependence of the dose. The SNRExample_3.m does the following: first of all, we have to change to the sub-directory SNR, where eight DICOM files named chicken1.dcm to chicken8.dcm can be found. The size of the headers is stored in a vector named headersize. A vector snrs, which will hold all the signal-to-noise ratios, is defined as well:

```
 1:> cd SNR
 2:> headersize=zeros(8,1);
 3:> headersize(1,1)=1384;
 4:> headersize(2,1)=1402;
 5:> headersize(3,1)=1390;
 6:> headersize(4,1)=1386;
 7:> headersize(5,1)=984;
 8:> headersize(6,1)=988;
 9:> headersize(7,1)=984;
10:> headersize(8,1)=988;
11:> snrs=zeros(8,1);
```

Next, we have to read the images and the signal-free sub-area where the standard deviation of the detector is determined:

```
12:> for i=1:8
13:> signalFreeArea=zeros(350,300);
14:> img=zeros(2364,2964);
15:> fname=sprintf('chicken%d.dcm',i);
16:> fp=fopen(fname);
17:> fseek(fp,headersize(i,1),'bof');
18:> img(:)=fread(fp,(2364*2964),'short');
19:> fclose(fp);
20:> img=transpose(img);
21:> for j=100:450
22:> for k=200:500
23:> signalFreeArea(j-99,k-199)=img(j,k);
24:> end
25:> end
26:> sigmaSignalFree=std(signalFreeArea(:));
27:> snrs(i)=mean(mean(img))/sigmaSignalFree;
28:> end
```

What has happened? The eight files were opened just as we did in Example 3.7.2, and the image matrix was transposed in order to keep a sufficient image orientation compared to the GIMP program, where the signal-free area was defined (see Figure 3.23). The signal-free area was stored in a separate matrix signalFreeArea. The standard deviation for the elements in the matrix signalFreeArea was computed using the command std.

By now, we have a vector snrs containing the SNR of images snr1.jpg ... snr8.jpg; it would be a nice idea to sort those SNRs. Practically, this is a linked list since we want to know which image has the best SNR. Such a hash table can be programmed – but it is cumbersome and usually slow. Therefore we may use a nasty little trick. We encode the file name into the values. The SNRs have values between 107.03 to 363.39; these values can be rounded to integer values without loss of information:

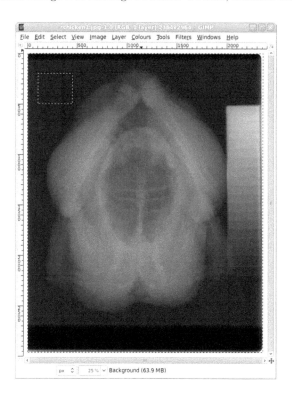

FIGURE 3.23: Selection of an appropriate signal-free area of the image using GIMP. For this example, an area defined by the rectangular section in the upper left of the screenshot was used. The actual coordinates are given in the lower left of the dialog.

```
29:> snrs=round(snrs);
```

Now comes the ugly part. In the following section, we *encode* the ordinal number of the image in the decimal area of the values, and we sort the vector; this is a trick to circumvent a hash-table – a linked list of paired values, where one of the entries is sorted. Such structures are usually computationally expensive. Therefore we add the ordinal number of the image that belongs to the SNR as the decile rank to an otherwise integer number:

```
30:> for i=1:8
31:> snrs(i)=snrs(i)+i/10;
32:> end
33:> ssnrs=sort(snrs)
34:> cd ..
```

From the output, we see that the images, sorted by SNR, are given as `chicken3.dcm`, `chicken4.dcm`, `chicken1.dcm`, `chicken2.dcm`, `chicken7.dcm`, `chicken8.dcm`, `chicken5.dcm`, and `chicken6.dcm`. Finally, we return to the parent directory.

Additional Tasks

Compute the CNR of the image series.

The MATLAB function `sort` also returns a permutation from the original vector to the sorted version. Use this to sort the images by their SNR.

3.8 SUMMARY AND FURTHER REFERENCES

Two- and three dimensional images are, strictly speaking, scalar mathematical functions defined on two- or three dimensional grid structures. The single 2D picture element, which is represented as a coordinate, an area, and an associated gray value, is called a pixel. The 3D equivalent is a volume element or voxel. Color images are similar to gray scale images; each color channel is stored in a separate gray scale image – however, color does not play a very important role in medical imaging. Images can be saved in various uncompressed and compressed formats. The most important format for 2D and 3D medical image data is DICOM, which does not only consist as a method of storing pixels and voxels, but also of communication, storage methods and more.

Literature

J. D. Murray, W. van Ryper: Encyclopedia of Graphics File Formats, O'Reilly, (1996)

O. S. Pianykh: Digital Imaging and Communications in Medicine (DICOM): A Practical Introduction and Survival Guide, Springer, (2008)

http://medical.nema.org/

A. Oppelt (ed.): Imaging Systems for Medical Diagnostics: Fundamentals, Technical Solutions and Applications for Systems Applying Ionizing Radiation, Nuclear Magnetic Resonance and Ultrasound, Wiley VCH, (2006)

E. Berry: A Practical Approach to Medical Image Processing, CRC Press, (2007)

CHAPTER 4

Operations in Intensity Space

Wolfgang Birkfellner

CONTENTS

4.1	The intensity transform function and the dynamic range	91
4.2	Windowing	93
4.3	Histograms and histogram operations	95
4.4	Dithering and depth	98
4.5	Practical lessons	98
	4.5.1 Linear adjustment of image depth range	98
	4.5.1.1 A note on good MATLAB® programming habits .	99
	4.5.2 Composing a color image from grayscale images	100
	4.5.3 Improving visibility of low-contrast detail – taking the logarithm	102
	4.5.4 Modelling a general nonlinear transfer function – the Sigmoid	104
	4.5.5 Histograms and histogram operations	105
	4.5.6 Automatic optimization of image contrast using the histogram	107
	4.5.7 Intensity operations using *ImageJ* and *3DSlicer*	112
4.6	Summary and further references	113

4.1 THE INTENSITY TRANSFORM FUNCTION AND THE DYNAMIC RANGE

We have already seen that not all types of gray values are suitable for direct display. For instance, in the case of the MR or CT images decoded in Example 3.7.2, the easiest way to get a suitable range of gray scales for display is a *linear transform* of the gray values ρ so that the maximum and the minimum of the image fit with the data range of the pixels to be displayed. If we look at the `BRAIN_CT` DICOM file, it turns out that the minimum data value of this CT slice is -1057, and the maximum value is 1440, whereas a conventional gray scale image format like PGM usually expects a range $\rho \in \{0 \ldots 255\}$; the `colormap(gray)`– command of MATLAB only displays 64 shades of gray, which is equivalent to a 6-bit depth.

The easiest way to transform image intensities is a linear transform, which is given as

$$\rho' = \frac{\rho - \rho_{\min}}{\rho_{\max} - \rho_{\min}} \omega_{\text{target}} + \rho'_{\min} \tag{4.1}$$

ρ' ... transformed pixel intensity

ρ ... original pixel intensity

$\rho_{\min}, \rho_{\max}$ ... minimum and maximum gray values in the original image

ω_{target} ... range of the target intensity space

Here, every gray value ρ in the original image is transformed to fit into the range of the target image; if the data type for the target image is, for instance, `signed char`, the possible gray values ρ' can take values between -127 and 127. Here, the range ω_{target} is 0 ... 255, and $\rho'_{\min}$ is -127. One issue of practical relevance must be emphasized here – if you apply an intensity scaling operation, you have to take care that the image depth of your target image stays in range. For instance, it does not make sense to scale an image to 16 bit depth and storing it as `char`.

In Section 3.2.2, we learned that the eye can distinguish approximately 100 shades of gray. However, it is possible to transform the gray levels in an image in a non-linear order. When shifting the gray values in an image to influence brightness and contrast, one can visualize the relationship between gray values in the original image and the modified image using an *intensity transfer function* (ITF), which is simply a curve that conveys gray scale ranges; an example of the MR-file from Section 3.7.2 can be found in Figure 4.1.

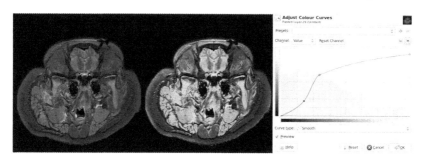

FIGURE 4.1: The original image from Section 3.7.2 (left), and a version with optimized gray scale representation (middle). The contrast transform function is shown to the right; it is actually a screen shot of the corresponding dialogue in GIMP. The original intensity range is shown on the x-axis of the intensity transform (ITF). The curve shows how a gray value in the original image is translated to an optimized gray scale range (which can be found on the y-axis of the ITF).

Basically, the ITF is a transform from one gray scale range to another. Here we find an analogy to the world of photography and x-ray detector characteristics. The *dynamic range* of a detector or chip is the range where a change in incident energy is translated in a different gray value. If the energy impacted on the detector is too high, the image is overexposed, and the intensity range is *saturated*. If the energy impacted is insufficient, the detector remains dark, and the image is underexposed. The range between these two extreme cases is the dynamic range, and it is characterized by the tangent of the angle between the x-axis and a straight line that approximates the response curve best (Figure 4.2); this value is generally referred to as the γ-value.

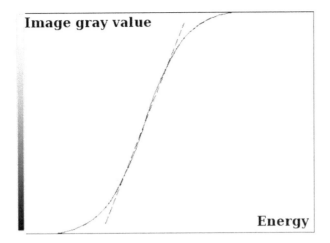

FIGURE 4.2: A general concept of a response curve. The x-axis gives the energy impacted on some sort of image detector. On the left side, there is not enough energy to evoke a response from the detector. On the right side, the energy flux on the detector is so high that it can no longer respond by a proportional gray value (or a similar signal). The gradient of the linear approximation in the dynamic range determines the γ-value of the detector.

When looking at Figure 4.2, the correspondence between the ITF as shown in Figure 4.1 and Figure 4.2 becomes obvious; the ITF transforms gray values to other gray values, whereas the response curve transforms energy to gray values, which can, for instance, be modelled as a so-called *Sigmoid function* (also referred to as *Logistic function*). A model of a Sigmoid-based ITF which transforms gray scale images of unsigned 8-bit depth is given in Equation 4.2:

$$S(\rho) \quad = \quad 255\frac{1}{1 + e^{-\frac{\rho - \omega}{\sigma}}} \tag{4.2}$$

ρ ... 8 bit gray value

ω ... Center of the gray value distribution; for 8-bit images, choose $\omega = 127$

σ ... Width of the gray value distribution

Figure 4.3 shows the impact of the parameters ω and σ on an unsigned 8-bit gray scale. A Sigmoid-shaped ITF can be used to achieve smooth and linear intensity transitions, or for modelling the characteristics of a detector in an imaging device.

4.2 WINDOWING

We know that the eye can only distinguish approximately 100 shades of gray, whereas it is possible to store a medical image in more depth. CT-images, for instance, have a depth of 12 bit and therefore contain up to 4096 shades of gray. This figure is linked to the units associated with the units associated with CT, the Hounsfield–scale. Air, which does not absorb x-ray radiation to a notable extent, has a density of -1000 HU. On the image, this density is black. The radio opaque structures of the body, such as bone, have a Hounsfield density of 700 and more HU. Some figures are given in Table 4.1.

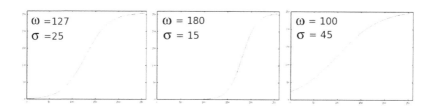

FIGURE 4.3: Three Sigmoid curves, defined on an 8 bit gray scale range $\rho \in \{0 \ldots 255\}$. The parameters from Eq. 4.2 were slightly varied. The impact of these modeled ITF curves will be demonstrated in Section 4.5.4.

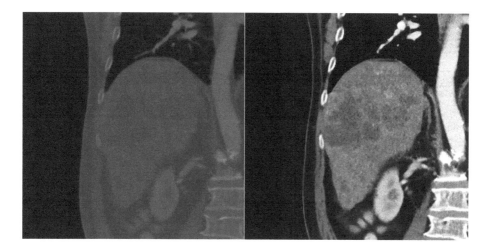

FIGURE 4.4: A clinical example that shows the importance of choosing proper window levels; the left image shows a liver CT in coronal orientation, without windowing. At first, the organ looks unssupicious, at least to a layman. The right image shows the same slice with appropriate windowing – large lesions, caused by a malignant disease, become clearly visible.

For visualization of subtle details, it is recommended not to scale the whole range of gray shades to 8 bit. Rather, the images should be windowed. Here, a *window center* is chosen; if the anatomical structure of interest is, for instance, soft tissue, it is advisable to choose the window center as the typical HU-value of that type of soft tissue according to Table 4.1. Then, a *window width* is selected; the window width delineates the maximum and minimum range of pixels that are displayed correctly; pixels outside the window width are either black (if their HU-value is smaller than the lower boundary of the pixel) or white (if the HU-value is beyond the upper limit of the window width). The clinical value of this visualization method cannot be overestimated. Basically, all CT-volumes undergo windowing (often as part of their acquisition and storage) in order to provide maximum information for the given diagnostic task. The process of windowing can also be described by an ITF. All gray values within the window transform linearly, whereas the others are either suppressed or displayed as saturated pixels. An illustration of the general shape of such an ITF is given in Figure 4.6; the similarity to Figure 4.3 is evident – windowing is actually an artificial change of the dynamic range. An example is given in Figure 4.7. It cannot be emphasized enough

Tissue	HU
Air	-1024
Lung	-900 ... -200
Water	0
Blood	20 ... 60
Liver	20 ... 60
Bone	50 ... 3072
Kidney	40 ... 50
Cortical Bone	> 250

TABLE 4.1: Typical Hounsfield units of some materials and tissue types. Data are taken from A. Oppelt (ed.): Imaging Systems for Medical Diagnostics, Wiley VCH, (2006).

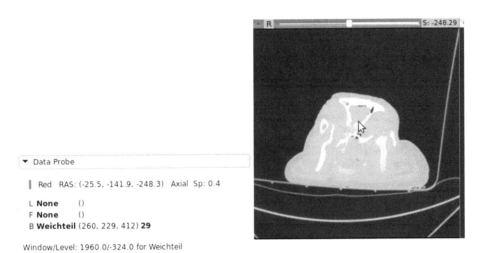

FIGURE 4.5: A screenshot of the windowing operation in *3DSlicer*. Windowing is a standard feature here and is controlled by moving the cursor while pressing the mouse button. Window width and window center (named "Window" and "Level") are given in the lower left part of the screenshot.

that windowing is a visualization method – it reveals information that was not perceptible before.

4.3 HISTOGRAMS AND HISTOGRAM OPERATIONS

In Chapter 3, we saw how important the actual gray scale value ρ of a pixel is – an image may contain an incredible amount of information that cannot be perceived if its gray values cannot be differentiated by the eye. This is somewhat of an analogy to the electromagnetic spectrum, which contains a lot of visual information (for instance infrared light) which cannot be perceived since the retina is only susceptible to radiation with wavelengths in the range of 430 – 680 nm – see also Section 1.2. In terms of image processing, it is therefore possible to provide the viewer with an entirely black (or white) image that does contain relevant information. It is also possible that this image does not contain any information at all. Therefore, it is of great interest to obtain an overview of the gray values ρ. An example

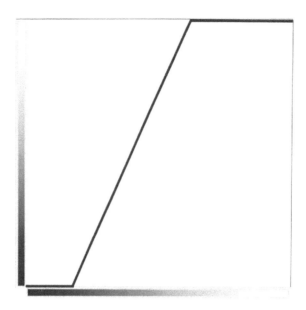

FIGURE 4.6: The general shape of an ITF for windowing. The difference between the higher and lower intensity values on the abscissa at the location of the sharp kinks in the ITF gives the window width; the window center lies in the middle of this window.

of such a distribution of gray values is given in Figure 4.1; the CTF is shown together with a histogram, which represents the actual distribution function of gray values.

For many image processing operations, it is essential to get an idea of the histogram, which is formed by sorting the gray values into predefined classes. These classes can be thought of as bins; one goes through every pixel (or voxel) in the image and selects the bin that is suitable for the particular gray value ρ. Subsequently, the amount of entries in this bin is increased by one. After finishing this operation, the histogram is represented by columns whose area represents the number of gray values in this bin. Two important rules for designing a histograms bin width exist:

> The histogram has to be complete and unambiguous; for each gray value ρ there is one and only one bin to which it belongs.

> The histogram bins should be of the same width; this is, however, not always feasible, for instance if outliers are present. Therefore, the area of the column is the relevant value which represents the frequency of occurrence for a certain range of gray values, not its height. In image processing, however, bins of varying width are uncommon and should be avoided.

The choice of the number of bins is arbitrary; for 8-bit images, it may be feasible to choose the number of bins to be equal to the number of the possible 256 gray values. This is, however, not recommended. General trends in gray value distribution may become obstructed by missing values, which lead to gaps in the histogram; for images of higher depth, the number of bins may also become too large. Figure 4.8 gives an illustration of the impact of bin width on the general shape of the histogram. The MATLAB-script for generating this output is given in Section 4.5.5. Connected to the number of bins and image

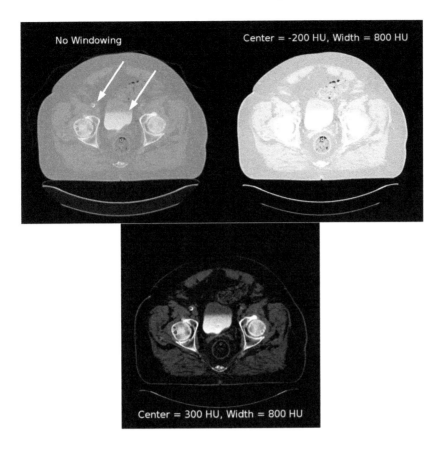

FIGURE 4.7: The effect of windowing a 12 bit CBCT–image. Two combinations of window center/window width are chosen, one giving optimum soft tissue contrast, the other showing details of bony structure. Interesting details are the liquid level of contrast agent in the bladder, which is of higher specific gravity than the urine, and a calcification of the right femoral artery (both marked by arrows in the first image). A ring artifact can also be seen in the bladder – more on ring artifacts can be found in Chapter 10. Image data courtesy of the Dept. of Radiation Oncology, Medical University Vienna.

depth is the width of a single bin, which can be simply computed as

$$\text{Bin Width} = \frac{\text{Image Depth}}{\# \text{ of bins}} \tag{4.3}$$

The applications of histograms are numerous; when confronted with image data in raw format, it is very handy to have a histogram that shows where the majority of gray values ρ can be found. Based on this information, one can choose the optimum data type and range for an initial intensity transform. Example 4.5.6 gives an example of how a deep 16-bit image with very broad variation of intensity values can be optimized automatically based on the histogram content. If one chooses to segment the bony content of an x-ray image, an initial guess for an optimum threshold can be taken from the histogram. Finally, it may be necessary to design an intensity transformation in such a manner that two histograms match each other; this process, usually referred to as *histogram equalization*, may be a necessary step prior to registration of two data sets. Furthermore, we will learn that histograms can

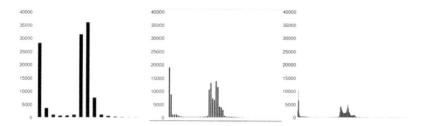

FIGURE 4.8: The histogram of the original abdomen CT-slice given in Figure 4.15, computed using 16 bin, 64 bins, and 256 bins (which is equivalent to the image depth). Note that the general shape of the histogram is preserved, whereas the height of its columns varies. In fact, it is the area occupied by the histogram bars that gives an idea of the values inside each bin, not its height – which is obvious since a larger number of bins will cause a lower count rate in a single bin. The output was generated using the script from Section 4.5.5. Strictly speaking, this figure has a flaw. In a histogram, bars should be placed next to each other, without any spacing. For the sake of simplicity – these graphs were generated using a spreadsheet program from the exported output of MATLAB – we generously neglect this requirement.

also be used to design similarity measures for image registration, as in the case of the *mutual information* algorithm, which we will encounter in Chapter 9.

4.4 DITHERING AND DEPTH

The task of reducing the depth of gray scale images is rather easy; one can either scale the range of data, or use a windowing function to fine tune visible detail. The issue gets more complicated when reducing the depth of color images. This process, usually referred to as dithering, reduces the color space to a smaller amount of possible colors, which can be given as a LUT. A classical algorithm is *Floyd-Steinberg dithering*, but numerous other algorithms exist. The good news is that in medical imaging, we barely ever encounter color images; even the colorful images provided by PET and SPECT are the result of color encoding of count rates from a nuclear decay process. This color coding is achieved by means of a LUT. However, the literature on general image processing gives numerous details about different dithering methods.

4.5 PRACTICAL LESSONS

4.5.1 Linear adjustment of image depth range

First, it would be great if we were able to apply a linear ITF to the images read in Section 3.7.2; for this purpose, we have to determine ρ_{max} and ρ_{min}, and apply Equation 4.1. Here, we transform the MR-image from the PIG_MR from its original gray values to an unsigned 6 bit image for good display using the MATLAB image function. The script is named LinearIntensityTransform_4.m. First, we have to load the image again:

```
1:> fpointer = fopen('PIG_MR','r');
2:> fseek(fpointer,8446,'bof');
3:> img = zeros(512,512);
4:> img(:) = fread(fpointer,(512*512),'short');
```

```
5:> img = transpose(img);
```

Next, the minimum and maximum values of the image are determined, and the whole image has to be transformed according to Equation 4.1. Again, we have to call `max` and `min` in order to get the maximum component of the `img` matrix. The result can be found in Figure 4.9, and now it looks pretty familiar compared to Figure 3.15.

```
6:> rhomax = max(max(img))
7:> rhomin = min(min(img))
8:> newimg=zeros(512,512);
9:> newimg = (img-rhomin)/(rhomax-rhomin)*64;
10:> colormap(gray)
11:> image(newimg)
```

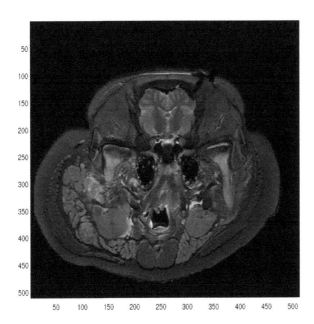

FIGURE 4.9: The output from `LinearIntensityTransform_4.m`. The MR-image already known from Example 3.7.2 is now displayed using an appropriate gray scale range.

Additional Tasks

Repeat the same procedure with the data set `PIG_CT`, but transform it to `unsigned 8 bit` and save it as a PGM.

4.5.1.1 A note on good MATLAB® programming habits

You may replace the double call to the `max` and `min` function in lines 6 and 7 of `LinearIntensityTransform_4.m` by a single function call:

```
6:> rhomax = max(img(:));
7:> rhomin = min(img(:));
```

The impact on algorithm performance is, however, negligible.

4.5.2   Composing a color image from grayscale images

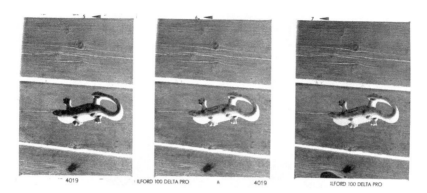

FIGURE 4.10: The original 60 × 45 mm analog black-and-white film used in Example `ComposeColorImage_4.m`. We see a small ceramic salamander, photographed three times using a red, green and blue filter. As proof that this is not simply a digital decomposition of a color image, one may notice that on the rightmost blue frame also a part of my toe can be seen.

Now, we can try to reproduce the efforts of the photographer who made the image from Figure 3.4. For this purpose, we need three grayscale images of a colorful object, each one taken through a red, green or blue filter. While black-and-white photography using film is no longer a widespread activity, one can still obtain B&W film, developer, fixing agents, and I had a camera at hand. In the given case, it is a medium format camera. I have three images of a ceramic salamander, a non-medical (but colorful) object. One intensity operation introduced here deserves special mentioning; sometimes, it makes sense to *invert* an image. The photographs taken here are negatives. In the days of analog photography, the film was used to expose photographic paper, and this production of a print resulted in inverted images. In this case, we have to do this by ourselves. Let us take a look at `ComposeColorImage_4.m`, which is to be found in your `LessonData` folder:

```
1:> clear
2:> imgr=double(imread('salamanderred.jpg'));
3:> imgg=double(imread('salamandergreen.jpg'));
4:> imgb=double(imread('salamanderblue.jpg'));
5:> cimg=double(zeros(400,400,3));
```

As always, we cleared all variables in the workspace, and we read three images `salamanderred.jpg`, `salamandergreen.jpg` and `salamanderblue.jpg`, which represent the three color channels. In this case, it is important to make sure that all gray values in the image are stored as floating point numbers, therefore we cast them using the command `double`. These scans of the exposures can also be found in Figure 4.10. From this scan, the three single images were taken. We also reserved some memory for the resulting color image `cimg`.

Next, we determine the maximum gray value of our three color channel images `imgr`, `imgg` and `imgb`. What follows is the image inversion step – we turn the negatives into positives by subtracting the image gray values from the maximum gray value in each channel.

This is possible since our images do not feature any negative gray values; therefore, black is equivalent to zero in the range of gray values. After this operation, the negative has turned into a positive image. Figure 4.11 shows the result of inverting the three single images `salamanderred.jpg`, `salamandergreen.jpg` and `salamanderblue.jpg`.

```
 6:> maxintr=max(max(imgr));
 7:> maxintg=max(max(imgg));
 8:> maxintb=max(max(imgb));
 9:> for i=1:400
10:> for j=1:400
11:> imgr(i,j)=maxintr-imgr(i,j);
12:> imgg(i,j)=maxintg-imgg(i,j);
13:> imgb(i,j)=maxintb-imgb(i,j);
14:> end
15:> end
```

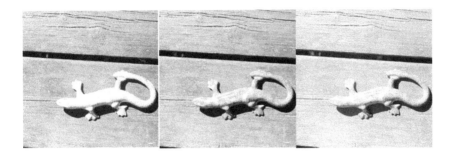

FIGURE 4.11: The three images `salamanderred.jpg`, `salamandergreen.jpg` and `salamanderblue.jpg` used in Example 4.5.2 after inversion. We see from left to right the red, green and blue channel.

In order to display the color image, we have to scale all intensities in the color channel images to an interval $0 \ldots 1$. Each color is therefore represented as a floating-point number where 0.0 is black and 1.0 is white. After this intensity scaling, we can copy the three images `imgr`, `imgg` and `imgb` to the color image `cimg`, which has three color layers. Remember Example 3.7.4, where we read a color image and MATLAB produced a three-dimensional matrix. Here, we go in the different direction. Finally, the image is displayed. For display of color images, we do not need to load a lookup table by calling `colormap`, as we did before. The result can be found in Figure 4.12. It is, admittedly, a little bit pale. If you want to cope with that problem, you may take a closer look at the additional task.

```
16:> imgr=imgr/maxintr;
17:> imgg=imgg/maxintg;
18:> imgb=imgb/maxintb;
19:> for i=1:400
20:> for j=1:400
21:> cimg(i,j,1)=imgr(i,j);
22:> cimg(i,j,2)=imgg(i,j);
23:> cimg(i,j,3)=imgb(i,j);
24:> end
25:> end
```

```
26:> image(cimg)
```

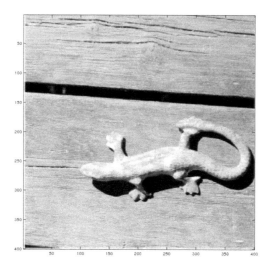

FIGURE 4.12: The composite resulting from combining the single B&W photographs. A color version of this illustration can be found on the accompanying CD.

Additional Tasks

What is not taken into account here is the fact that film (and the photographic paper is intended for) does not feature a strictly linear γ-curve. Therefore, the image is a little bit pale; we can improve this by manipulating the intensity transfer function for all three color channels simultaneously – this operation is also somewhat connected to *lightness*. The easiest way to operate on all three color channels is to save the resulting color image from `ComposeColorImage_4.m` (or to open the corresponding image from your CD that comes with this volume) with a program like GIMP and to manipulate an intensity transform. Figure 4.13 shows an example of what this could look like.

4.5.3 Improving visibility of low-contrast detail – taking the logarithm

In `LogExample_4.m.`, we will learn about a very simple way to improve the visibility of low-contrast detail. A simple method to enhance the visibility of low contrast detail is to take the logarithm of the image prior to intensity scaling. Remember that the logarithm is a function $y = \log(x)$ that is zero for $x = 1$, $-\infty$ for $x = 0$, and becomes shallow for growing values of x. Applying the logarithm $\rho' = \log(\rho + 1)$ to a 12 bit DICOM image should therefore result in an image where the dark, low contrast parts of the image appear enhanced – given that the intensity range of the image starts with 0 since the logarithm of a negative number is complex. If we want to apply the logarithm to a standard CT, it is advisable to compute $\log(\rho + 1025)$ in order to compensate for the possible negative values

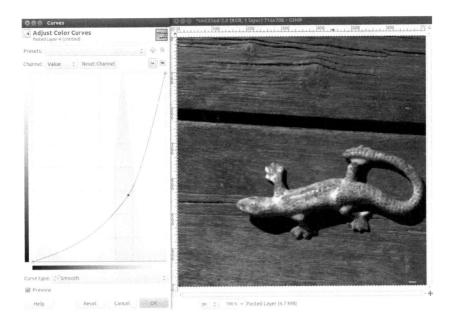

FIGURE 4.13: The overall impression of the color composite from Figure 4.12 can be changed by changing the intensity transfer function for all three color channels simultaneously. This screenshot shows how an improvement of the initial appearance of the composite image from `ComposeColorImage_4.m` – which is a little bit pale – can be achieved by applying a non-linear ITF using GIMP. The function used can be localized in the menu "Color → Curves...".

in the Hounsfield scale. Denote that, as opposed to Equation 4.1, this transformation is not linear.

First, we open a DICOM image from CT showing an axial slice; we transform the range of gray values from $\{\min, \dots, \max\}$ to $\{1, \dots, \max - \min + 1\}$ just to avoid the pole of $\log(0)$. Next, the logarithm is taken and the result is scaled to 6 bit image depth and displayed. Figure 4.14 shows the result.

```
1:> fp=fopen('SKULLBASE.DCM', 'r');
2:> fseek(fp,1622,'bof');
3:> img=zeros(512,512);
4:> img(:)=fread(fp,(512*512),'short');
5:> img=transpose(img);
6:> fclose(fp);
7:> minint=min(min(img));
8:> img=img-minint+1;
9:> img=log(img);
10:> maxint=max(max(img));
11:> img=img/maxint*64;
12:> colormap(gray)
13:> image(img)
```

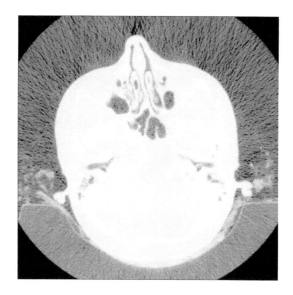

FIGURE 4.14: Taking the logarithm of an image emphasizes low-contrast detail; in this example, both CT reconstruction artifacts as well as radiolucent structures such as the hair of the patient are emphasized whereas diagnostic detail vanishes. Image data courtesy of the Dept. of Radiology, Medical University Vienna.

Additional Tasks

Can you think of a similar non-linear transform that emphasizes high-contrast detail? Modify `LogExample_4.m` to achieve this.

4.5.4   Modelling a general nonlinear transfer function – the Sigmoid

In `SigmoidIntensityTransform_4.m`, we demonstrate the impact of the ITF-curves modelled as the sigmoid function $S(\rho)$ from Equation 4.2 on a sample 8 bit CT-slice. First, we have to assign the working volume again, and load the image `ABD_CT.jpg` using `imread`. The JPG-image was saved as gray scale, therefore only one layer is available (as opposed to Example 3.7.4). Finally, the width and height of the read image is determined using `size`. The result is 435 pixels width and 261 pixels height.

```
1:> oimg = imread('ABD_CT.jpg');
2:> size(oimg)
```

In the next step, a vector containing the values for $S(\rho)$ is defined and filled; the parameters `pomega` and `psigma` ($= \omega$ and σ in Equation 4.2) have to be defined as well. Again, the suffix ; is important in the `for`–loop. Indexing a vector like `sigmoid` starts from 1, but the gray scale values ρ start from zero – therefore the running independent variable ρ has to be augmented by 1 for indexing `sigmoid`.

```
3:> pomega = 127;
4:> psigma = 25;
5:> sigmoid = zeros(256,1);
6:> for rho=0:255
7:> sigmoid(rho+1,1) =
```

```
    64*1/(1+exp(-((rho-pomega)/psigma)));
    8:> end
```

We can now take a look at the curve $S(\rho)$, $\rho \in \{0 \ldots 255\}$ using the plot–command, which generates output similar to Figure 4.3. The interesting concept here is that sigmoid is indeed a mathematical function represented by numbers that belong to discrete pivot points. In the next steps, the original values of image gray value ρ are transformed using the vector sigmoid, which translates these gray values according to the modelled ITF. Denote that we use a little trick here: being a function defined as discrete values, the Sigmoid is saved as pairs $(x, f(x))$. However, we only have a simple vector sigmoid that holds all the dependent values from Equation 4.2; the independent variable is the index of the vector here. Therefore we can determine the gray value rho in the original image and replace it with the value of the sigmoid vector at position rho+1 since the gray values range from 0 to 255, but indices in MATLAB are given as $1 \ldots 256$.

```
    9:> plot(sigmoid)
    10:> transimage = zeros(261,435);
    11:> for i=1:261
    12:> for j=1:435
    13:> rho = oimg(i,j);
    14:> transimage(i,j)=sigmoid(rho+1,1);
    15:> end
    16:> end
```

After calling colormap(gray), image(transimage) and image(oimg) show the transformed and the original image.

Additional Tasks

Repeat the procedure for parameter pairs $w/\sigma = 180/15$ and $100/45$. Results are shown in the images in Figure 4.15. Try it!

The basic method in windowing is to cut off the intensity values that are outside the window, and to scale the remaining pixels. Therefore, *windowing* is a simplification of the sigmoid-shaped ITF in a sense that the dynamic range is a given as a linear function. The general shape of a linear function is given as

$$f(x) = a * x + b$$

where a is the gradient of the linear function, and b gives the value for $f(0)$. Implement a windowing operation. Do you see a correspondence of pomega and psigma and the window center and width?

4.5.5 Histograms and histogram operations

As a first example in Histogram_4.m, we will derive a number of histograms of varying bin number from the example CT-slice ABD_CT.jpg. We define the working directory, read the image, determine its depth of gray values, and allocate memory for a number of histograms of varying bin width.

```
    1:> img = imread('ABD_CT.jpg');
    2:> depth = max(max(img))-min(min(img))
    3:> hist16 = zeros(16,1);
```

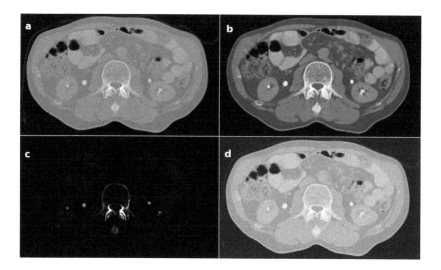

FIGURE 4.15: The impact of the three sigmoid functions $S(\rho)$ from Figure 4.3 on an 8-bit CT slice of the abdomen (upper left, denoted as **a**). The first function with $\omega = 127$ and $\sigma = 25$ gives a well balanced image where the extreme dark and extreme bright areas are slightly suppressed, and the middle gray values translate more or less linear (upper right, denoted as **b**). A sigmoid function with $\omega = 180$ and $\sigma = 15$ suppressed the darker areas and highlights only the extremely intense image content such as cortical bone or contrast-agent filled vessels (lower left, denoted as **c**). Finally, a wide and shallow sigmoid ($\omega = 100$ and $\sigma = 45$) gives a dull image. Dark areas appear brighter, revealing additional low contrast detail (such as the patients clothing), whereas high-contrast detail is darker and less intense (lower right, denoted as **d**). The sigmoid functions can also be considered a model for detector efficiency – for instance in x-ray imaging – if the original gray values are considered to be an equivalent of incident energy. Image data courtesy of the Dept. of Radiation Oncology, Medical University Vienna.

We have found that our image has a depth of 8 bit, and we have allocated a vector `hist16`, which will be our histogram with 16 bins. The next step is to determine the minimum gray value of the image, which is the starting point for the first bin, and the bin width; in order to cover a range of 256 gray values, we need a bin width of 16 for a histogram with 16 bins according to Equation 4.3. We can now sort the gray values ρ into the histogram bins. The image has a width of 435 pixels and a height of 261 pixels; we design the `for`-loops accordingly:

```
4:> for i = 1:261
5:> for j = 1:435
6:> rho = img(i,j);
7:> b16 = floor(rho/17.0)+1;
8:> hist16(b16,1)=hist16(b16,1)+1;
9:> end
10:> end
```

We have used a nasty little trick for determination of the appropriate bin; the result of the division $\rho/(\text{Bin Width}+1)$ is rounded to the lower integer by using `floor`. This operation should result in the appropriate bin number, ranging from 0 to the number of bins minus one. Since indices in Octave and MATLAB range from 1 to the maximum number of bins, the bin number has to be increased by 1. In the next step 1 was added to the resulting bin. For a visualization of the histograms, the following command is helpful:

```
11:> bar(hist16)
```

The output from `Histogram_4.m` can be found in Figure 4.16.

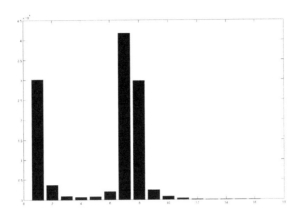

FIGURE 4.16: The output from `Histogram_4.m`, where a histogram of 16 bins is computed from the 8 bit image `ABD_CT.jpg`.

For visualization of the histogram using a spreadsheet program, one can also save the histogram as a text file, and import it into a standard spreadsheet program; the command to be used is `save`; the visualization of such histograms in a spreadsheet program such as *Microsoft Excel* or *OpenOffice* can be found in Figure 4.8.

```
12:> save('Histogram16.txt','hist16','-ascii');
```

Additional Tasks

Generate a histogram with 64 and 256 bins.

Compute a histogram with 64 bins for the 12 bit dataset `PROSTATE_CT`. It is a single DICOM slice of 512×512 pixels, 16 byte depth, and a header of 980 bytes.

Use the MATLAB function `hist` to draw the histograms.

4.5.6 Automatic optimization of image contrast using the histogram

A powerful application of histogram analysis is automated contrast optimization. As many of our images are of 16 bit depth, it is not clearly defined which numerical value ρ is black since the measurement provided by an image detector may only consume a small part of the possible gray values. This is, for instance, quite common in digital x-ray images provided by amorphous silicon detectors. When scaling the range of gray values for display, the simple linear intensity transfer of the original image range, defined by ρ_{max} and ρ_{min} in Equation

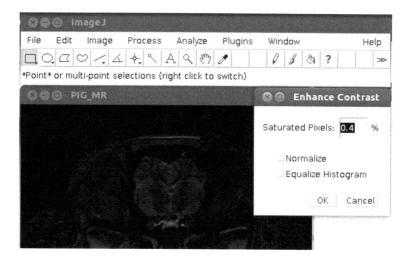

FIGURE 4.17: The dialog of *ImageJ* shown after clicking the "Enhance Contrast" menu item. The dialog asks for a percentage of "Saturated Pixels". This function clips the extreme parts of the histogram and sets the pixels that contain such extreme gray values to a slightly higher level. The script `OptimizeContrast_4.m` illustrates this method.

4.1 to the desired depth (usually 8 bit or, as in many of our samples here, 6 bit), detail can be lost since a cluttered histogram may lead to too dark or too bright an image. *ImageJ* provides a function named "Enhance Contrast", to be found under the "Process" menu. Figure 4.17 shows the dialog that pops up. This contrast enhancement is automatic once a small percentage of the histogram area is identified. The darkest and brightest pixels that fall into that area of the histogram are set to a slightly higher or lower value, which defines the new margins of the histogram. Noise of single extremely bright or dark pixels, which can be a result of a faulty detector, no longer affects the overall contrast of the image.

If we try to optimize the contrast of the well-known `PIG_MR` DICOM file from your `LessonData` folder using *ImageJ* with a saturation level of 0.4% – therefore, the 0.2% that belongs to the brightest part of the image and the 0.2% of the darkest part of the image is set to its lowest value – we get a result like the one shown in Figure 4.18. Fine details on this process are provided in the `OptimizeContrast_4.m` script given in this section later on.

Let us investigate `OptimizeContrast_4.m`, a script that implements such a function. As usual, it can be found in your `LessonData` folder. It comes with two DICOM images named `LungCT.dcm` and `LungCT_WithSpot.dcm`. First, we clear all variables from the workspace and open the file the usual way. Denote that we skip the header this time in a very elegant fashion – we determine the amount of data necessary for holding the raw image and go back from the end of file (`eof`) before reading the data.

```
1:> clear;
2:> fp = fopen('LungCT.dcm');
3:> fseek(fp,(-512*512*2),'eof');
4:> img=zeros(512,512);
5:> img(:)=fread(fp,(512*512),'short');
6:> img=transpose(img);
7:> fclose(fp);
```

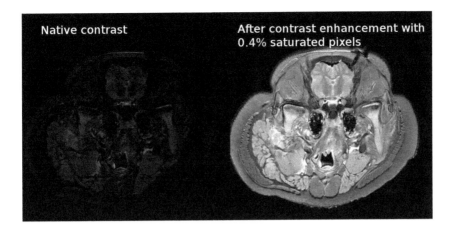

FIGURE 4.18: The result of contrast enhancement on the `PIG_MR` dataset given in the `LessonData`-folder in *ImageJ*. 0.4% pixel saturation was chosen.

Next, we store the maximal and minimal intensity values in two variables named `minoriginal` and `maxoriginal`. The range of gray values – which is equivalent to the width of the histogram – is stored in a variable `depth`. The image is then copied to `oimg`, which is scaled to 6 bit and is displayed. That is the look of the original image with 6 bit depth. Finally, an old-school statement halts the script until we press the ENTER key on our keyboard.

```
8:> minoriginal=min(min(img))
9:> maxoriginal=max(max(img))
10:> depth=maxoriginal-minoriginal;
11:> colormap(gray)
12:> oimg=img;
13:> oimg=round((oimg-minoriginal)/(depth)*64);
14:> image(oimg)
15:> foo=input('Press ENTER to proceed ...
to the histogram...');
```

In the next step, the histogram `hist` is computed. We choose the number of bins equivalent to the range of gray values – each value ρ therefore gets its own bin. The process is therefore slightly simplified compared to Section 4.5.5. The histogram is plotted using the `bar` function of MATLAB. Again, the script is halted until we press the ENTER key.

```
16:> hist = zeros(depth+1,1);
17:> for i = 1:512
18:> for j = 1:512
19:> hindex = img(i,j)-minoriginal+1;
20:> hist(hindex,1)=hist(hindex,1)+1;
21:> end
22:> end
23:> bar(hist)
24:> foo=input('Press ENTER to proceed to the ...
contrast-enhanced image...');
```

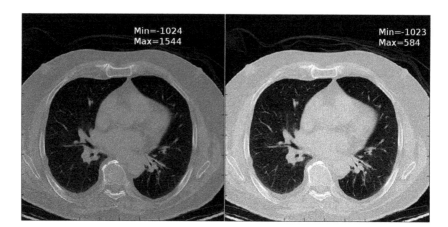

FIGURE 4.19: The result of `OptimizeContrast_4.m` on the image `LungCT.dcm`. The left image shows the original image, scaled to 6 bit from an original range of -1024 . . . 1544 HU. The right image is the result after removal of 0.8% of the most extreme histogram content. The range now is -1023 . . . 584 HU; however, the impact on the image is miniuscule since the histogram is rather compact.

Now, we determine a percentage of the total histogram area that contains pixels that are extremely dark or extremely bright – we might even call them outliers. This percentage is defined using the variable `cutoff`. We want to remove 0.4% of the darkest and 0.4% of the brightest pixels. The number of pixels which are either too dark or too bright is computed by multiplying the total number of pixels with the variable `cutoff`:

```
25:> cutoff=0.004;
26:> border=round(512*512*cutoff);
```

Here comes the major part of the algorithm; we determine the lower boundary for the new, contrast-enhanced histogram. For this purpose, we add up the number of pixels in each bin in a variable `noOfPixels` until this number exceeds the value `border`, which was defined above. The number of histogram bins is stored in `count`. This value defines the new minimal gray value in the contrast enhanced image; it is given by the appropriate bin `lowerHistBoundary` in the histogram.

```
27:> belowLeftBorder=1;
28:> count=1;
29:> noOfPixels=0;
30:> while belowLeftBorder==1
31:> noOfPixels=noOfPixels+hist(count,1);
32:> count=count+1;
33:> if noOfPixels > border
34:> belowLeftBorder=0;
35:> end
36:> end
37:> lowerHistBoundary=count-1;
```

Now, we repeat the same procedure for the upper part of the histogram, truncating it to the bin given as `upperHistBoundary`. Since the bin width is equivalent for each possible gray value in the image, this is also the new highest gray value to be found in the histogram.

```
38:> count=depth+1;
39:> noOfPixels=0;
40:> aboveRightBorder=1;
41:> while aboveRightBorder==1
42:> noOfPixels=noOfPixels+hist(count,1);
43:> count=count-1;
44:> if noOfPixels > border
45:> aboveRightBorder=0;
46:> end
47:> end
48:> upperHistBoundary=count+1;
```

The image is a CT – its minimal gray value is usually -1024 HU. However, the histogram `hist` starts at 1. In order to re-establish the proper gray values in Hounsfield units, we have to shift the gray values at the boundary back to the Hounsfield-scale:

```
49:> newmin=lowerHistBoundary+minoriginal
50:> newmax=upperHistBoundary+minoriginal
```

Now, we do the intensity transform. All gray values in the image that are lower than `newmin` are set to `newmin` – these are the pixels that formerly belonged to the lowest 0.4% of the histogram area. The pixels with gray values above `newmax` are set to `newmax`:

```
51:> for i = 1:512
52:> for j = 1:512
53:> if img(i,j) < newmin
54:> img(i,j)=newmin;
55:> end
56:> if img(i,j)>newmax
57:> img(i,j)=newmax;
58:> end
59:> end
60:> end
```

Finally, we scale the new image to 6 bit and display it. The result, alongside with the original image, is shown in Figure 4.19.

```
61:> img=round((img-newmin)/(newmax-newmin)*64);
62:> image(img)
```

Additional Tasks

Another image – `LungCT_WithSpot.dcm` in the `LessonData` folder is a manipulated version of `LungCT.dcm` which was used in this example. Utilizing almost the full range of 16 bit, I added a few white spots with a gray value of 30000 in the upper left part of the image. The effect on image display is devastating, as one can see from Figure 4.20. Due to the extreme width of the populated histogram, the image content more or less disappears as can be seen on the left image. After contrast enhancement, the relevant image content re-appears. This is the true power of histogram based contrast enhancement – it allows us to concentrate on the major part of the image in terms of histogram content. Inspect the output of `OptimizeContrast_4.m` yourself!

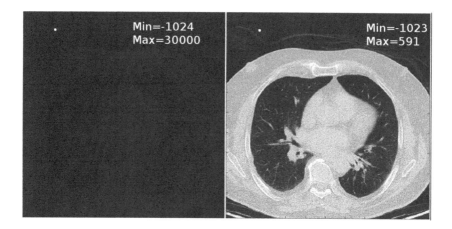

FIGURE 4.20: An example of an image with an extremely cluttered histogram. The data type is signed 16 bit. The major content of the image is found in the Hounsfield range (-1024 - 3072). However, a small artificial spot in the upper left corner of the image with an intensity of 30000 makes the linear intensity scaling to 6 bit unusable (left image). After contrast enhancement using `OptimizeContrast_4.m` on that image, the relevant image content reappears (right image).

4.5.7 Intensity operations using ImageJ and 3DSlicer

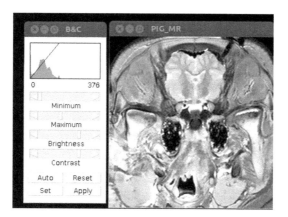

FIGURE 4.21: A linear intensity adjustment in ImageJ. By changing the sliders named "Minimum" and "Maximum", we carry out a similar procedure as we did in Section 4.5.1. The linear ITF is, of course, a windowing function.

Let us take a quick look at intensity scaling in ImageJ – we already know how to open a DICOM image from Section 3.7.3. Let's open `PIG_MR` again. In dependence on your monitor settings, you will see a rather dark image. If you got to the menu "Image → Adjust → Brightness/Contrast", you will see a small dialog similar to the one shown in Figure 4.21. The menu "Image → Adjust → Window/Level" performs a similar operation, as shown in Figure 4.22.

In 3DSlicer, Windowing is implemented in the standard manner which can be found in

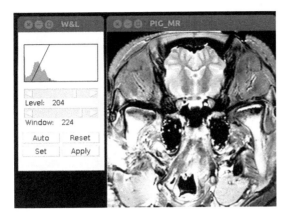

FIGURE 4.22: Similar to the dialog shown in Figure 4.21, the linear intensity transform can also be defined as a windowing function in ImageJ. The only difference is the definition of parameters for the linear ITF, which are given here as window center and window width. Here, the center is named "Level" and the width is called "Window".

most medical imaging workstations. If you load a DICOM file, you can change the windowing parameters by moving your mouse to the images as shown in Figure 3.20. Moving the mouse with the left mouse button pressed in a left/right direction changes the window width, and moving the mouse (again with the left button pressed) up or down changes the window center. The result can be found in Figure 4.5.

4.6 SUMMARY AND FURTHER REFERENCES

Transformations in intensity space play an extremely important role in medical image processing and image display in general, especially since medical images are usually recorded with an image depth beyond human perception. Transformations can range from applying rather simple analytical functions like taking the logarithm to more sophisticated models such as parameterized sigmoid curves or special windowing operations, which enhance the details visible within the signal range of a certain tissue type. The distribution of gray values is represented by a histogram.

Literature

R. C. Gonzalez, R. E. Woods: Digital Image Processing, Prentice-Hall, (2007)

A. Oppelt (ed.): Imaging Systems for Medical Diagnostics: Fundamentals, Technical Solutions and Applications for Systems Applying Ionizing Radiation, Nuclear Magnetic Resonance and Ultrasound, Wiley VCH, (2006)

W. Burger, M. J. Burge: Digital Image Processing – An Algorithmic Introduction using Java, Springer, (2008), http://www.imagingbook.com

CHAPTER 5

Filtering and Transformations

Wolfgang Birkfellner

CONTENTS

5.1   The filtering operation 116
    5.1.1   Kernel based smoothing and sharpening operations 118
    5.1.2   Differentiation and edge detection 121
    5.1.3   Helpful non-linear filters 126
5.2   The Fourier transform 128
    5.2.1   Basic linear algebra and series expansions 128
    5.2.2   Waves – a special orthonormal system 131
    5.2.3   Some important properties of the Fourier transform 137
    5.2.4   Image processing in the frequency domain 137
    5.2.5   Modelling properties of imaging systems – the PSF and the
             MTF 139
5.3   Other transforms 140
    5.3.1   The Hough transform 141
    5.3.2   The distance transform 142
5.4   Practical lessons 143
    5.4.1   Kernel – based low pass and high pass filtering 143
    5.4.2   Basic filtering operations in *ImageJ* 145
    5.4.3   Numerical differentiation 145
        5.4.3.1   A note on good MATLAB® programming habits . 148
    5.4.4   Unsharp masking 148
    5.4.5   The median filter 149
    5.4.6   Some properties of the Fourier-transform 150
        5.4.6.1   Spectra of simple functions in k-space 150
        5.4.6.2   More complex functions 152
        5.4.6.3   Convolution of simple functions 158
        5.4.6.4   Differentiation in k-space 159
    5.4.7   Frequency filtering in Fourier-space on images 161
    5.4.8   Applied convolution – PSF and the MTF 162
    5.4.9   Determination of system resolution of an Anger-camera using
             a point source 164
    5.4.10   The Hough transform 167

     5.4.11 The distance transform 172

5.5   Summary and further references 174

5.1 THE FILTERING OPERATION

A *filter* in mathematics or signal processing describes a *function* that *modifies an incoming signal*. Since images are two- or three dimensional signals, a filter operation can, for instance, remove noise or enhance the contrast of the image. In this chapter, we will learn about some basic filtering operations, the basics of signal processing, and we will encounter a powerful tool in signal processing.

In order to get a systematic overview of filtering operations, a completely non-medical example might prove useful. We know that a convex lens, made of a material that changes the speed of light, can focus incoming light. Crown glass, with a refractive index $n = 1.51$, is the most common material for lenses. The focusing of incoming rays of light (which are the normals to the wavefront) is achieved by the fact that at least one boundary layer between air and glass is curved. The rays that intersect the lens surface on the outer diameter have a shorter travel through the glass, whereas the ray that intersects the middle of the lens (the so-called paraxial ray) has to stay within the glass for a longer period of time. Since the speed of light changes in the optically dense medium, the paraxial ray lags behind his neighbors, and as a consequence, the rays (which are, again, normals to the wavefront) merge in the focus. The angle of the ray is determined by the *law of refraction*.[1]

A mirror can also focus light; here, the more simple *law of reflection* governs the formation of the focus. Each incoming ray is reflected by an angle of the same absolute value as the angle of incidence. In a spherical mirror (which bears its name because it is part of a sphere), all rays emerging from the center of curvature (COC) are reflected back to the COC; in this case, the COC is the focus of the mirror. When rays come from a different position than the COC, the reflected rays are no longer focused in a single spot – rather than that, the rays close to the paraxial ray have a different focus than the rays which hit the mirrors edge. Figure 5.1 illustrates this behavior, which is called *spherical aberration*. The consequences are clear; if we mount an image detector such as a CCD, we will not get a sharp image since the rays emerging from a point-shaped object (such as, star) are not focused to a single spot. A spherical mirror is therefore not a very good telescope.

We can model this optical aberration using a so-called *ray tracing program*. It is already apparent that these programs for the design of optical systems do something similar to the rendering algorithm we will encounter in Chapter 8. One of these raytracing programs is OSLO (Sinclair Optics, Pittsford, NY), which we will use to model the extent of the spherical aberration in a spherical mirror of 150 mm diameter and a focal length of 600 mm. The task in optical design is to optimize the parameters of the optical elements in such a manner that the optical systems deliver optimum image quality. This is achieved by simulating the paths of light rays through the optical system. The laws of reflection and refraction are being taken into account. The optical system is considered optimal when it focuses all possible rays of light to a focus as small as possible. OSLO computes a spot diagram, which is a slice of the ray cone at its minimal diameter; the spot diagram therefore

---

[1]The law of refraction, also called Snell's law, reads $n_1 \sin \theta_1 = n_2 \sin \theta_2$ where n_i is the refractive index of the material that contains the ray, and θ_i is the angle of incidence associated.

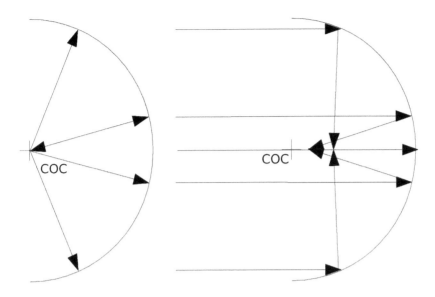

FIGURE 5.1: An illustration of the spherical aberration in a mirror. If a single point source of light is located at the center of curvature (COC), all rays of light will be reflected back to the COC, which is also the location of the focus in this case. This situation is illustrated in the left part of the image. If the point source is located at infinity, all rays come in parallel; in this case, the rays closer to the center of the mirror form a different focus than the distal rays. In other words, the light from the point source is not focused to a single spot – the image will be unsharp.

gives us an idea of what the image of the point source of light will look like after it passes the spherical mirror. We assume a single monochromatic point source of light at infinity. The resulting spot diagram can be found in Figure 5.2.

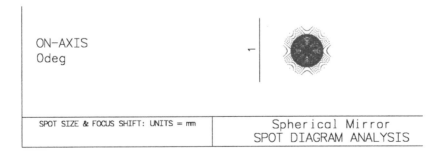

FIGURE 5.2: The spot diagram of a spherical mirror of 150 mm diameter and 600 mm focal length. OSLO simulates a point light source located at infinity here. As we can see, the smallest image possible of this point source on an image detector is a blob of approximately 1 mm diameter. The spot diagram is a representation of the point-spread function, which is the general concept of modelling signal transfer by an arbitrary signal processing system.

Here ends our excursion into optics; the mirror is, in fact, a filter – it modifies the original signal to something else. If we want a perfect telescope (or another imaging system), we should take care that the image provided is as identical as possible to the original. The way to describe the performance of such a signal transferring system is actually the performance on a single, point like source. The result of the filter on this point-like signal is called the *Point Spread Function* (PSF). If we want to know about the looks of the whole image, we simply have to apply the PSF to every single point in the original image. The process of blending the PSF with the original image is called *convolution*. In the convolution operation, the PSF is applied to every pixel, which of course might also affect the surrounding pixels in the resulting image. The convolution operation is denoted using the $\star$ sign. Many textbooks in image processing introduce the various image processing operations by providing small matrices, which represent a *convolution kernel*. Subsequently, this kernel, which can be considered a PSF, is applied to every single pixel and re-distributes the gray values ρ in order to achieve the desired outcome. In this course, we will try to avoid this formulation in favor of a more strict (and simple) formalism for convolution, which will be introduced in Section 5.2.2.

5.1.1 Kernel based smoothing and sharpening operations

A common task in image processing is the smoothing and sharpening of images; an image corrupted by noise – which can be considered ripples in the landscape of gray values ρ – may be improved if one applies an operation that averages the local surrounding of each pixel. Such a kernel K can, for instance, take the following form:

$$K_{\text{blur}} = \frac{1}{10} \begin{pmatrix} 1 & 1 & 1 \\ 1 & 2 & 1 \\ 1 & 1 & 1 \end{pmatrix}. \tag{5.1}$$

So what happens if this kernel is convolved with an image? In fact, a weighted average of the gray values surrounding each pixel in the original images is assigned to the same pixel position in the new image. Small fluctuations in the gray values are reduced by this averaging operation. However, the central pixel position is emphasized by receiving a higher weight than the others. Example 5.4.1 illustrates this simple operation; a detail of the outcome is also given in Figure 5.3. In data analysis, this is referred to as a moving average. Another interesting detail of this kernel is also the fact that it is normalized by multiplying every component of K_{blur} with the factor $\frac{1}{10}$. It is clear that a blurring PSF like K_{blur}, which essentially does something similar to the spherical mirror, cannot add energy to a signal – and therefore, the total sum of elements in the kernel is one. It is of the utmost importance to emphasize that kernels such as the blurring kernel given in Equation 5.1 are indeed *functions*, just like the images they are convolved with.

Let's go back to the spherical telescope. A star emits energy; a small fraction of this energy hits the mirror, which focuses this energy onto an image detector. Due to spherical aberration, the image is blurred, therefore the energy is distributed over more than one pixel of our image detector. As we may recall from Chapter 4, the gray value is proportional to the energy as long as we stay within the dynamic range of the detector. There is no obvious reason why the telescope should add energy to the signal. K_{blur} should not do so, either. If a kernel changes the sum of all gray values ρ, one might consider normalizing the whole image by a simple global intensity scaling to the same value $\sum_{i,j} \rho_{i,j}$ found in the original image.

The opposite of smoothing is an operation called *sharpening*; in a sharpening operation,

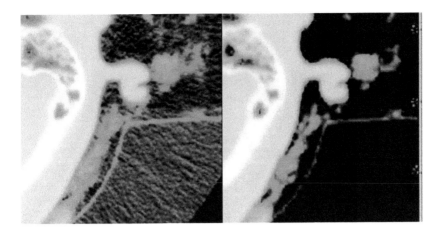

FIGURE 5.3: A detail from the SKULLBASE.DCM before and after the smoothing operation carried out in Example 5.4.1. The whole image (a CT slice in the vicinity of the skull base) is shown in Figure 5.24. On the left side, we see some reconstruction artifacts in the air surrounding the head. The smoothing filter K_{blur} successfully removes these artifacts by weighted averaging. For visualization purposes, the image intensities were transformed here in order to improve the visibility of low contrast details. Image data courtesy of the Dept. of Radiology, Medical University Vienna.

it is desired to emphasize edges in the images. Edges can be considered an abyss in the landscape of the image. A sharpening operator therefore does merely nothing if the surrounding of a pixel shows a homogeneous distribution of gray values. If a strong variation in gray values is encountered, it emphasizes the pixels with high intensity and suppresses the low intensity pixels. The classic sharpening operator looks like this:

$$K_{\text{sharp}} = \begin{pmatrix} -1 & -1 & -1 \\ -1 & 9 & -1 \\ -1 & -1 & -1 \end{pmatrix} \tag{5.2}$$

It strongly weights the pixel it operates on, and suppresses the surrounding. The region from SKULLBASE.DCM from Figure 5.3 after applying K_{sharp} is shown in Figure 5.4. An interesting effect from applying such a kernel can, however, be observed in Example 5.4.1; the strong weight on the central pixel of K_{sharp} causes a considerable change in the shape of the histogram. Still, K_{sharp} preserves the energy stored in a pixel. The change in image brightness is a consequence of the scaling to 6 bit image depth – check Example 5.4.1 for further detail.

Both smoothing and sharpening operations are widely used in medical imaging. A smoothing operator can suppress image noise, as can be seen from Figure 5.3. In modalities with a poor SNR, for instance in nuclear medicine, this is quite common. Sharpening, on the other hand, is a necessity in computed tomography to enhance the visibility of fine detail, as we will see in Chapter 10. Figure 5.5 shows two CT slices of a pig jaw; one is not filtered after reconstruction, the other one was filtered using the software of the CT. Besides the improvement in detail visibility and the increased visibility of reconstruction artifacts, we also witness a change in overall image brightness – a phenomenon we have already seen in Figure 5.4. It is also an intensity scaling artifact.

A large number of other kernels can be defined, and they usually just represent different

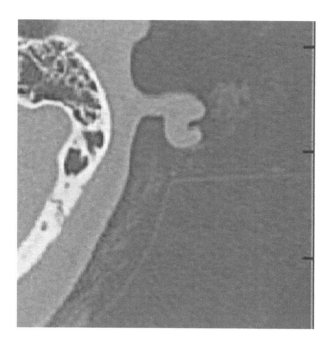

FIGURE 5.4: The same detail from the SKULLBASE.DCM already shown in Figure 5.3 after a sharpening operation using the K_{sharp} kernel. Fine details such as the spongeous bone of the mastoid process are emphasized. Image data courtesy of the Dept. of Radiology, Medical University Vienna.

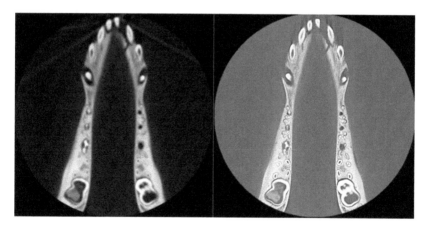

FIGURE 5.5: Two CT slices of a dry mandible of a pig. The left image was reconstructed without the use of a sharpening operator, the right slice was sharpened. Both images were directly taken from the DICOM-server connected to the CT and not further processed. Again, the change in overall image brightness from the use of the sharpening operator is clearly visible. This is, however, an intensity scaling artifact. Image data courtesy of the Dental School Vienna, Medical University Vienna.

types of PSFs. K_{blur}, for instance, is a simple numerical approximation of a two-dimensional Gaussian curve. In numerical mathematics, we have already seen that functions are simply represented as vectors of discrete values, which represent the result of a function (see, for instance, Example 4.5.4). If we want to use more precise kernels, we may simply increase the number of pivoting values. For instance, a more sophisticated Gaussian kernel with five instead of three pivoting elements in each dimension looks like this:

$$K_{5\times 5\,\text{Gauss}} = \frac{1}{256} \begin{pmatrix} 1 & 4 & 6 & 4 & 1 \\ 4 & 16 & 24 & 16 & 4 \\ 6 & 24 & 36 & 24 & 6 \\ 4 & 16 & 24 & 16 & 4 \\ 1 & 4 & 6 & 4 & 1 \end{pmatrix} \tag{5.3}$$

The single elements of the kernel $K_{5\times 5\,\text{Gauss}}$ are approximated from the well known analytic expression for the Gaussian curve. However, the more precise a kernel gets, the more time consuming the actual implementation is.[2] As already announced in the introduction to this chapter, a more convenient formalism for convolution with complex kernel functions exists, therefore we will now close this section.

5.1.2 Differentiation and edge detection

Since images can be considered mathematical functions, one can of course compute derivatives of these images. We know that the derivative of a function gives a local gradient of the function. However, the problem in image processing lies in the fact that we cannot make assumptions about the mathematical properties of the image such as differentiability. The good news is that we can make numerical approximations of the derivation process. The differential expression $\frac{df(x)}{dx}$ for a function $f(x) = \rho$ becomes a finite difference:

$$\frac{df(x)}{dx} = \frac{\rho_{i+1} - \rho_i}{\Delta x} \tag{5.4}$$

In this special case, we are dealing with a *forward difference* since the numerator of the differential is defined as the difference between the actual value ρ_i and its next neighbor ρ_{i+1}. There is also a *backward difference* and a *central difference*, which we will encounter in the next sections. In Example 5.4.3, we will apply this operation to a simple rectangular function; the result can be found in Figure 5.6.

A function that maps from two or three coordinates to a scalar value (such as an image) features a derivative in each direction – these are the *partial derivatives*, denoted as $\frac{\partial I(x,y,z)}{\partial x}$, $\frac{\partial I(x,y,z)}{\partial y}$ and so on if our function is the well known functional formulation $I(x, y, z) = \rho$ as presented in Chapter 3. The forward difference as presented in Equation 5.4, again, is the equivalent of the partial derivative: $\frac{\partial I(x,y,z)}{\partial x} = \rho_{x+1,y,z} - \rho_{x,y,z}$, where $\rho_{x,y,z}$ is the gray value at voxel position $(x, y, z)^T$; the denominator Δx is one, and therefore it is already omitted. If we want to differentiate an image, we can define a kernel that produces the forward difference after convolution with the image. Such a kernel for differentiation in the x-direction is given as:

$$K_{\text{x-forward}} = \begin{pmatrix} 0 & 0 & 0 \\ 0 & -1 & 1 \\ 0 & 0 & 0 \end{pmatrix} \tag{5.5}$$

---

[2] As for all kernels presented in this chapter, it is necessary to emphasize that we assume isotropic image data.

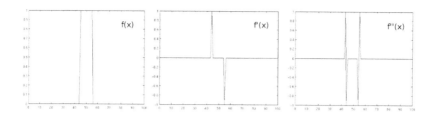

FIGURE 5.6: The results from Example 5.4.3. In the first plot, we see a simple rectangle function $f(x)$. The first derivative $\frac{df(x)}{dx}$, computed by forward differentiation, is named $f'(x)$ in this illustration. As we can see, the derivative takes a high value if something rapidly changes in $f(x)$, and it becomes zero if neighboring values of $f(x)$ are similar. The same holds true for the second derivative $f''(x)$. In image processing, differentiation yields the edges of an image, whereas areas of similar gray values become black.

The correspondence between $K_{\text{x-forward}}$ and Equation 5.4 is obvious. The kernel subtracts the gray value $\rho_{x,y}$ located at the central pixel from the gray value $\rho_{x+1,y}$ located to the right. $K_{\text{x-forward}}$ therefore computes the partial forward difference of an image $I_{x,y}$. The effects of $K_{\text{x-forward}}$ are also presented in Example 5.4.3. The result of applying forward differentiation on the already well-known SKULLBASE.DCM image is shown in Figure 5.7. Apparently, all the homogeneous gray value information is lost, and only the edges in the image remain. Due to the forward differentiation, the whole image shows some drift to the right hand side. $K_{\text{x-forward}}$ is also known as the *bas-relief kernel*; SKULLBASE.DCM looks a little bit like a lunar landscape since it shows shadows in the positive x-direction, and the whole image is also pretty flat. While $K_{\text{x-forward}}$ is an edge-detection filter in its simplest form, the dullness of the whole image is somewhat disturbing. The cause of this low contrast can be guessed from the middle image showing the first derivative of the rectangle function in Figure 5.6 – when proceeding from a low value of $f(x)$ to a high value, the derivative takes a high positive value; if $f(x)$ is high and $f(x+1)$ is low, the derivative yields a high negative value. However, when detecting edges, we are only interested in the sudden change in image brightness – we are not interested in the direction of the change. A modification of $K_{\text{x-forward}}$ is the use of the absolute value of the gradient. This is an additional task for you in Example 5.4.3, and the result is found in the right image in Figure 5.7.

Given the rather trivial structure of $K_{\text{x-forward}}$, the result of this operation as presented in Figure 5.7 is not that bad for a first try on an *edge detection* filter. Only two problems remain. First, only the partial derivative for the x-direction is computed, whereas the y-direction is neglected. And the forward-direction of $K_{\text{x-forward}}$ gives the image a visual effect that simulates a flat relief. Both issues can easily be resolved.

If we want to know about the gradient – the direction of maximal change in our image $I(x, y, z) = \rho$ – we have to compute all partial derivatives for the independent variables x, y, and z, and multiply the result with the unit vectors for each direction. Mathematically speaking, this is the nabla operator $\nabla = \left(\frac{\partial}{\partial x}, \frac{\partial}{\partial y}, \frac{\partial}{\partial z} \right)^T$; it returns the gradient of a function as a vector. Computing the norm of the nabla operator and $I(x, y, z)$ gives the absolute value of the maximal change in the gray scale ρ.

$$||\nabla I(x, y, z)|| = \sqrt{\left(\frac{\partial I(x, y, z)}{\partial x} \right)^2 + \left(\frac{\partial I(x, y, z)}{\partial y} \right)^2 + \left(\frac{\partial I(x, y, z)}{\partial z} \right)^2} \tag{5.6}$$

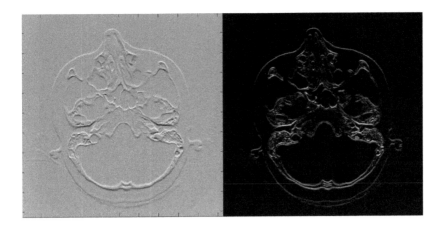

FIGURE 5.7: Some more results from Example 5.4.3. The left image shows the effects of $K_{\text{x-forward}}$ on the SKULLBASE.DCM-image. It is pretty evident why this filter is also called the bas-relief filter. When computing the absolute value of the convolution of $K_{\text{x-forward}}$ with SKULLBASE.DCM, the image on the right is produced. It does always give a positive value, no matter whether the image edges change from bright to dark pixel values or vice versa. In can also be seen that vertical edges like the skin surface close to the zygomatic arch is not emphasized; the x- and y-axis are swapped - this is a direct consequence of the matrix indexing conventions in MATLAB, where the first index is the column of the matrix image. Image data courtesy of the Dept. of Radiology, Medical University Vienna.

What looks mathematical and strict is in fact very simple; it is the length of the gradient. The fact that this gradient length is always positive also makes the use of the absolute value of a differentiation kernel as proposed for $K_{\text{x-forward}}$ unnecessary. The asymmetric nature of the forward differentiation from Equation 5.4 can be replaced by the average of the forward- and the backward difference. This so-called *central difference* is given by

$$\frac{df(x)}{dx} = \frac{1}{2}\Big(\underbrace{\rho_{i+1} - \rho_i}_{\text{Forward } \Delta} + \underbrace{\rho_i - \rho_{i-1}}_{\text{Backward } \Delta}\Big) \tag{5.7}$$

for a stepwidth of $\Delta x = 1$. This expression can be rewritten as $\frac{df(x)}{dx} = \frac{1}{2}(\rho_{i+1} - \rho_{i-1})$. This central difference yields the following 2D convolution kernels for derivations in x and y

$$K_{\text{x-central}} = \frac{1}{2}\begin{pmatrix} 0 & 0 & 0 \\ -1 & 0 & 1 \\ 0 & 0 & 0 \end{pmatrix} \text{ and } K_{\text{y-central}} = \frac{1}{2}\begin{pmatrix} 0 & -1 & 0 \\ 0 & 0 & 0 \\ 0 & 1 & 0 \end{pmatrix} \tag{5.8}$$

Therefore, the result of the operation

$$\sqrt{\big(K_{\text{x-central}} \star I(x,y)\big)^2 + \big(K_{\text{y-central}} \star I(x,y)\big)^2},$$

which is actually the length of the gradient of the image $I(x,y)$ should give a rather good edge detection filter. In Example 5.4.3, you are prompted to implement that operation.

The $K_{\text{x-central}}$ and $K_{\text{y-central}}$ kernels obviously provide a nice edge detection filter, as we can see from Figure 5.8. We can, of course, widen the focus of the kernels. For instance, it is possible to add more image elements to the kernel, as we have seen in Equation 5.3,

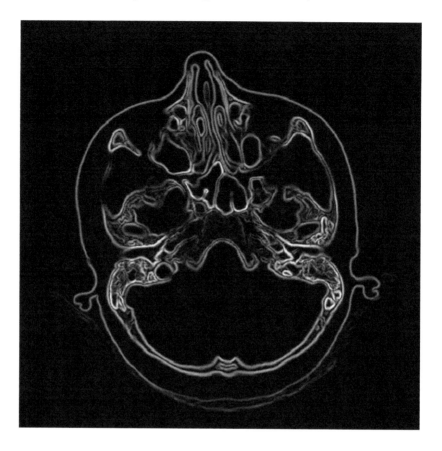

FIGURE 5.8: The effects of computing the length of the resulting gradient after convolution result of $K_{\text{x-central}}$ and $K_{\text{y-central}}$ with SKULLBASE.DCM. This is already a pretty satisfying edge detector; due to the use of central differences, no shadowing effects appear. The use of the total differential does respect changes in all directions, and the gradient length only yields positive results for the derivation result. Image data courtesy of the Dept. of Radiology, Medical University Vienna.

where our simple smoothing kernel K_{blur} was enhanced by modelling a Gaussian curve over a 5×5 kernel. The general concept of *connectedness* can be introduced here; a pixel has four next neighbors – these are the *four-connected* pixels. Beyond that, there are also the *eight-connected* neighbors. If we add the contributions of the next but one neighbors to the center of the kernel, we are using the eight-connected pixels as well. $K_{\text{x-central}}$ and $K_{\text{y-central}}$ only utilize the four-connected neighbors, whereas K_{sharp} and K_{blur} are eight-connected. Figure 5.9 gives an illustration. From this illustration it also evident that the neighbors on the corners of the kernel are located at a distance $\sqrt{2}\Delta x$ from the center of the kernel with Δx being the pixel spacing. Therefore the weight of these image elements that are distant neighbors is lower. The concept of connectedness can of course be generalized to 3D. The equivalent to a four connected neighborhood is a six connected kernel (which also uses the voxel in front of and behind the central voxel), and if we also use the next but one voxels to construct our kernel, we end up with 26 connected voxels.

A more general formulation of the kernels from Equation 5.8 including the next and next

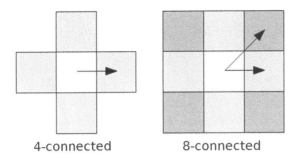

4-connected   8-connected

FIGURE 5.9: The four-connected and eight-connected neighborhood of a pixel. The contribution from the neighboring pixels depends on their distance; the pixels on the corner are at a distance that is larger by a factor $\sqrt{2}$ compared to the 4-connected neighbors. If a kernel utilizes information from these next but one neighbors, there has to be assigned a lower weight than to the nearest neighbors.

but one neighboring pixels (while omitting the factor $\frac{1}{2}$) and assigning appropriate weights (rounded down to integer numbers) to the next and next but one pixels would be:

$$K_{\text{Sobel}_x} = \begin{pmatrix} -1 & 0 & 1 \\ -2 & 0 & 2 \\ -1 & 0 & 1 \end{pmatrix} \text{ and } K_{\text{Sobel}_y} = \begin{pmatrix} -1 & -2 & -1 \\ 0 & 0 & 0 \\ 1 & 2 & 1 \end{pmatrix} \tag{5.9}$$

As the subscript already shows, these are the *Sobel-kernels*, which are among the best known edge detection operators in image processing.

Many more kernels can be designed, and many of them are virtually redundant and can be constructed as linear combinations of the kernels presented. However, blurring, sharpening, and edge detection are among the most common and important operations in medical imaging. What all kernels presented until now have in common is the fact that they are linear; the kernel can be applied to the whole image, or one can divide the kernel in parts and apply the filter subsequently to the image. After fusing the outcome, the result is the same. If an image $I(x, y) = I_1(x, y) + s * I_2(x, y)$ is convolved with an arbitrary linear kernel K, the following identity is true:

$$K \star I(x, y) = K \star I_1(x, y) + s * K \star I_2(x, y) \tag{5.10}$$

Another similarity of all the kernels presented so far is the fact that they are constant; the weights in the kernel are always the same, no matter what gray value ρ is encountered by the central pixel of the kernel. A somewhat adaptive technique that bears its name from analog photography is *unsharp masking*. Originally designed to cope with the limited dynamic range of photographic paper, the analog unsharp masking operation consists of exposing a photographic plate with a defocused image from negative film. If the plate has the same size as the photographic paper, one can expose the focused image of the negative through the developed photographic plate onto photographic paper. Both a sharpening effect and a suppression of overexposed areas is the result; while dynamic range is no longer that big an issue in digital imaging, the sharpening effect is still widely used, and the procedure from analog photography – exposition of the unsharp mask and summation of the unsharp mask and the focused image – can directly be transferred to the world of digital image processing.

First, we need the unsharp mask, which can be derived using blurring kernels such as $K_{5 \times 5 \, \text{Gauss}}$ or K_{blur}; subsequently, the unsharp mask is subtracted from the original image. Therefore, an unsharp masking kernel $K_{\text{Unsharp Mask}}$ using the simple smoothing filter K_{blur} looks like this:

$$K_{\text{Unsharp Mask}} = \underbrace{\begin{pmatrix} 0 & 0 & 0 \\ 0 & 1 & 0 \\ 0 & 0 & 0 \end{pmatrix}}_{\text{Unity operator}} - w * K_{\text{blur}} \tag{5.11}$$

The unity operator is the most trivial kernel of all; it simply copies the image. Example 5.4.4 implements this operation. w is a scalar factor that governs the influence of the low pass filtered image on the resulting image. Denote that the convolution operation by itself is also linear: $K_1 \star I(x,y) + s * K_2 \star I(x,y) = (K_1 + s * K_2) \star I(x,y)$. We can therefore generate all kinds of kernels by linear combination of more simple kernels.

5.1.3   Helpful non-linear filters

While most filters are linear and fulfill Equation 5.10, there are also non-linear filters. The most helpful one is the median filter. The median of a set of random variables is defined as the central value in an ordered list of these variables. The ordered list of values is also referred to as the rank list. Let's take a look at a list of values x_i for an arbitrary random variable, for instance $x_i \in 5, 9, 12, 1, 6, 4, 8, 0, 7, 9, 20, 666$. The mean of these values is defined as $\bar{x} = \frac{1}{N} \sum_i x_i$, where N is the number of values. In our example, $\bar{x}$ is 62.25. This is not a very good expectation value since most values for x_i are smaller. However, we have an outlier here; all values but the last one are smaller than 21, but the last value for x_i screws everything up. The median behaves differently. The rank list in our example would look like this: $x_i \in 0, 1, 4, 5, 6, 7, 8, 9, 9, 12, 20, 666$. Since we have twelve entries here, the central value lies between entry #6 and #7. The median of x_i is 7.5 – the average of the values x_6 and x_7 in the ordered rank list. The strength of the median is its robustness against outliers. As you can see, the median differs strongly from the average value $\bar{x}$. But it is also a better expectation value for x. If we pick a random value of x_i, it is more likely to get a result close to the median than a result that resembles $\bar{x}$.

A median filter in image processing does something similar to a smoothing operation – it replaces a gray value ρ at a pixel location $(x,y)^T$ with an expectation value for the surrounding. It is remarkable that the median filter, however, does not change pixel intensities in an image – it just replaces some of them. As opposed to K_{blur} and $K_{5 \times 5 \, \text{Gauss}}$, it does not compute a local average, but it uses the median of a defined surrounding. In general, the median filter for 3D and a kernel of dimension $n \times m \times o$ is defined in the following way:

Record all gray values ρ for the image elements in a surrounding of dimension $n \times m \times o$.

Sort this array of gray values.

Compute the median as the one gray value located in the middle of the sorted vector of gray values.

Replace the original pixel by this median.

Example 5.4.5 gives an implementation of a 5×5 median filter. Compared to linear smoothing operators, the median filter retains the structure of the image content to a larger extent by preserving image edges while being very effective in noise suppression. A comparison of smoothing and median filters of varying kernel size is given in Figure

5.10. The power of the median filter is demonstrated best when taking a look at "salt and pepper" noise, that is images stricken with black or white pixels, for instance because of defective pixels on the image detector. A median filter removes such outliers, whereas a simple blurring operation cannot cope with this type of noise.

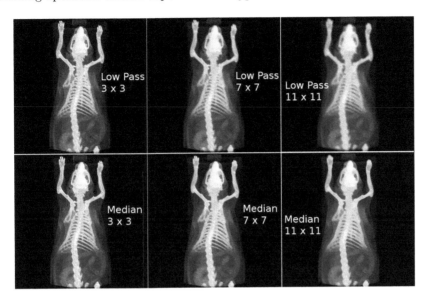

FIGURE 5.10: A topogram of a mouse from MicroCT with 733×733 pixels. The upper row shows the effects of low-pass filtering with varying kernel sizes. For comparison, the same image underwent median filtering with similar kernel sizes, which is shown in the lower row of images. While the median filter is a low-pass filter as well, the visual outcome is definitively different. The images can also be found on the CD accompanying this book in the JPGs folder. Image data courtesy of C. Kuntner, AIT Seibersdorf, Austria.

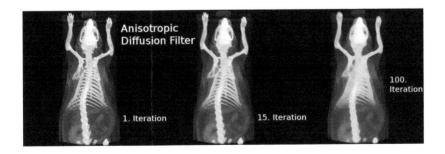

FIGURE 5.11: The same topogram as in Figure 5.10 after anisotropic diffusion filtering. As the diffusion process proceeds (as indicated by the number of iterations), one can see how the images get more blurred; still, structure is largely retained. The anisotropic diffusion filter is another example for a non-linear lowpass filter. Here, the large number of parameters allow for a very fine tuning of the degree of blurring and noise reduction. Image data courtesy of C. Kuntner, AIT Seibersdorf, Austria.

Not all non-linear filters are based on sorting or selection processes; an interesting filter that yields similar results compared to the median filter as a smoothing filter that retains general image structure is the *anisotropic diffusion filter*, which will be introduced as an example for a whole class of iterative filters. Imagine a glass of water with an oil layer covering it. If you release a drop of ink in the water layer, the ink will slowly diffuse within the water layer, but not the oil layer. Over time we will see nothing but a slightly tinted water layer. This process, which is based on the Brownian motion of the water molecules, is called diffusion. Mathematically, it is described by a *partial differential equation* (PDE). While the PDE itself is always the same for all possible substances, the outcome is governed by various parameters such as the viscosity of the fluid, the concentration of the substances and so on. The PDE can be solved numerically. If we consider an image to be a distribution of different substances, with ρ being a measure of the concentration, we can define a filter that simulates the diffusion of the image intensities over time. The various boundary conditions and the number of time steps chosen allow for a very fine tuning of the filter. In fact, the anisotropic diffusion filter is a very powerful tool for noise suppression. The effects of the filter are shown in Figure 5.11, which was generated using the AnalyzeAVW 9.1 software (Biomedical Imaging Resource, Mayo Clinic, Rochester/MN).

5.2 THE FOURIER TRANSFORM

5.2.1 Basic linear algebra and series expansions

Throughout this book, we tried to make the mathematics of medical image processing as tangible as possible. Therefore we restrict ourselves to a few equations and rely on the illustrative power of applied programming examples. Now, we will proceed to a chapter that is of immense importance for signal processing in general; however, it is also considered sometimes to be difficult to understand. We are now talking about the *Fourier transform*, which is based on the probably most important *orthonormal functional system*. And it is not difficult to understand, although the introduction given here serves only as a motivation, explanation, and reminder. It cannot replace a solid background in applied mathematics.

We all know the representation of a vector in a Cartesian coordinate system[3]: $\vec{x} = (x_1, x_2)^T$. That representation is actually a shorthand notation. It only gives the components of the vector in a Cartesian coordinate system, where the coordinate axes are spanned by unit vectors $\vec{e}_x = (1, 0)^T$ and $\vec{e}_y = (0, 1)^T$. The vector $\vec{x}$ is therefore given by the sum of unit vectors, multiplied with their components x_1 and x_2: $\vec{x} = x_1 \vec{e}_x + x_2 \vec{e}_y$. Figure 5.12 shows a simple illustration. We can invert this formulation by using the *inner product* (also referred to as *scalar product* or *dot product*). The inner product of two arbitrary 3D vectors $\vec{y} = (y_1, y_2, y_3)^T$ and $\vec{z} = (z_1, z_2, z_3)^T$ is defined as:

$$\vec{y} \bullet \vec{z} = \begin{pmatrix} y_1 \\ y_2 \\ y_3 \end{pmatrix} \bullet \begin{pmatrix} z_1 \\ z_2 \\ z_3 \end{pmatrix} = y_1 z_1 + y_2 z_2 + y_3 z_3 = ||\vec{y}|| ||\vec{z}|| \cos(\alpha) \qquad (5.12)$$

α is the angle enclosed by the two vectors $\vec{y}$ and $\vec{z}$, and the $|| \ldots ||$ operator is the norm of the vector – in this case, the vector's length. A geometrical interpretation of the inner product in three dimensional space is the projection of one vector onto the other times the length of both – see the last equality in Equation 5.12 . However, one has to be aware that Equation 5.12 is only valid if the coordinate system is *orthonormal* – all unit vectors have to be orthogonal to each other and their length has to be 1. Mathematically speaking, it is

---

[3]Throughout this book, we use column vectors. However, for the sake of readability, we usually *transpose* such a column vector if it occurs within text; by doing so, we can write the vector as a row-vector.

required that the inner product of two unit vectors $\vec{e}_i$ and $\vec{e}_j$ is one if i equals j and zero otherwise:

$$\vec{e}_i \bullet \vec{e}_j = \delta_{ij} \qquad (5.13)$$

δ_{ij} is the so-called Kronecker-function, defined as

$$\delta_{ij} = \begin{cases} 1 \text{ if } i = j \\ 0 \text{ if } i \neq j \end{cases} . \qquad (5.14)$$

The most important consequence of this property of a coordinate system lies in the fact that the components of a vector, given in such an orthogonal coordinate system, are built by inner products. So let's look at a vector in a new manner; suppose we have a vector

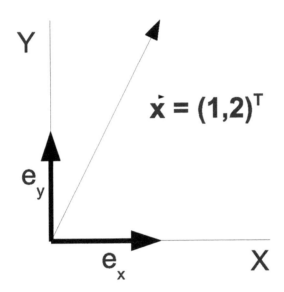

FIGURE 5.12: The representation of a vector $\vec{x} = (1,2)^T$ in a Cartesian coordinate system. The coordinate system is spanned by two unit vectors $\vec{e}_x$ and $\vec{e}_y$, which are of length 1 and define the coordinate axes. The components of the vector $\vec{x}$ are given as the inner product of the vector and the unit vectors: $\vec{x} \bullet \vec{e}_x = x$ and $\vec{x} \bullet \vec{e}_y = y$.

$\vec{x}$, and a Cartesian coordinate system spanned by orthonormal vectors $\vec{e}_i$. If we want to know about the components x_1 and x_2 of this vector, we have to form the inner products $\vec{x} \bullet \vec{e}_i = x_i$. As far as the example in Figure 5.12 is concerned, one may easily verify this. In general it is an immediate consequence of Equation 5.13 and the linearity of the inner product:

$$\vec{x} = \sum_i x_i \vec{e}_i$$

$$\vec{x} \bullet \vec{e_k} = \left(\sum_i x_i \vec{e}_i \right) \bullet \vec{e_k} = \sum_i x_i \vec{e}_i \bullet \vec{e_k} \qquad (5.15)$$

$$= \sum_i x_i \delta_{ik} = x_k$$

So far, all of this is pretty trivial. One may also ask oneself why one should retrieve the components of a vector if they are already known from the standard notation $\vec{x} = (x_1, x_2)^T$. The key issue is the fact that giving the components only makes sense if a coordinate system, defined by the unit vectors $\vec{e}_i$. Figure 5.13 illustrates this – the vector $\vec{x}$ is the same in both sketches, but the different orientation of orthonormal unit vectors results in different components. Let's change our way of thinking, and the whole thing will make sense.

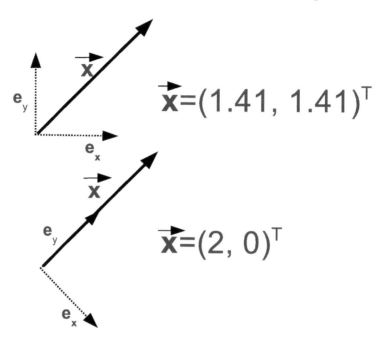

FIGURE 5.13: An illustration on the dependency of the components of a given vector $\vec{x}$ on the choice of unit vectors $\vec{e}_i$. While the vector $\vec{x}$ does not change in the upper and lower illustration, the unit vectors span a different coordinate system, resulting in different components of the very same vector.

Let's consider an arbitrary function $f(x_1, \ldots, x_n)$ a vector in a coordinate system spanned by an infinite number of base functions $e_i(x_1, \ldots, x_n)$. It may be hard to imagine a coordinate system of infinite dimension spanned by functions. I can't do that either. But it is also not necessary since a few things remain valid for such a coordinate system. If it is to be orthonormal, the base functions have to fulfill Equation 5.13. We can then compute the contribution of each base function $e_i(x_1, \ldots, x_n)$ to the function $f(x_1, \ldots, x_n)$ by computing the inner product of the two. The question that remains is the definition of an *inner product for functions*. A possible definition is the integral of a product of functions:

$$f(x_1, \ldots, x_n) \bullet g(x_1, \ldots, x_n) = \int_{-\infty}^{\infty} dx_1 \ldots dx_n f(x_1, \ldots, x_n) g^*(x_1, \ldots, x_n) \qquad (5.16)$$

$g^*(x_1, \ldots, x_n)$ is the complex conjugate of $g(x_1, \ldots, x_n)$; we will learn more about this operation in Section 5.2.2. The orthogonality requirement from Equation 5.13 can therefore be rewritten as

$$\int\limits_{-\infty}^{\infty} dx_1 \ldots dx_n e_i(x_1,\ldots,x_n)e_j^*(x_1,\ldots,x_n) = \delta_{ij} \tag{5.17}$$

After decomposing the function $f(x_1,\ldots,x_n)$ to its components – let's call them c_i as the x_i are the variables – the function can be written as:

$$f(x_1,\ldots,x_n) = \sum_{i=0}^{\infty} c_i e_i(x_1,\ldots,x_n) \tag{5.18}$$

We can compute the coefficients c_i like in Equation 5.15:

$$c_i = \int\limits_{-\infty}^{\infty} dx_1 \ldots dx_n f(x_1,\ldots,x_n)e_i^*(x_1,\ldots,x_n) \tag{5.19}$$

Usually, we hope that the components c_i of higher order i do not contribute much, and that the series can be truncated after a while.

A large number of different functions fulfilling Equation 5.17 exists, and one can even design special ones. If we have such a functional system, we can always decompose an arbitrary function $f(x_1,\ldots,x_n)$ into its components in the coordinate system spanned by the base functions $e_i(x_1,\ldots,x_n)$. The usefulness of such an operation lies in the choice of the base function set $e_i(x_1,\ldots,x_n)$. Remember that mathematical problems can be simplified by choosing the appropriate coordinate system such as polar coordinates. Here, it is just the same. A function that shows radial symmetry can be expanded in a series of base functions that exhibit a radial symmetry themselves; since base functions are very often polynomials, a simplification of the mathematical problem to be tackled is usually the consequence.

One may object that computing the integral from Equation 5.16 will be extremely cumbersome – but we are talking about image processing here, where all functions are given as discrete values. Computing an integral in discrete mathematics is as simple as numerical differentiation. The integral is simply computed as the sum of all volume elements defining by the function. The mathematical $\int$ sign becomes a $\sum$, and ∞ becomes the domain where the function is defined. Things that look pretty scary when using mathematical notation become rather simple when being translated to the discrete world.

So what is the purpose of the whole excursion? In short terms, it can be very helpful to describe a function in a different frame of reference. Think of the Cartesian coordinate system. If we are dealing with a function that exhibits a rotational symmetry, it may be very helpful to move from Cartesian coordinates with components x_i to a polar or spherical coordinate system, where each point is given by r – its distance from the origin of the coordinate system – and ϕ, the angle enclosed with the abscissa of the coordinate system (or two angles if we are talking about spherical coordinates). The same holds true for functions, and in Section 5.2.2, we will examine a set of extremely useful base functions in a painstaking manner.

5.2.2 Waves – a special orthonormal system

Jean Baptiste Joseph Fourier, orphan, soldier and mathematician, studied the problems of heat transfer, which can be considered a diffusion problem. In the course of his efforts, he formulated the assumption that every periodical function can be decomposed into a series of sines and cosines. These *Fourier Series* are built like in Equation 5.18, using $\cos kx$, $k =$

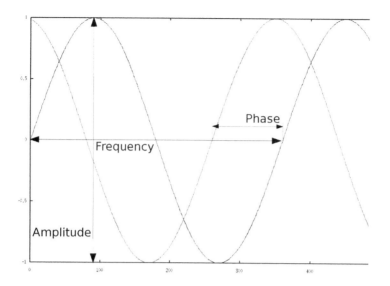

FIGURE 5.14: Two sines, which may be considered simple plane waves; the two variables that influence the shape of the sine are its *frequency*, and its *amplitude*. Furthermore, we have a second sine here with identical frequency and amplitude, but with a different *phase*. Periodical signals can be composed out of such simple waves with different frequencies, amplitudes and phases. The Fourier-transformation is a mathematical framework to retrieve these components from such a superimposed signal. Images can be considered 2D or 3D signals, and therefore it is possible to decompose them to simple planar signals as well. The sum of all frequencies and amplitudes is the *spectrum* of the signal.

$0, 1, \ldots$ and $\sin kx$, $k = 0, 1, \ldots$ as base functions. The inner product is defined similarly to Equation 5.16 by $f(x) \bullet g(x) = \int_{-\pi}^{\pi} dx f(x) g(x)$. Orthogonality relations like Equation 5.17 can be proven, and we end up with the series expansion

$$f(x) = \frac{a_0}{2} + \sum_{k=1}^{\infty} a_k \cos kx + \sum_{k=1}^{\infty} b_k \sin kx \qquad (5.20)$$

with Fourier coefficients

$$a_k = \frac{1}{\pi} \int_{-\pi}^{\pi} dx f(x) \cos kx, \; b_k = \frac{1}{\pi} \int_{-\pi}^{\pi} dx f(x) \sin kx \qquad (5.21)$$

A few more things are necessary to unveil the power and the beauty of the Fourier-expansion; first of all, we should remember complex numbers. Real numbers have a blemish. For each operation like addition and multiplication, there exists an inverse operation. When carrying out the multiplication operation $ab = c$ on real numbers a and b, we can invert the operation: $\frac{c}{a} = b$. The same holds true for addition. But multiplication also features a pitfall. When computing the square of a real number – let's say d^2, we do also have an inverse operation (the square root), but the result is ambiguous. If d is negative, we won't get d as the result of $\sqrt{d^2}$ – we will get $|d|$. In general, it is even said sometimes (by the timid and weak such as cheap hand-held calculators) that one cannot compute the square root of a negative number. This is, of course, not true. We just have to leave the realm of real numbers, just as we had to move from natural numbers to rational numbers when dealing with fractions. Man has known this since the sixteenth century when *complex numbers* were introduced. A central figure in complex math is the *complex unit* **i**. It is defined as the square root of -1. A complex number c is usually given as $c = a + \mathbf{i}b$. In this notation, a is referred to as the *real part*, and b is the *imaginary part* of c; a complex number is therefore represented as a doublet of two numbers, the real and the imaginary part.

Complex numbers have a number of special properties; the most important ones are listed below:

Addition is carried out by applying the operation to the real and imaginary part separately.

Multiplication is carried out by multiplying the doublets while keeping in mind that $\mathbf{i}^2 = -1$.

Complex conjugation, of which you already heard in Section 5.2.1. It is a very simple operation which consists of switching the sign of **i**, and it is denoted by an asterisk. In the case of our complex number c, the complex conjugate reads $c^* = a - \mathbf{i}b$.

The *norm* of a complex number: $||c|| = \sqrt{a^2 + b^2}$. The norm operator yields a real number.

The *Real and Imaginary operator*. These return the real and the imaginary part separately.

The one identity that is of the utmost importance for us is the following; it is called *Euler's formula*:

$$e^{i\phi} = \cos\phi + \mathbf{i}\sin\phi \tag{5.22}$$

Complex numbers can be represented using a Cartesian coordinate system in the plane; the real part is displayed on the x-axis, whereas the y-axis shows the imaginary part. The length r of the vector is the norm. In the representation $c = a + \mathbf{i}b$ for a complex number, a and b represent the Cartesian coordinates; in polar coordinates, where r and ϕ – the angle enclosed with the abscissa – are given to represent a complex number, c can be rewritten as $c = re^{\mathbf{i}\phi}$ using Equation 5.22. This representation in the *complex plane* is also shown in Figure 5.15.

Equation 5.22 is of great importance, since it allows for a complex representation of the Fourier series using the inner product $f(x) \bullet g(x) = \int_{-\pi}^{\pi} dx f(x)g^*(x)$ and the base functions $e^{\mathbf{i}kx}$, $k = -\infty, \ldots \infty$, which represent actually the plane waves.

$$f(x) = \frac{1}{\sqrt{2\pi}} \sum_{k=-\infty}^{\infty} c_k e^{\mathbf{i}kx} \tag{5.23}$$

with Fourier coefficients

$$c_k = \frac{1}{\sqrt{2\pi}} \int_{-\pi}^{\pi} dx f(x) e^{-\mathbf{i}kx} \tag{5.24}$$

As you may see we have a little mess with our prefactors. In Equation 5.21 it was $\frac{1}{2\pi}$, now

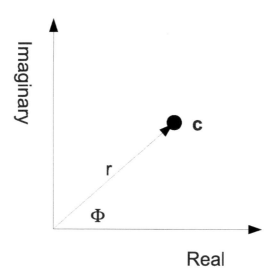

FIGURE 5.15: The representation of a complex number $c = a + \mathbf{i}b$ in the complex plane, where the real part a is represented on the abscissa and the imaginary part b lies on the ordinate. Switching to polar coordinates using r and ϕ and using Equation 5.22 we get another representation for a complex number: $c = re^{\mathbf{i}\phi}$.

it is $\frac{1}{\sqrt{2\pi}}$, but both in front of the sum Equation 5.23 and the Fourier coefficients Equation 5.24. The prefactors are chosen to get simpler formulas, but are unfortunately not consistent in the literature (as we know, beauty is in the eye of the beholder).

With a limiting process, which we cannot describe in detail, the sum in Equation 5.23 becomes an integral, the sequence c_k becomes a function $c(k)$ (which we will denote by $\hat{f}(k)$ from now on), and the limits of the integrals in Equation 5.24 become $-\infty$, and ∞. We can therefore define the Fourier-transform of an arbitrary function $f(x)$ as:

$$\hat{f}(k) \quad = \quad \frac{1}{\sqrt{2\pi}} \int_{-\infty}^{\infty} dx\, f(x) e^{-\mathbf{i}kx} \qquad (5.25)$$

$$f(x) \quad = \quad \frac{1}{\sqrt{2\pi}} \int_{-\infty}^{\infty} dk\, \hat{f}(k) e^{\mathbf{i}kx} \qquad (5.26)$$

$$k \quad \dots \quad \text{Wave number}$$

The similarity to Equation 5.23 and therefore to Equation 5.19 is obvious. The Fourier transformation is an inner product of the function $f(x)$ with the base functions $e^{-\mathbf{i}kx}$. The *wave number* k is related to the *wavelength* λ of a wave by $k = \frac{2\pi}{\lambda}$; the wavelength by itself is related to the *frequency* ν as $\lambda = \frac{c}{\nu}$ where c is the propagation speed of the wave. A particular wave number k_n is therefore the component of the function $f(x)$ that is connected to a wave $e^{-\mathbf{i}k_n x}$. The Fourier-transformation is therefore a transformation to a coordinate system where the independent variable x is replaced by a complex information on frequency (in terms of the wave number) and phase. The space of the Fourier transform is therefore also referred to as *k-space*.

If we want to use the Fourier-transformation for image processing, we have to take two further steps. First of all, we will replace the integrals by sums. This is called the *discrete Fourier transformation* (DFT). Second our images are of finite size – they are not defined on a domain from $-\infty$ to ∞. This problem can be resolved by assuming that the images are repeated, just like tiles on a floor. This is illustrated in Figure 5.16. This assumption also has visible consequences, for instance in MR-imaging. In an MR-tomograph, the original signal is measured as waves (in k-space), and is transformed to the spatial domain (the world of pixels and voxels) by means of a Fourier-transform. Figure 5.17 shows an MR image of a wrist. The hand moves out of the field-of-view of the tomograph. What occurs is a so called *wraparound artifact*. The fingers leaving the image on the right side reappear on the left side of the image. The principle of the discrete Fourier transformation is also shown in Figure 5.16.

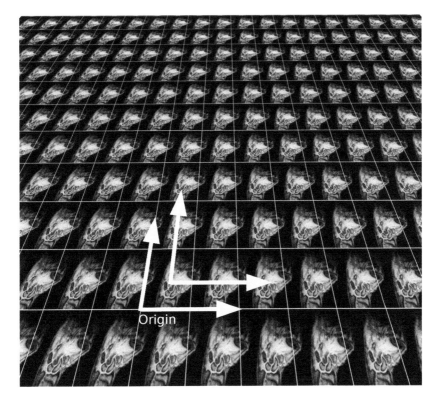

FIGURE 5.16: When applying a Fourier transformation to an image of finite size, it is assumed that the image is repeated so that the full spatial domain from $-\infty$ to ∞ is covered. An image, however, has a coordinate origin in one of the image corners; in order to establish symmetry, MATLAB provides a function called `fftshift`. This function shifts the origin of the coordinate system to the center of the image.

When applying a DFT, Equations 5.25 and 5.26 are expressed as discrete sums, rather than the clumsy integrals. Fortunately, this was already handled in a procedure called the *Fast Fourier Transformation* (FFT), which became one of the most famous algorithms in computer science. We can therefore always perform a Fourier transformation by simply calling a library that does a FFT, and there is quite a number of them out there. In MATLAB, a discrete FFT of a 2D function $I(x, y)$ is carried out by the command `fft2`. Equation 5.26 is performed by calling `ifft2`. Example 5.4.6.1 gives a first simple introduction to the

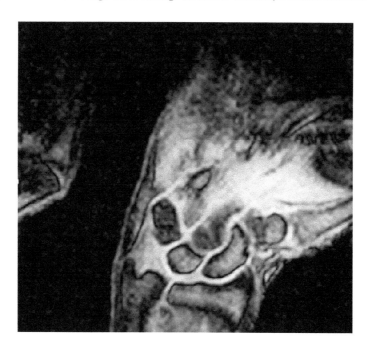

FIGURE 5.17: A wraparound artifact in MRI. In this dynamic sequence of a wrist in motion, a part of the hand lies outside the field-of-view. Since reconstruction of volumes in MR takes place using a Fourier transformation of the original signal, the image continues like a tile so that the transformation is defined on the whole spatial domain from $-\infty$ to ∞ – see also Figure 5.16. The right part of the hand therefore re-appears on the left side of the image. Image data courtesy of the Dept. of Diagnostic Radiology, Medical University Vienna.

Fourier-transformation, where a sine is overlaid by a second sine of higher frequency. As you can see from Figure 5.29, the two frequencies of the two sines show up as four spikes, with their amplitude governing the height of the k-value in the Fourier domain. It is four spikes since a sine of negative frequency may also produce the same signal – furthermore, our initial signal, which is defined on a domain $x \in [0, 2\pi]$ has to be shifted to $x \in [-\pi, \pi]$ since the Fourier transformation is defined on an interval $-\infty \dots \infty$, not on $0 \dots \infty$. This is done by calling the `fftshift` function whose principle is illustrated in Figure 5.16.

After all these theoretical considerations, we may get to business. We know what the Fourier transformation is, and we know how to compute it. So what is the merit of the Fourier transform in image processing? Since an image is a function defined on the 2D or 3D domain, it can be decomposed to plane or spherical waves; noise, for instance, is a signal with a high frequency. If we want to get rid of noise, we may reduce the weight of the higher frequencies (the components with a large value of the wave number k). If we want to sharpen the image, we can emphasize the higher frequencies. These operations are therefore obviously equivalent to K_{blur} and K_{sharp}, which were already called high-pass and low-pass filters. The advantage of blurring and sharpening in the Fourier domain, however, is the possibility to tune the operations very specifically. We can select various types of noise and remove it selectively, as we will do in Example 5.4.6.1. Furthermore, the Fourier transformation has some remarkable properties, which are extremely handy when talking about filtering operations beyond simple manipulation of the image spectrum.

5.2.3 Some important properties of the Fourier transform

The Fourier transformation has some properties of particular interest for signal and image processing; among those are:

Linearity: $w * f + g \mapsto w * \hat{f} + \hat{g}$.

Scaling: Doubling the size of an image in the spatial domain cuts the amplitudes and frequencies in k-space in half.

Translation: $f(x + \alpha) \mapsto \hat{f}(k)e^{ik\alpha}$. A shift in the spatial domain does not change the Fourier transform $\hat{f}(k)$ besides a complex phase. This property is also responsible for so-called ghosting artifacts in MR, where motion of the patient during acquisition causes the repetition of image signals (see also Figure 5.18).

Convolution: $f(x) \star g(x) \mapsto \sqrt{2\pi} * \hat{f}(k) * \hat{g}(k)$. As you may remember from the introduction to this chapter, it was said that the convolution operation by mangling kernels into the image will be replaced by a strict and simple formalism. Here it is. In k-space, the convolution of two functions becomes a simple multiplication. Therefore, it is no longer necessary to derive large kernels from a function such as the Gaussian as in Equation 5.3.

Differentiation: $\frac{d^n}{dx^n} f(x) \mapsto (\mathbf{i}k)^n \hat{f}(k)$. Computing the derivative of a function $f(x)$ is apparently also pretty simple. Again it becomes a simple multiplication.

The Gaussian: The Gaussian $G(x)$ retains its general shape in k-space. Under some circumstances, is even an *eigenfunction* of the Fourier transform;[4] in general, however, $\hat{G}(k)$ is a Gaussian as well.

Parseval's Theorem: The total energy in the image, which can be considered the sum of squares of all gray values ρ, is maintained in k-space. Another formulation is $f \bullet g \mapsto \hat{f} \bullet \hat{g}$.

Another important theorem that is connected to the DFT is the *Nyquist-Shannon Sampling Theorem*. In the DFT, the sampling frequency has to be double the highest frequency of the signal to be reconstructed – if, for instance in an audio signal, the highest frequency is 20 kHz (which is the maximum frequency man can hear), the sampling frequency has to be 40 kHz for a lossless reconstruction of the signal.

From this little excursion, it should be clear why the Fourier transformation is considered such a powerful tool in signal processing. In the next sections, we will learn how to apply the Fourier transform to medical images. A first example on the conditioning of signals named Rect_5.m can be found in the **LessonData** folder. The power spectrum of a more complex function – the mouse topogram from Figs. 5.10 and 5.11 – is given in Figure 5.19.

5.2.4 Image processing in the frequency domain

From Example 5.4.6.1, we will see that we can get rid of image noise with a known frequency. In medical imaging, such periodical artifacts may also occur, for instance in MR – imaging,

---

[4]It is noteworthy that the terms *eigenspace, eigenvector,* and *eigenfunction* are not named after a person. It is a loan word from German; its direct translation would be something like *own function.* Eigenvectors and eigenfunctions span a sub-space – the eigenspace – of elements which are invariant to a given transformation. We will learn more about eigenvectors and eigenvalues in Chapter 7.

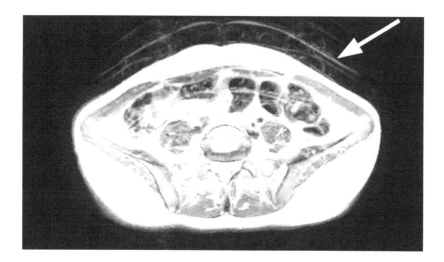

FIGURE 5.18: The translation property of the Fourier transform at work. As said before, the MR signal is acquired in k-space and transformed to the spatial domain for volume reconstruction. When patient motion during image acquisition occurs, the result is the repetition of image structures in the reconstructed volume (see arrow). This T2-weighted image of the pelvis was windowed in such a manner that the ghosting artifact – the repetition of the abdominal wall in the upper part of the image – becomes prominent. Ghosting artifacts in this area of the body are common due to breathing motion. Image data courtesy of the Dept. of Radiology, Medical University Vienna.

or in CR plates, which may be stricken by discretization artifacts. An example of a band-stop filter, which removes some of the middle frequencies in the image, is given in Example 5.4.7. Of course, we can also introduce blurring and sharpening by removing the high or low frequencies in the image (Figure 5.36). The maximum wave number k, which represents the highest frequency in the image, is defined by the resolution of the image since the smallest signal given in the image is a single point.

Another important property of the Fourier-transformation is the convolution-operation; remember Section 5.1.1, where small 2D-functions like K_{blur} were convolved with the image. In k-space, convolution becomes a multiplication. We can convolve kernels of all kinds (some of them have names such as Hann, Hamming, Butterworth and so on) by simply transforming both the kernel and the image to k-space, and multiply the two. After re-transformation to the spatial domain, we get the effect of the convolution operation. This may look like artificially added complexity, but the operation is actually way more simple than convolution in the spatial domain when it comes to more complicated kernels. One may remember $K_{5\times5\,\mathrm{Gauss}}$ from Equation 5.3, where a simple 5×5 kernel already requires 25 operations per pixel for convolution. Furthermore, we can invert the convolution operation; if we know the exact shape of our PSF, we can apply the inverse process of the convolution operation in k-space, which is actually a multiplication with the inverse of the PSF. This process is called *deconvolution* or resolution recovery.

Next, we know that translation of the image just introduces a complex phase in k-space. When taking a look at the norm of a shifted function $f(x + \alpha)$ in k-space, we will have to compute $\hat{f}(k)e^{ik\alpha}\left(\hat{f}(k)e^{ik\alpha}\right)^{*}$ – the product of the transformed function $\hat{f}e^{ik\alpha}$ and its

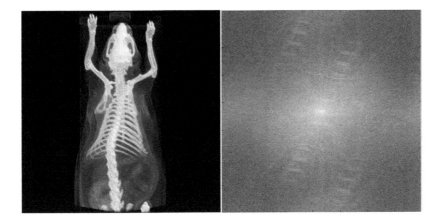

FIGURE 5.19: The topogram of a mouse taken from small animal CT, and the absolute value of the Fourier-spectrum after a logarithmic intensity transform. Some of the details in the left image from the spatial domain leave a recognizable trace in the spectrum on the right-hand side. For instance, the low frequencies in the y-direction are more dominant than in the x-direction since the mouse occupies more space in the y-direction. Furthermore, the ribcage gives a significant signal of high intensity at a higher frequency, and the bow-shaped structures in the medium frequency range indicate this. Image data courtesy of C. Kuntner, AIT Seibersdorf, Austria.

complex conjugate. For complex conjugation, the identity $(c_1 c_2)^* = c_1^* c_2^*$ is true. The norm of a shifted function in k-space therefore reads $\hat{f}\hat{f}^*$ – the complex phase introduced by the shift in the spatial domain disappears. An image and a shifted image can therefore be identified as one and the same besides the shift if one compares the norm of the Fourier-transforms of the image. This is especially handy in image registration, which will be introduced in Chapter 9.

5.2.5   Modelling properties of imaging systems – the PSF and the MTF

Let us go back to the introduction, where an optical system was introduced as a filter. The quality of the PSF, as we may recall, gives an idea of the overall performance of the system since it can be convolved with an arbitrary signal; if we leave the domain of medical images, we can encounter an excellent example in Figure 5.20. This is the globular cluster M13 in the constellation of Hercules, a collection of old stars at the edge of our galaxy. It contains hundreds of thousands of stars. From a signal processing perspective, the image of each star is the result of the convolution with the PSF of the telescope. The interesting question is – how does the PSF, or the optical quality of the telescope, affect the resolution of the image? How close can two stars, which are pretty perfect examples for distant point light sources, be in order to be resolved as separate? The ability to distinguish two point sources depending on their distance is given by the so-called *modulation transfer function* (MTF). The MTF gives a score whether the two images overlap as a function of the spatial frequency that separates the two PSF-like images in term of *cycles over range*. It is obvious that a bad optical system with a large PSF such as the spherical mirror introduced in Figure 5.2 will not resolve nearby objects since the PSFs would overlap. Figure 5.21 shows the MTF of the

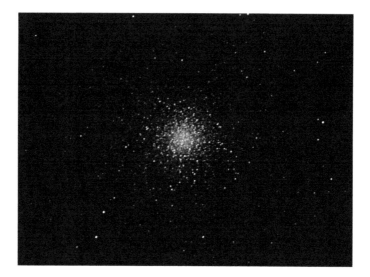

FIGURE 5.20: M13, the great globular cluster in the Hercules constellation. The ability to resolve two stars as separated depends on the PSF of the optical system used. In a poor optical system like the spherical mirror presented in the introduction, the image would not look like that since the amount of overlap between two images of the nearby stars would fuse them. The ability to distinguish two close objects is measured by the modulation transfer function, the MTF.

spherical mirror that gives the PSF from Figure 5.2. The question therefore is – what is the exact relationship of the PSF and the MTF?

The answer is not very surprising. The MTF is the absolute value of the Fourier-transform of the PSF. This is illustrated in Example 5.4.8. The mouse image `MouseCT.jpg`, already misused many times for all types of operations, is convolved with Gaussian PSFs of varying width. A narrow Gaussian will not distort the image a lot – fine detail will remain distinguishable; therefore the MTF is wide. While the Fourier-transform of a narrow Gaussian is still a Gaussian, it becomes a very wide distribution. Figure 5.39 illustrates this. If we apply a wide Gaussian PSF, the MTF will become narrow since fine details vanish. In Example 5.4.8, this will be demonstrated. It is noteworthy that a measurement of the PSF is a common task in the maintenance of medical imaging systems such as CTs, where dedicated phantoms for this purpose exist. Example 5.4.9 illustrates such an effort.

5.3 OTHER TRANSFORMS

An infinite number of orthonormal base function systems $e_i(x_1, \ldots, x_n)$, which are usually polynomials, can be constructed. Whether a transform to these systems makes sense depends on the basic properties. If it is of advantage to exploit the rotational symmetry of an image, one may compute the representation of the image in a base system that shows such a symmetry. Jacobi polynomials are an example for such a base system. Another example of a particularly useful transformation is real-valued subtype of the discrete Fourier transform, the discrete cosine transform (DCT). The DCT is, for instance, used in JPG-compression (see also Chapter 3). For now, we will stop dealing with these types of transformations,

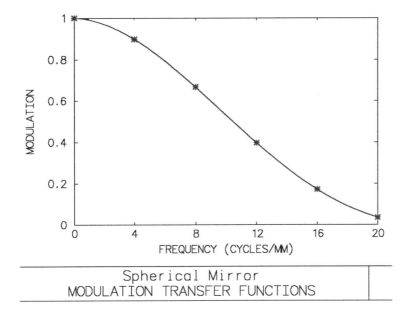

FIGURE 5.21: The modulation transfer function of the spherical mirror from Figure 5.2. The graph was, again, produced using the OSLO optical design software. The MTF gives a figure of the capability of a signal-transducing system to resolve two point-shaped objects. The higher the spatial frequency (given in cycles/mm in the image plane in this example), the lower the resolution of the system. The MTF is coupled to the PSF by means of the Fourier-transformation; a wide PSF gives a narrow MTF and vice versa.

and we will introduce two important transforms that are not based on orthonormal base functions.

5.3.1 The Hough transform

The *Hough transform* is a transformation that can be used for any geometrical shape in a binary image that can be represented in a parametric form. A classical example for a parametric representation is, for instance, the circle. A circle is defined by the fact that all of its points have the same distance r from the center of the circle (M_x, M_y). A parametric representation of a circle in a Cartesian coordinate system is given as:

$$\sqrt{(x - M_x)^2 + (y - M_y)^2} = r.$$

Center coordinates M_x, M_y and radius r are the parameters of the circle. We will make use of this representation in a number of examples, for instance Example 6.8.5 and 7.6.4. As a parametric representation of a straight line we choose the *Hesse normal form*. It is simply given by the normal vector of the line which intersects with the origin of a Cartesian coordinate system. An illustration is given in Figure 5.22. The parameters are the polar coordinates of this normal vector $\vec{n}$. The Hough transform inspects every non-zero pixel in a binary image and computes the polar coordinates of his pixel, assuming that the pixel is part of a line. If the pixel is indeed part of a line, the transform to polar coordinates will produce many similar parameter pairs.

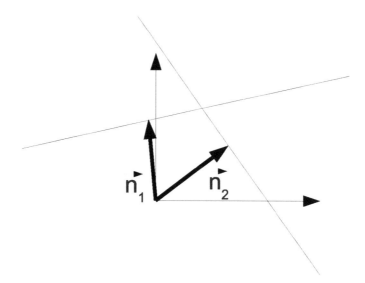

FIGURE 5.22: The Hesse normal form representation of lines in a Cartesian coordinate system. Each line is represented by a normal vector $\vec{n}$ that intersects the origin of the coordinate system. The polar coordinates of the intersection point of $\vec{n}$ and the line are the parameters of the line.

The trick in the case of the Hough transform is to plot the parameters of the shape in a new coordinate system which is spanned by the two parameters of the normal form, the length r of the normal vector $\vec{n}$ and the angle ϕ enclosed by $\vec{n}$ and the x-axis. Pixels belonging to a line will occupy the same location in Hough-space. Since the Hough transform acts only on binary images, the varying brightness of points in Hough-space is a measure of the number of pixels with the same normal vector. In Example 5.4.10, we will apply the Hough-transform to the image shown in Figure 5.44.

The result of the transformation to the parameter space can be found in Figure 5.46. The pixels that lie on a line appear as bright spots in the image. By setting all pixels below a given threshold to zero, only the bright spots in the parameter image remain. Next, one can define a so-called accumulator cell; this is a square in parameter space which assigns a single parameter pair to the area in the parameter space covered by the accumulator, thus narrowing down the number of possible parameters. While the detection of lines is a classical example of the Hough-transform, the principle is applicable to every shape that can be modeled in a parameter representation. In Chapter 10, we will encounter a very similar transformation. In medicine, the Hough transform can also be very helpful in identifying structures in *segmented* images, for instance when identifying spherical markers in x-ray images. A simplified application of the Hough-transform in segmentation can be found in Example 6.8.8.1.

5.3.2 The distance transform

Another transformation that we will re-encounter in Chapter 9 is the *distance transform*. It also operates on binary images; here, the nearest black pixel for each non-black pixel is sought. The value of the non-black pixel is replaced by the actual distance of this pixel to the next black pixel. A very simple example can be found in Figure 5.23, which is the output of Example 5.4.11.

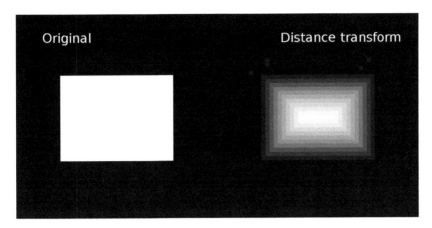

FIGURE 5.23: The result of the distance transform as carried out in Example 5.4.11. The innermost pixels of the rectangle are those with the greatest separation to the border of the rectangle; therefore they appear as bright, whereas the pixels closer to the border become darker.

5.4 PRACTICAL LESSONS

5.4.1 Kernel – based low pass and high pass filtering

In the `SimpleLowPass_5.m` script, a single CT slice in DICOM format named `SKULLBASE.DCM` is opened, and a simple smoothing filter K_{blur} is applied. The results of this script can be seen in Figs. 5.3, 5.4, and 5.24. The DICOM-file is read in the same manner as in Example 3.7.2. In order to cope with the indexing conventions of MATLAB and Octave, the image is transposed. Finally, memory for a second image `lpimg` is allocated.

```
1:> fp=fopen('SKULLBASE.DCM', 'r');
2:> fseek(fp,1622,'bof');
3:> img=zeros(512,512);
4:> img(:)=fread(fp,(512*512),'short');
5:> img=transpose(img);
6:> fclose(fp);
7:> lpimg=zeros(512,512);
```

Next, we will visit each pixel and convolve the image with the smoothing kernel K_{blur}. In order to avoid indexing conflicts, we leave the edges of the image untouched. Finally, the image intensities are shifted and scaled for an optimum representation, just like in Example 4.5.1.

```
8:> for i=2:511
9:> for j=2:511
10:> lpimg(i,j) = 0.1*(img((i-1),j) + 2*img(i,j) +
img((i+1),j) + img(i,(j-1)) + img(i,(j+1)) +
img((i-1),(j-1)) + img((i-1),(j+1)) +
```

```
        img((i+1),(j-1)) + img((i+1),(j+1)));
11:> end
12:> end
13:> minint=min(min(lpimg));
14:> lpimg=lpimg-minint;
15:> maxint=max(max(lpimg));
16:> lpimg=lpimg/maxint*64;
17:> colormap(gray);
18:> image(lpimg)
```

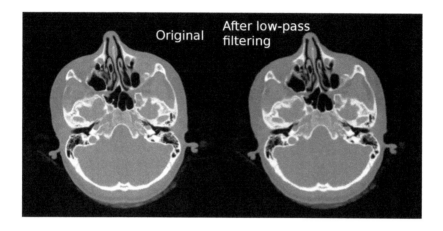

FIGURE 5.24: The original image SKULLBASE.DCM, and the result of the filtering operation in SimpleLowPass_5.m. Noise such as the reconstruction artifacts visible in the air surrounding the head is suppressed. Since the details are subtle and are hard to recognize in print, you may also inspect the JPG-images used for this illustration. These can be found in the LessonData folder for this chapter, and are named SKULLBASE_Filtered.jpg and SKULLBASE_Original.jpg. Image data courtesy of the Dept. of Radiology, Medical University Vienna.

Additional Tasks

Modify SimpleLowPass_5.m in such a manner that it utilizes the 5×5 Gaussian kernel from Equation 5.3, and compare the results.

Modify SimpleLowPass_5.m to sharpen the image using the K_{sharp} kernel from Equation 5.2. A detail from the result can be found in Figure 5.4. A high pass filter can be somewhat difficult for images with negative pixel values like CT image data due to the negative values in the K_{sharp} kernel.

As one may see from this script, a generalization to the 3D domain is pretty straightforward and simple. The kernel K_{blur} can easily be generalized to average the gray values in neighboring voxels. What would a 3D-equivalent of K_{blur} look like?

It was already stated in the introduction, a prerequisite for applying kernels like K_{blur} is an isotropic image. Can you think of a kernel that properly operates on an image where the pixels are stretched by a given ratio?

5.4.2 Basic filtering operations in ImageJ

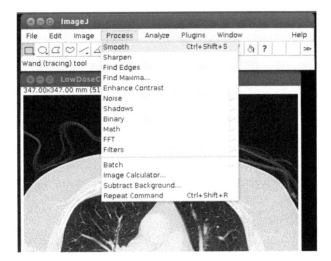

FIGURE 5.25: Screenshot of ImageJ; in the "Process" menu, basic operations such as smoothing, sharpening and edge detection using Sobel-kernels can be found.

One of the strengths of ImageJ is the fact that it can be easily expanded by plugins. The built-in functionality is therefore somewhat limited; however, the basic filtering operations that can be found in ImageJ are smoothing, sharpening and edge detection using the length of the image gradient as determined by a Sobel filter (see also Figure 5.25). Basically, the three filtering operations that can be found under the Menu topics "Process → Smooth", "Process → Sharpen" and "Process → Find Edges" correspond to the application of the kernels K_{blur} – Equation 5.1, K_{sharp} – Equation 5.2 and the length of the gradient as determined by K_{Sobel_x} and K_{Sobel_y} – Equation 5.9 to the image LowDoseCT.tif from the LessonData folder. The image is a slice from a whole-body CT scan taken in the course of a PET-CT exam; since the dose applied in a PET-CT exam is considerable (up to 25 mSv), the CT is a so-called low-dose CT with considerable image noise. This is especially evident after using the sharpening and the edge-detection filter (see Figure 5.26).

5.4.3 Numerical differentiation

In this example, we are dealing with two scripts. The first one illustrates numerical forward differentiation on a simple one dimensional rectangle function. It is named NumericalDifferentiation_5.m.

```
1:> rect=zeros(100,1);
2:> for i=45:55
3:> rect(i,1)=1;
4:> end
5:> plot(rect);
6:> foo=input('Press RETURN to proceed to the
first derivative');
```

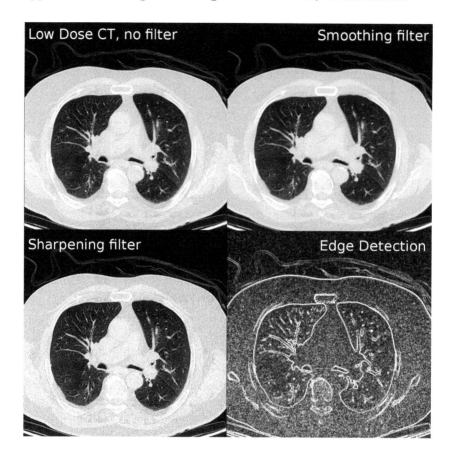

FIGURE 5.26: Effect of blurring (or "smoothing"), sharpening, and edge detection on the image file `LowDoseCT.tif` from the `LessonData` folder. The image is part of a PET-CT scan; since the whole patient was scanned, the radiologist in charge chose a low dose CT protocol, which results in considerable noise in the image. The design of the filter kernels used here is similar to the kernels presented in Section 5.1.1. Image data courtesy of the Dept. of Radiology, Medical University Vienna.

`rect` is the vector containing the dependent variable of the rectangle function, which is zero for $x \in 1 \ldots 44$ and $x \in 56 \ldots 100$, and one otherwise. This function is plotted, and after an old-fashioned command line prompt, the script proceeds:

```
7:> drect=zeros(100,1);
8:> for i=1:99
9:> drect(i,1)=rect(i+1)-rect(i);
10:> end
11:> plot(drect)
12:> foo=input('Press RETURN to proceed to the
second derivative');
```

The first derivative, $\frac{df(x)}{dx}$, is computed. As you can see, it is a simple forward difference. The $df(x)$ term becomes a finite difference, $f(x_{i+1}) - f(x_i)$, and the denominator is 1 since we are dealing with discrete values for x that increment by one. The second derivative,

$\frac{d^2 f(x)}{dx^2}$, is computed in the same manner. The forward differences of the `drect` vector yield a vector `ddrect`, which contains the second derivative.

```
13:> ddrect=zeros(100,1);
14:> for i=1:99
15:> ddrect(i,1)=drect(i+1)-drect(i);
16:> end
17:> plot(ddrect)
```

The output of this operation can be found in Figure 5.6. Interpreting the derivative is simple. Whenever the slope of the original function $f(x)$ is steep, the numerical value of the derivative is high. If we encounter a descent in the function, the derivative has a high negative value.

In terms of image processing, edges in the image are steep ascents or descents; forming the derivatives will give sharp spikes at these edges, visible as very dark or very bright lines in the resulting image. Numerical differentiation is therefore the easiest way to detect edges in images. The second script, named `ForwardDifference_5.m`, implements the simple differentiation kernel $K_{\text{x-forward}}$ from Equation 5.5. Otherwise, it is largely identical to `SimpleLowPass_5.m`.

```
1:> fp=fopen('SKULLBASE.DCM', 'r');
2:> fseek(fp,1622,'bof');
3:> img=zeros(512,512);
4:> img(:)=fread(fp,(512*512),'short');
5:> img=transpose(img);
6:> fclose(fp);
7:> diffimg=zeros(512,512);
```

Since we are computing a forward difference, the indexing may start from `i=1`, as opposed to the `SimpleLowPass_5.m` script. The result of the convolution operation, `diffimg` is, as usual, scaled to 6 bit depth and displayed. The result can be found in Figure 5.7.

```
8:> for i=1:511
9:> for j=1:511
10:> diffimg(i,j) = -img(i,j) + img(i+1,j);
11:> end
12:> end
13:> minint=min(min(diffimg));
14:> diffimg=diffimg-minint;
15:> maxint=max(max(diffimg));
16:> diffimg=diffimg/maxint*64;
17:> colormap(gray);
18:> image(diffimg)
```

Additional Tasks

Implement $K_{\text{y-forward}}$, and inspect the result.

What would $K_{\text{x-backward}}$ look like? Implement it and compare the result to the outcome of `ForwardDifference_5.m`.

Since we are interested in edges only, we can also implement a version of $K_{\text{x-forward}}$

which takes absolute values of the derivative only. The result should look like the right hand image in Figure 5.7.

Implement the operation for total differentiation using Equation 5.8. The result is found in Figure 5.8. The `Sobel_5.m` script in the `LessonData` folder implements a Sobel filter. Compare the outcome, which can also be found in Figure 5.27 by subtracting the resulting images from each other prior to scaling the images to 6 bit depth.

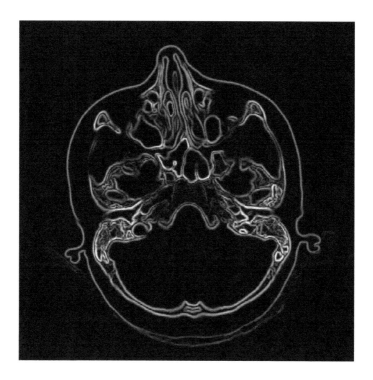

FIGURE 5.27: The result of applying a Sobel-filter to `SKULLBASE.DCM`. The reader is encouraged to compare this image to the corresponding image in Figure 5.8. Image data courtesy of the Dept. of Radiology, Medical University Vienna.

5.4.3.1   A note on good MATLAB® programming habits

By using MATLABs vector notation, lines 2 − 4 in `NumericalDifferentiation_5.m` can be replaced by:

```
...:> rect(45:55,1)= 1;
```

5.4.4   Unsharp masking

The `UnsharpMask_5.m` script is mainly derived from `SimpleLowPass_5.m` script; it implements the kernel for unsharp masking as given in Equation 5.11. The beginning of the script looks familiar. Besides the low pass filtered image `lpimg`, we reserve the memory for a second image `uming`, and a constant factor `weight` is defined:

```
1:> fp=fopen('SKULLBASE.DCM', 'r');
2:> fseek(fp,1622,'bof');
3:> img=zeros(512,512);
4:> img(:)=fread(fp,(512*512),'short');
5:> img=transpose(img);
6:> fclose(fp);
7:> lpimg=zeros(512,512);
8:> umimg=zeros(512,512);
9:> weight=1;
```

Now, the low pass filtered image using K_{blur} is computed, and the unsharp masking kernel is applied according to Equation 5.11.

```
10:> for i=2:511
11:> for j=2:511
12:> lpimg(i,j) = 0.1*(img((i-1),j) + 2*img(i,j) +
img((i+1),j) + img(i,(j-1)) + img(i,(j+1)) +
img((i-1),(j-1)) + img((i-1),(j+1)) +
img((i+1),(j-1)) + img((i+1),(j+1)));
13:> umimg(i,j) = img(i,j) - weight*lpimg(i,j);
14:> end
15:> end
```

Finally, the whole image is scaled to 6 bit depth as we have done so many times before.

```
16:> minint=min(min(umimg));
17:> umimg=umimg-minint;
18:> maxint=max(max(umimg));
19:> umimg=umimg/maxint*64;
20:> colormap(gray);
21:> image(umimg)
```

Additional Tasks

Experiment with different constants `weight` and inspect the image.

We have learned that the convolution operation is linear – therefore it should be possible to compute $K_{\text{Unsharp Mask}}$ as a single kernel, and apply that kernel to the image instead of computing `lpimg`. Derive the kernel and implement it. Does the result look the same as from `UnsharpMask_5.m`?

5.4.5 The median filter

In the `MedianFiveTimesFive_5.m` script, a median filter is implemented. The beginning is similar to the other scripts in this chapter. Again, `SKULLBASE.DCM` is read, and a matrix for the resulting image is reserved:

```
1:> fp=fopen('SKULLBASE.DCM', 'r');
2:> fseek(fp,1622,'bof');
3:> img=zeros(512,512);
4:> img(:)=fread(fp,(512*512),'short');
```

```
5:> img=transpose(img);
6:> fclose(fp);
7:> mfimg=zeros(512,512);
```

Next, a vector `rhovect` is reserved, which holds all the gray values ρ in the 25 pixels which form the kernel of the 5×5 median filter. These values are stored, and the vector is sorted by calling the `sort` function of MATLAB (whose function is self-explaining). After sorting the vector `rhovect`, the median is computed as the central element of this rank list. Since we have 25 entries in `rhovect`, the central element is located at position 13. The weak may be tempted to use the `median` function of MATLAB, which does essentially the same:

```
8:> rhovect = zeros(25,1);
9:> for i=3:510
10:> for j=3:510
11:> idx = 1;
12:> for k = -2:2
13:> for l = -2:2
14:> rhovect(idx)=img((i+k),(j+l));
15:> idx = idx + 1;
16:> end
17:> end
18:> rhovect=sort(rhovect);
19:> mfimg(i,j) = rhovect(13,1);
20:> end
21:> end
```

Finally, we will again scale the image to 6 bit depth, and display the result using the `image` function; Figure 5.28 shows the result.

```
22:> minint=min(min(mfimg));
23:> mfimg=mfimg-minint;
24:> maxint=max(max(mfimg));
25:> mfimg=mfimg/maxint*64;
26:> colormap(gray);
27:> image(mfimg)
```

Additional Tasks

Enhance the filter to an 11×11 median filter.

Can you imagine what a maximum and a minimum filter is? Implement them based on `MedianFiveTimesFive_5.m`.

5.4.6 Some properties of the Fourier-transform

5.4.6.1 Spectra of simple functions in k-space

In order to become familiar with the Fourier transform, we will take a closer look at the effects of the FFT on a well known function, the sine. The script `Sine_5.m` can be found in the `LessonData` folder. First, a sine function for angles x from 0 to 360 degrees is plotted; we do, of course, use radians. A second sine `wxx` with a frequency hundred times higher, but

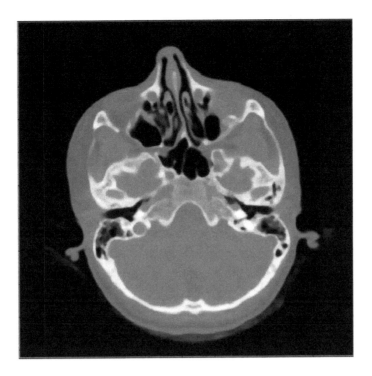

FIGURE 5.28: The result of a 5×5 median filter as performed in Example 5.4.5. The median filter suppresses noise and does also blur the image like a linear low-pass filter. However, it is robust to outliers by definition, and it tends to retain overall structural information to a larger extent compared to linear smoothing filters, as already shown in Figure 5.10. Image data courtesy of the Dept. of Radiology, Medical University Vienna.

with only a tenth of the amplitude of wx is generated as well and added to the sinusoidal signal wx, resulting in a signal y. Again, the good old command-line prompt halts the script until you are satisfied inspecting the resulting function in the spatial domain.

```
1:> x=1:360;
2:> wx=sin(x*pi/180);
3:> rattlefactor = 0.1;
4:> wxx=rattlefactor*sin(x*100*pi/180);
5:> y=wx+wxx;
6:> plot(y)
7:> foo=input('Press RETURN to see the spectrum ...');
```

The signal y is transformed to k-space using the built-in fft command, and shifted to a symmetric origin using fftshift. The absolute value of the complex spectrum is displayed, and the script is halted again.

```
8:> fy=fft(y);
9:> fys=fftshift(fy);
10:> plot(abs(fys))
11:> foo=input('Press RETURN to see the
     filtered spectrum...');
```

By removing the part of the spectrum that contains the additional signal wxx, we get the signal of the original sine signal wx. Again, the absolute value of the complex spectrum is displayed.

```
12:> for i=70:90
13:> fys(i)=0;
14:> fys(200+i)=0;
15:> end
16:> plot(abs(fys))
17:> foo=input('Press RETURN to see the
filtered sine in the spatial domain...');
```

Finally, we transform the cleaned spectrum back to the spatial domain, and look at the result, which is a sine function without added noise. The function to perform an inverse Fourier transformation in MATLAB is called ifft. Since we also have to re-establish the origin of the image coordinate system, the inverse operation for fftshift called ifftshift has to be carried out. We have not yet scaled the k-space properly, therefore the values on the k-axis of the plots for the spectra are not correct. Figure 5.29 shows the four plots generated by the script.

```
18:> rsine=ifft(ifftshift(fys));
19:> plot(real(rsine))
```

5.4.6.2 More complex functions

Spectra in 1D – decomposing a chord In this example, we will apply the Fourier-transform to a sound. That is a very obvious application since sounds are, technically speaking, periodic fluctuations of air density. A sound is therefore composed out of an overlay of several waves. In your LessonData folder, you find in the sub-folder 5_Filtering three sounds named c_piano.wav, c_aguitar.wav and c_eguitar.wav. These were also stored in MPG format, and you can listen to them on your computer. All three files are recordings of the same chord – a simple C major chord. A simple major chord consists of a triad of three single notes. The first one is the root note, followed by the major third and the fifth. In the case of C major, we are talking about the notes C, e and g. These notes are generated in a different fashion on different instruments; therefore, a chord sounds different when being played on a piano or a guitar.

For the sake of simplicity, we have also converted the .wav sound files to a raw format. The sounds are read by MATLAB using the ChordSpectrum_5.m script in the usual manner, just like we did with the DICOM files in earlier examples – the sound consists of a series of numbers with 16 bit, and these values are read into a vector called chord after opening the raw data file:

```
1:> clear;
2:> fp = fopen('c_piano.raw','r');
3:> chord=zeros(240630,1);
4:> chord(:)=fread(fp,240630,'short');
5:> fclose(fp);
6:> plot(chord)
7:> ylim([-22000 22000]);
8:> foo=input('Now proceed to the spectrum of the ...
chord played on piano...');
```

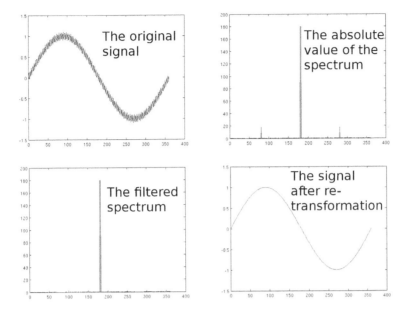

FIGURE 5.29: The four plots generated by the Sine_5.m script. The first plot shows the initial signal y – a sine overlaid by a smaller sine with higher frequency. The second and third plot show the absolute value of the spectrum. The frequency of the wx signal, which has a higher amplitude, is found in the middle of the plot. The higher frequency of the noise wxx is further to the left and the right of the origin of the coordinate system – it is lower since the amplitude of wxx is smaller. After removal of the contributions of wxx to the spectrum, the transformation back to the spatial domain shows the signal wx without the ripple added by wxx.

The command ylim (and the command xlim, which we will encounter in the next few lines of code) makes sure that the scaling of the x- and y-axis does not change when displaying the different chords. The signal now undergoes a Fourier-transform, just as we did before with other signals:

```
9:> kpchord=abs(fftshift(fft(chord)));
10:> plot(kpchord);
11:> xlim([100000 140000])
```

The remainder of the script is very straightforward; we repeat the same procedure for the C major chord played on acoustic guitar and on a mighty electric guitar. The result can be found in Fig. 5.30.

```
12:> foo=input('Now look at the chord...
played on acoustic guitar...');
13:> fp = fopen('c_aguitar.raw','r');
14:> chord=zeros(239616,1);
15:> chord(:)=fread(fp,239616,'short');
16:> fclose(fp);
17:> plot(chord)
```

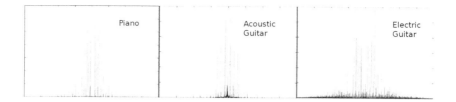

FIGURE 5.30: The results of `ChordSpectrum_5.m`, where a C major chord played on piano, acoustic and electric guitar is displayed as a power spectrum. The differences – showing the different contributions in amplitude and harmonics – are clearly visible. The audible result is the different sound of the chord, which is also stored as an audio file in the `LessonData` folder.

```
18:> ylim([-22000 22000]);
19:> foo=input('Now proceed to the spectrum of the...
chord played on acoustic guitar...');
20:> kagchord=abs(fftshift(fft(chord)));
21:> plot(kagchord);
22:> xlim([100000 140000])
23:> foo=input('Now look at the chord played ...
on electric guitar...');
24:> fp = fopen('c_eguitar.raw','r');
25:> chord=zeros(239616,1);
26:> chord(:)=fread(fp,239616,'short');
27:> fclose(fp);
28:> plot(chord)
29:> ylim([-22000 22000]);
30:> foo=input('Now proceed to the spectrum of the ...
chord played on acoustic guitar...');
31:> kegchord=abs(fftshift(fft(chord)));
32:> plot(kegchord);
33:> xlim([100000 140000])
```

From the spectra we see the subtle difference – we have decomposed the chords into their components, and we see the different contributions from the higher harmonics, which result in a different sound, despite the fact that the three chords are identical.

A Rectangle function In the `Rect_5.m` script, the rect-function also known from Figure 5.6 is transformed to k-space. The rect-function does not have a single frequency like the sine from `Sine_5.m`. Rather than that, it is composed out of many plane waves with different frequencies and amplitudes:

```
1:> rect=zeros(100,1);
2:> ffrect=zeros(100,1);
3:> for j=45:55
4:> rect(j,1)=1;
5:> end
6:> frect=fft(rect);
7:> frect=fftshift(frect);
```

In the next few lines, we remove the higher frequencies in steps of ten up to all hundred frequencies and transform the remainder back to the spatial domain. The result is the approximation of the rect-function up to a given order, just as indicated in Equation 5.18. Subsequently, the single steps are displayed using the `plot` function. Since the Fourier transform is complex valued, the inverse Fourier-transform yields complex numbers; however, the imaginary part of these complex numbers is zero, therefore we can use the `real` operator to retrieve the real part of these values in the spatial domain. The `ylim` command takes care of the proper scaling of the y-axis:

```
8:> for j = 1:4
9:> klimlow=50-j*10
10:> klimhigh=50+j*10
11:> for k=1:100
12:> if (k < klimlow) | (k > klimhigh)
13:> ffrect(k,1) = 0;
14:> else
15:> ffrect(k,1)=frect(k,1);
16:> end
17:> end
18:> rrect=ifft(ifftshift(ffrect));
19:> plot(real(rrect))
20:> ylim([-0.2 1.5])
21:> foo=input('Press RETURN to proceed
to the next rectangle pulse');
22:> end
```

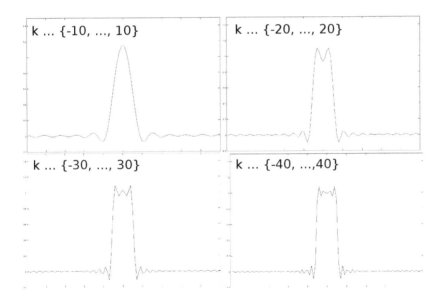

FIGURE 5.31: The output from script `Rect_5.m`. We see how the original rect-function is low-pass filtered from the Fourier spectrum. The lower the maximum order i (which is called `klimlow` and `klimhigh` in the script), the more massive the low-pass filtering.

Additional Tasks

Implement a simple high-pass filter based on the `Rect_5.m` script.

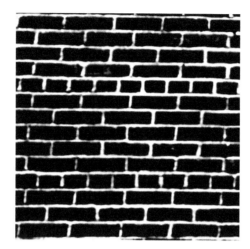

FIGURE 5.32: Another not-so-medical example (it is at least a hospital wall) of a 2D image with very few frequencies. We see bricks and mortar joints here, pretty well aligned in horizontal and vertical direction. In this example, we can filter frequencies in the direction of the coordinate axes using the `WallFourier_Y_LP_5.m` script from the `LessonData`-folder.

Filtering a simple 2D image   Let us now proceed to twodimensional signals. Figure 5.32 shows a simple black and white photography of a brickwall. To some extent, this image is similar to the 1D-rectangle function. Let us apply a 2D-Fourier transform to this image. The script is called `WallFourier_Y_LP_5.m`, and as usual, it can be found in the `LessonData` folder. First, we clear all variables from the workspace, we allocate a matrix for the 512×512 image `brickwall.jpg`, and we carry out a 2D Fourier transform, followed by a `fftshift` command that establishes a symmetry around the center of the image:

```
1:> clear;
2:> img=zeros(512,512);
3:> img = imread('brickwall.jpg');
4:> fimg = fft2(img);
5:> fimg= fftshift(fimg);
```

Next, we set all the frequencies to the left and the right of a line that is parallel to the y-axis and passes through the center of the image to zero. What remains are the major frequencies in the y-direction. As a matter of fact, all elements of the image that have a major component in the x-direction are removed, leaving only the horizontal mortar joints in the image.

```
6:> for i=1:512
7:> for j=1:254
8:> fimg(i,j)=complex(0,0);
9:> end
10:> end
```

```
11:> for i=1:512
12:> for j=258:512
13:> fimg(i,j)=complex(0,0);
14:> end
15:> end
```

The only thing that is left for us is to transform the image back to the spatial domain, to scale the image intensities to 6 bit, and to display the image. The result can be found in Figure 5.33:

```
16:> lpimg=zeros(512,512);
17:> lpimg = real(ifft2(ifftshift(fimg)));
18:> minint=min(min(lpimg));
19:> lpimg=lpimg-minint;
20:> maxint=max(max(lpimg));
21:> lpimg=lpimg/maxint*64;
22:> colormap(gray);
23:> image(lpimg)
```

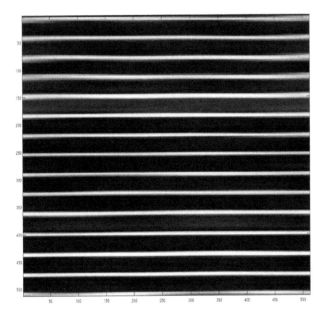

FIGURE 5.33: The output of `WallFourier_Y_LP_5.m`. All the vertical details visible in Figure 5.32 were removed by setting the frequencies that contribute in the x-direction of the image to zero.

The spectrum of a 2D image A more complex function is the mouse, already known from Figs. 5.10 and 5.11. The script `MouseSpectrum_5.m` performs a two-dimensional Fourier transform of the `MouseCT.jpg` image. The image is read, transformed using the `fft2` command, and the low frequencies are shifted to the center of the matrix containing the k-values.

```
1:> img=zeros(733,733);
2:> img = imread('MouseCT.jpg');
3:> fimg = fft2(img);
4:> fimg = fftshift(fimg);
5:> psimg=zeros(733,733);
```

Next, we compute the norm of the power spectrum using the `abs` function; in order to visualize the low contrast detail in the resulting image, we apply a logarithmic transform to the resulting image, just as in Example 4.5.3, and display the result using the `image` command. The result can be found in Figure 5.19:

```
6:> for j=1:733
7:> for k=1:733
8:> psimg(j,k) = abs(fimg(j,k));
9:> end
10:> end
11:> psimg = log(psimg);
12:> minint=min(min(psimg));
13:> psimg=psimg-minint;
14:> maxint=max(max(psimg));
15:> psimg=psimg/maxint*64;
16:> colormap(gray);
17:> image(psimg)
```

5.4.6.3 Convolution of simple functions

Another example can be found in the `Simpleconvolution_5.m` script, where a rect-function and a sawtooth are convolved. We have already performed the convolution operation on images; mathematically speaking, a convolution of two functions $f(x)$ and $g(x)$ is an integral: $f \star g(x) = \int_{-\infty}^{\infty} dy f(y)g(x-y)$. According to the convolution theorem, we can as well transform the two functions to k-space and simply multiply them. The re-transformation yields the convolved function. First, we draw the two functions – the rect and the sawtooth – and plot them separately:

```
1:> rect=zeros(100,1);
2:> for i=35:65
3:> rect(i,1)=15;
4:> end
5:> saw=zeros(100,1);
6:> for i=1:15
7:> saw(i,1)=i-1;
8:> end
9:> for i=16:29
10:> saw(i,1)=29-i;
11:> end
12:> plot(rect)
13:> ylim([-1 20]);
14:> foo=input('Press RETURN to proceed to the
sawtooth to be convolved...');
15:> plot(saw)
```

```
16:> ylim([-1 20]);
17:> foo=input('Press RETURN to proceed...');
```

The `input` function causes a program halt until the `RETURN` key is pressed; the `ylim` function, which was already used earlier, takes care of a proper scaling of the ordinate.

Next, we transform `rect` and `saw` to k-space. The convolution takes place by a component-wise multiplication of the resulting complex vectors `fr` and `fs` using the `.*` operator. After this operation, the resulting function `fconv` is transformed back to spatial domain, and the resulting function `rconv` is displayed.

```
18:> fr=fft(rect);
19:> frs=fftshift(fr);
20:> fs=fft(saw);
21:> fss=fftshift(fs);
22:> fconv=frs.*fss;
23:> fconvs=ifftshift(fconv);
24:> rconv=ifft(fconvs);
25:> plot(real(rconv))
```

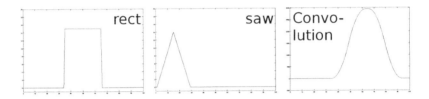

FIGURE 5.34: The result of the `Simpleconvolution_5.m` script, which convolves a rect-function and a sawtooth. The two dimensional counterpart of the rect function would be a bright spot with sharp edges, whereas the sawtooth resembles the K_{blur} kernel from Equation 5.1. We have not taken any care about proper scaling of the k values yet, therefore the absolute height of the convolved function is not correct.

5.4.6.4 Differentiation in k-space

Finally, we will give a simple example of differentiation in k-space. The `FourierDiffRect_5.m` script differentiates the rect function; the result of such an operation we have already seen in Figure 5.6. For the first time, we will try to do a proper mapping of the possible values of k. We remember that the maximum frequency (or the maximum *cycles over range*) are given by the number of pixels in an image, or the number of pivoting points when defining a function as a vector of numbers. First, a rect function `rect` is defined, just like in Example 5.4.3. The function is transformed to k-space and shifted in such a manner that the origin lies in the middle of the transformed function.

```
1:> rect=zeros(100,1);
2:> for j=45:55
3:> rect(j,1)=1;
4:> end
5:> rect=transpose(rect);
```

```
6:> frect=fft(rect);
7:> frect=fftshift(frect);
```

Next, we have to derive the appropriate values for k; after the `fftshift` operation, these may assume negative values as well. We simply define a vector `k`, which is normalized and shifted as well:

```
8:> k=[(1:100)]/100;
9:> k=fftshift(k);
```

The only thing that is left to do is to perform the derivation by computing $-ik\hat{f}(k)$ using the component-wise multiplication `.*`; the result undergoes an inverse shifting and is transformed back to the spatial domain. The resulting vector `drect` is complex valued, but the imaginary part should be zero and is therefore omitted by using the `real` operator. The result can be found in Figure 5.35.

```
10:> drect=ifft(ifftshift(((-i*k)).*frect));
11:> plot(real(drect))
```

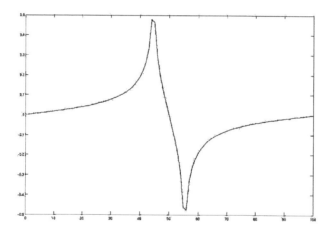

FIGURE 5.35: The result of computing the first derivative of a rect function in k-space. Due to the limited resolution (and the resulting low number of frequencies available), the result is not as clearly defined as its counterpart – the result of a numerical forward differentiation – in Figure 5.6.

Additional Tasks

In the `LessonData`-folder, you will find an improved version of `FourierDiffRect_5.m` named `BetterFourierDiffRect_5.m`. It does essentially the same but the outcome definitely resembles Figure 5.6 to a greater extent than Figure 5.35. Why?

5.4.7 Frequency filtering in Fourier-space on images

The script `MouseFourierLP_5.m` is derived from `MouseSpectrum_5.m`, and it implements a very simple low pass filter. In fact, all higher frequencies are cut off in a very rude manner, which leads to some artifacts in the resulting representation.

```
1:> img=zeros(733,733);
2:> img = imread('MouseCT.jpg');
3:> fimg = fft2(img);
```

Now, we remove the higher frequencies from the spectrum, and the result is displayed. Figure 5.36 shows the results when cutting off the frequencies for $k > 5$, $k > 15$, and $k > 25$; denote that the image in k-space is again shifted using `fftshift` in such a manner that the lowest frequency lies in the middle of the image. In order to implement a low-pass filter, we have to remove the frequencies whose absolute value is beyond a certain threshold. The lowest frequency is therefore found in the middle of the transformed image `fimg`, approximately at position $(366, 366)^T$.

```
4:> fimg= fftshift(fimg);
5:> for i=1:733
6:> for j=1:733
7:> crad=sqrt((i-366)^2+(j-366)^2);
8:> if crad > 10
9:> fimg(i,j)=complex(0,0);
10:> end
11:> end
12:> end
13:> lpimg=zeros(733,733);
14:> lpimg = real(ifft2(fimg));
15:> minint=min(min(lpimg));
16:> lpimg=lpimg-minint;
17:> maxint=max(max(lpimg));
18:> lpimg=lpimg/maxint*64;
19:> colormap(gray);
20:> image(lpimg)
```

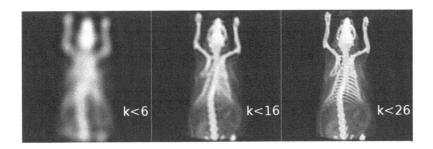

FIGURE 5.36: The output from script `MouseFourierLP_5.m`. Instead of smoothly suppressing higher frequencies like the K_{blur} kernel does, we simply cut off the frequencies, which leads to a lower image quality. A more sophisticated method would produce images just like Figure 5.3. Image data courtesy of C. Kuntner, AIT Seibersdorf, Austria.

Additional Tasks

Using the `MouseFourierLP_5.m` script, you can implement a simple high pass and band pass filter. A sample output can be found in Figure 5.37.

The basic operation in this script is actually the multiplication of the image in k-space with a function that is 1 in a circle of radius `crad` around the center of the image. Can you compute the PSF that would yield the same result by convolution in the spatial domain? A possible result can be found in Figure 5.38. Compare the image to Figure 5.31, and try to find some literature on *Gibbs phenomenon*.

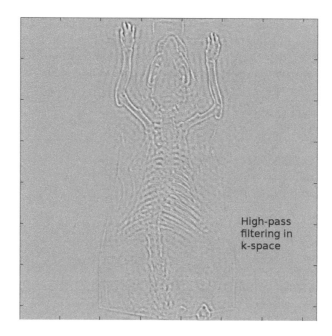

High-pass filtering in k-space

FIGURE 5.37: The results of a simple high pass filter in *k*-space applied to `MouseCT.jpg`. Image data courtesy of C. Kuntner, AIT Seibersdorf, Austria.

5.4.8 Applied convolution – PSF and the MTF

Finally, we will explore the full power of the convolution operation in *k*-space; the `MouseConvolve_5.m` script convolves a Gaussian with arbitrary standard deviation σ with the `MouseCT.jpg` image. Let's take a look at the code. First, we read the image and transform it to *k*-space, and we allocate some space for a Gaussian named `gs`; the Gaussian is then drawn into the center of the image. `sig` defines the width σ of the Gaussian:

```
1:> img=zeros(733,733);
2:> img = imread('MouseCT.jpg');
3:> fimg = fft2(img);
4:> fimg = fftshift(fimg);
5:> gs=zeros(733,733);
6:> sig=2;
7:> for j=1:733
```

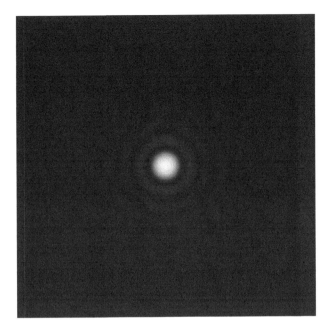

FIGURE 5.38: This PSF would give one of the blurred images from Figure 5.36. It can be derived by identifying the MTF in k-space and applying a Fourier-transform to it.

```
8:> for k=1:733
9:> gs(j,k)=exp(-((j-366)^2+(k-366)^2)/(2*sig^2));
10:> end
11:> end
```

The looks of the Gaussian can be found in Figure 5.39. Next, we transform the Gaussian to k-space – a step that is not necessary since a Gaussian stays a Gaussian when undergoing a Fourier-transformation[5] – and we convolve the two functions by component-wise multiplication using the .* operator. The absolute value for the transformed Gaussian is also shown in Figure 5.39.

```
12:> gs=fftshift(fft2(gs));
13:> fimg=gs.*fimg;
```

Next, we move back to the spatial domain; since our Gaussian was drawn in the center of the image to be convolved with MouseCT.jpg, we have to apply ifftshift twice. Finally, the image is scaled to 6 bit and displayed. The result of the operation using values $\sigma \in \{2, 4, 6\}$ is given in Figure 5.40.

```
14:> cimg=ifftshift(ifft2(ifftshift(fimg)));
15:> minint=min(min(cimg));
16:> cimg=cimg-minint;
17:> maxint=max(max(cimg));
18:> cimg=cimg/maxint*64;
19:> colormap(gray);
20:> image(real(cimg))
```

---

[5]Remember that the Gaussian retains its shape in k-space.

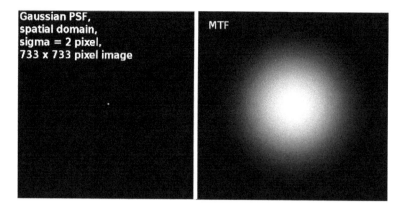

FIGURE 5.39: The left image shows the Gaussian kernel **gs** with width $\sigma = 2$ in the spatial domain; this represents the PSF for the filtering process. The PSF is rather sharp and narrow; its counterpart in the Fourier-domain is the MTF. A well-defined PSF allows for good resolution of fine detail; therefore the MTF is wide. One may also notice that the MTF on the right hand side has also a Gaussian shape.

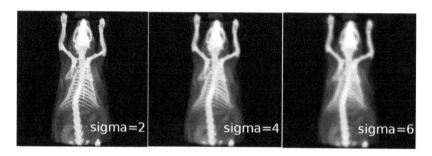

FIGURE 5.40: The results of the convolution operation with a Gaussian of width $\sigma = 2, 4,$ and 6 pixels. Image data courtesy of C. Kuntner, AIT Seibersdorf, Austria.

Additional Tasks

Display **gs** in the spatial domain, and **abs(gs)** in k-space, similar to Figure 5.39. What happens for large values of **sigma**?

5.4.9 Determination of system resolution of an Anger-camera using a point source

By using a point source, it is possible to derive the MTF directly from an image. In this example, we have such an image of a point source. A syringe was filled with ^{99m}Tc and positioned over the scintillator crystal of a γ-camera.. The camera allows to read out the image at various resolutions, ranging from 64×64 to 1024×1024 pixels. The dimension of the scintillator is 614×614mm^2. Two DICOM images named PSF64.dcm and PSF1024.dcm showing the needle tip can be found in your LessonData folder. The three subimages showing only the needle tip at the same scale can be found in Figure 5.41. The script ComputeMTF_5.m computes the MTF from these real life PSF images. Let us take a look at it. This version of the script reads the DICOM image taken with the lowest resolution of 64×64 pixels:

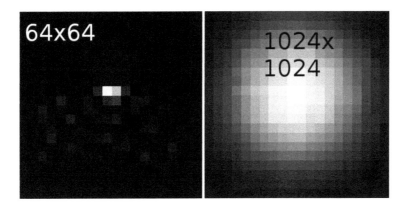

FIGURE 5.41: Two magnified images of a real life PSF in a γ camera. A syringe was filled with a small activity of ^{99m}Tc. These are the images of the needletip, all covering an area of 20×20 pixels, at two preset resolutions (64×64 and 1024×1024 pixels) of the γ camera. By computing the Fourier-transform of this PSF, it is possible to derive the overall system resolution of the γ camera. Image data courtesy of P. Schaffarich, University Clinic for Nuclear Medicine, Vienna General Hospital, Austria.

```
1:> clear;
2:> dimension=64;
3:> fp=fopen('PSF64.dcm','r');
4:> fseek(fp,-(dimension*dimension*2),'eof');
5:> img=zeros(dimension,dimension);
6:> img(:)=fread(fp,(dimension*dimension*2),...
'uint16');
7:> fclose(fp);
```

As usual, we clear all variables from our MATLAB-workspace, and since we are going to read the first image PSF64.dcm, which features a 64×64 matrix, we set the variable dimension to 64. Next, the file is opened, and we skip the DICOM header by simply starting 8192 bytes before the end of the file, denoted by the phrase 'eof', which stands for *end of file*. Then we assign an empty matrix of 64×64 pixels, we read the image data into that matrix, and we close the file again.

```
8:> thresh = 300;
9:> weights=0;
10:> centroid=zeros(2,1);
11:> for i=1:dimension
12:> for j=1:dimension
13:> rho=img(i,j);
14:> if rho > thresh
15:> weights=weights+rho;
16:> centroid=centroid+rho*[i j]';
17:> end
18:> end
19:> end
20:> centroid=round(centroid/weights);
```

```
21:> shift=[(centroid(1,1)-round(dimension/2))...
(centroid(2,1)-round(dimension/2))]';
```

This part of the code is not directly connected to the determination of the system resolution. Rather than that, we determine the center of gravity of the image. Each pixel with an intensity above a certain threshold `thresh` is inspected. The pixel locations, which contain a gray value above 300 (denote that the intensity range is 0...64555 since we are dealing with unsigned 16 bit images here, therefore everything below a gray value of 300 is considered plain black here), are added after scalar multiplication with their respective gray values, and the result is the center of mass of the image – in other words, we compute the weighted average of non-black pixels. The location of this center of mass is stored in a vector `shift`. More on the computation of centroids can be found in Chapter 6.

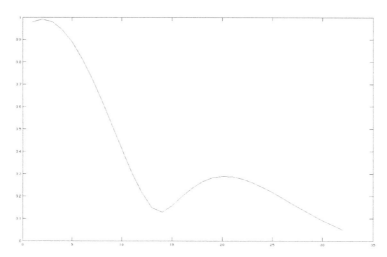

FIGURE 5.42: The result of `ComputeMTF_5.m`. We see a MTF for the PSF which is shown in the leftmost part of Figure 5.41. From this function it is evident that an Anger-camera with a field-of-view of 64×64 pixels can resolve up to 15 line pairs over the range of the scintillator – in general, it is said that a value of 0.1 still gives somes useful contrast. Since the width of the scintillator is 614 mm, 15 line pairs correspond to approximately 20 mm resolution.

```
22:> cimg=zeros(dimension,dimension);
23:> for i=1:dimension
24:> for j=1:dimension
25:> rho=img(i,j);
26:> if rho > thresh
27:> if (i-shift(1,1) > 0) && ...
(i-shift(1,1) < dimension) && ...
(j-shift(2,1) > 0) && (j-shift(2,1) < dimension)
28:> cimg((i-shift(1,1)),(j-shift(2,1)))=img(i,j);
29:> end
30:> end
31:> end
32:> end
```

Here, we assign a new matrix for an image `cimg`, which is of the same dimension as `img`. The pixels are all shifted by the vector `shift`. The purpose of this procedure is to make sure that the most important part of the PSF, given by the center of mass of the image since it does not contain anything but the PSF, is located in the center of the image. Next, we can compute the Fourier-transform of `cimg`, which should give us the MTF. The absolute value of the Fourier-transform is computed, and we scale the intensities in the absolute values of the spectrum to a range of $0 \ldots 1$:

```
33:> mtfimg = fft2(cimg);
34:> mtfimg=abs(fftshift(mtfimg));
35:> maxmtfimg=max(max(mtfimg));
36:> mtfimg=mtfimg/maxmtfimg;
```

Now we can derive a modulation transfer function plot like the one in Figure 5.21 from this image. Remember that we are only interested in the positive leg of the MTF, and that the MTF is radially symmetric since our PSF is also, at least in an idealized version, radially symmetric. Therefore, we simply save the intensities of the MTF in a line that is parallel to the x-axis of the image, and which starts in the middle of `cimg`:

```
37:> mtf=zeros(round(dimension/2),1);
38:> for i=1:round(dimension/2)
39:> mtf(i)=mtfimg(round(dimension/2),...
((round(dimension/2)-1) +i));
40:> end
41:> plot(mtf)
```

The result can be found in Figure 5.42. A matrix of 64×64 is pretty poor, and the result is not very impressive. The reason lies in the fact that the field-of-view is too small and limits the system resolution. Figure 5.43, which is connected to the *Additional Tasks* of this example, gives the MTF for a full resolution of 1024×1024 matrix.

Additional Tasks

Check `PSF128.dcm` and `PSF1024.dcm` using `ComputeMTF_5.m`. Both can be found in the `LessonData` folder. Is the improvement in resolution dramatic, or is there some "void resolution" due to the fact that the ability to resolve fine detail is not only limited by the matrix of the digital image?

5.4.10 The Hough transform

In `Hough_5.m`, a Hough transform is carried out on the image shown in Figure 5.44. First, we read the image, and then we scale it to binary values – just to make sure that we have nothing but 0s and 1s in the image:

```
1:> img = imread('evil.jpg');
2:> minint=min(min(img));
3:> img=img-minint;
4:> maxint=max(max(img));
5:> img=round(img/maxint);
```

Next, we allocate an image for the Hough-representation named `himg`. It is 360 pixels

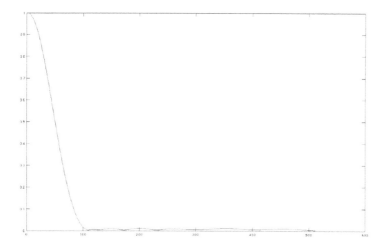

FIGURE 5.43: The result of `ComputeMTF_5.m` with the variable `dimension` set to 1024, and after reading in the file `PSF1024.dcm`. The resolution is no longer limited by the pixel resolution of the camera. The resolution in this diagram is given in "cycles over range" – therefore, 100 cycles over half the width of the scintillator results in a theoretical resolution of approximately 3 mm.

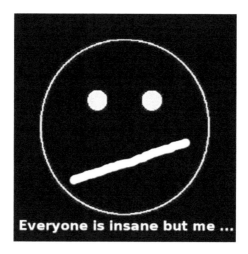

FIGURE 5.44: The binary image which will undergo a Hough-transform in Example 5.4.10. The representation in Hough-space can be found in Figure 5.46.

wide (for all possible angles θ) and the maximum radius is given as $310 \times \sqrt{2} = 439$ (because `size(img)=[310 310]`). Just to make sure, we allocate 442 pixel for the radius r. If a non-zero pixel is encountered, we go through all angles θ, convert them in radians and derive the appropriate distance $r = i \cos\theta + j \sin\theta$. These parameter pairs increment the counts of found parameters on a trigonometric curve in `himg`. Take a closer look at the computation of `r` – in fact, we map all possible normal vectors to Hough space. This is also illustrated in Figure 5.45:

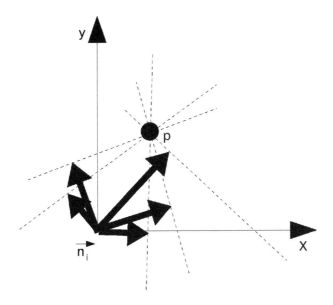

FIGURE 5.45: The basic principle of the Hough – transform is to store the parametric representation of the normal vectors $\vec{n}_i$ of lines that may pass a non-zero pixel **p**. If a series of pixels lies on a line, the location of the parameters for the normal vector of this very line will be densely populated. The parameters for less populated normal vectors are being disregarded prior to back-transformation.

```
6:> himg=zeros(360,442);
7:> for i=1:310
8:> for j=1:310
9:> if img(i,j) > 0
10:> for ang=1:360
11:> theta=ang*pi/180;
12:> r=round(i*cos(theta)+j*sin(theta));
13:> if r > 0
14:> himg(ang,r)=himg(ang,r)+1;
15:> end
16:> end
17:> end
18:> end
19:> end
```

Next, we have to reduce the number of parameters only to those spots in himg where most of the parameter pairs r, θ are found. This is done by thresholding the image (more on the subject can be found in Chapter 6). We introduce the threshold by a variable perc, which determines the percentage of the pixels below the maximum intensity maxint to be used. All pixels above that threshold are set to 64, all others are set to zero.

```
20:> perc=10;
21:> maxint=max(max(himg));
22:> for i=1:360
```

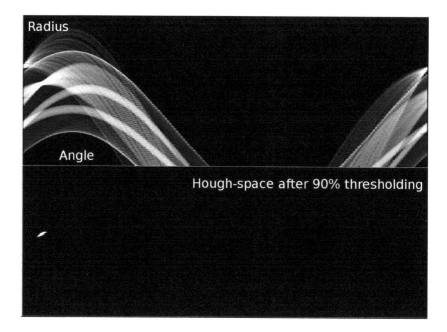

FIGURE 5.46: An intermediate result of `Hough_5.m`. The binary image from Figure 5.44 is transformed to Hough-space; after thresholding the resulting image, only the areas with the highest concentration of parameter pairs remain. In this representation, the abscissa represents the angles θ, and the ordinate is the parameter r.

```
23:> for j=1:442
24:> if himg(i,j) > maxint-maxint*perc/100
25:> himg(i,j) = 64;
26:> else
27:> himg(i,j) = 0;
28:> end
29:> end
30:> end
```

By now, we already have everything, but the re-transformation from parameter space to lines is a little bit cumbersome. What follows is a lot of code, but it is not difficult to understand. For all remaining points {`maxr`, `maxphi`} in the thresholded parameter space, we compute the Hesse normal vector $\vec{n}$, named `normalvect` by transforming `maxr` and `maxphi` back to Cartesian coordinates. A second vector, `unitvect`, is computed as the normal vector to $\vec{n} = (n_1, n_2)^T$ by setting its components to $(-n_2, n_1)$. As one may easily verify from computing the inner product of this vector with $\vec{n}$, the two vectors are normal. Finally, the vectors length is scaled to 1.

```
31:> transimg=zeros(310,310);
32:> for maxphi=1:360
33:> for maxr=1:442;
34:> if himg(maxphi,maxr) > 0
35:> normalvect=zeros(1,2);
36:> unitvect=zeros(1,2);
```

```
37:> normalvect(1,1)=maxr*cos((maxphi)*pi/180);
38:> normalvect(1,2)=maxr*sin((maxphi)*pi/180);
39:> unitvect(1,1)=-normalvect(1,2);
40:> unitvect(1,2)=normalvect(1,1);
41:> unitvect=unitvect/(sqrt(unitvect(1,1)^2...
+unitvect(1,2)^2));
```

We have now a unit vector unitvect that gives the direction of the line defined by the Hesse normal vector normalvect. In order to draw a line, we have to move this unitvect to the tip of $\vec{n}$, and draw a pixel to the top of this shifted vector; after that, we increase the length len of unitvect, and draw the next pixel until we leave the domain of the image.

```
42:> len=0;
43:> i=round(normalvect(1,1));
44:> j=round(normalvect(1,2));
45:> while (i > 1) & (i < 309) & (j > 1) & (j < 309)
46:> i=round(normalvect(1,1)+len*unitvect(1,1));
47:> j=round(normalvect(1,2)+len*unitvect(1,2));
48:> transimg(i,j)=64;
49:> len=len+1;
50:> end
```

The same procedure is repeated, but the direction of unitvect is reversed. Finally, everything is displayed.

```
51:> unitvect=-unitvect;
52:> len=0;
53:> i=round(normalvect(1,1));
54:> j=round(normalvect(1,2));
55:> while (i > 1) & (i < 309) & (j > 1) & (j < 309)
56:> i=round(normalvect(1,1)+len*unitvect(1,1));
57:> j=round(normalvect(1,2)+len*unitvect(1,2));
58:> transimg(i,j)=64;
59:> len=len+1;
60:> end
61:> end
62:> end
63:> end
64:> colormap(gray)
65:> image(transimg)
```

Additional Tasks

In the LessonData folder, you may find a more medical example named MosaicBone-EdgeBinary.jpg, which is the result of Sobel filtering and intensity thresholding of an x-ray image of a long bone. Modify Hough_5.m in such a manner that this image is processed. By modifying perc, you will be able to display a number of straight lines in the image. Besides changing the intensity threshold of the image in Hough-space – can you think of a way to reduce the number of lines in the image transformed back to Cartesian coordinates? A small hint: think of the resolution of parameters in Hough space.

FIGURE 5.47: The final outcome of `Hough_5.m`. Using only the brightest 10% of the image, Figure 5.46 is transformed back to the line representation in Cartesian coordinates. Only the mouth of our slightly frustrated character remains. However, it is not limited to its original boundaries since the retransform from Hough space does not care whether we deal with line segments or lines. In Section 6.8.8.1, we will encounter the Hough transform again, and there we will learn how this problem can be handled.

5.4.11 The distance transform

A simple little example illustrates the distance transform on the small binary rectangle from Figure 5.23, which also shows the result from the script `DistanceMap_5.m`. First, we load a 50×50 image of the rectangle, and we allocate some space for the transformed image. Next, we visit each pixel in the original image `img`. If such a pixel is not zero – remember that we are operating on binary images – we search for the nearest black pixel in the whole image. In order to find the correct distance, three conditions have to be met:

The nearest pixel in question has to be within the image domain.

It has to be zero.

And its distance must be smaller than the previously found distance; `mindist` is initialized as the maximum distance possible within the image. In the end, the smallest distance `mindist` is plotted in the image `distImg` and displayed as usual.

```
1:> img=imread('dtrect.jpg');
2:> distImg=zeros(50,50);
3:> for i=1:50
4:> for j=1:50
5:> mindist=71;
6:> if img(i,j)>0
```

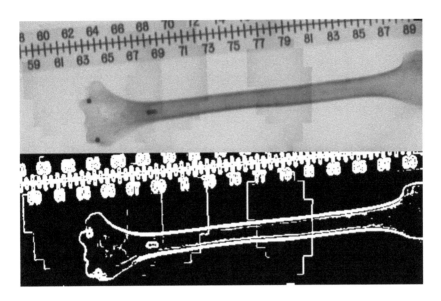

FIGURE 5.48: The original x-ray image of a long bone, together with a ruler. This image is actually the result of *mosaicing* – it was assembled from several x-ray images acquired with a mobile x-ray unit. The lower image can also be found in the LessonData folder; a modification of Hough_5.m will produce an image similar to Figure 5.47. Image data courtesy of Z. Yaniv, ISIS Center, Department of Radiology, Georgetown University.

```
7:> for k=-49:49
8:> for l=-49:49
9:> if (i+k)>0 && (i+k)<51 && (j+l)>0 && (j+l)<51
10:> if img((i+k),(j+l)) == 0
11:> dist=round(sqrt(k*k+l*l));
12:> if dist < mindist
13:> mindist=dist;
14:> end
15:> end
16:> end
17:> end
18:> end
19:> distImg(i,j)=mindist;
20:> end
21:> end
22:> end
23:> maxint=max(max(distImg));
24:> distImg=distImg/maxint*64;
25:> colormap(gray)
26:> image(distImg)
```

Until now, we have little use for this simple transformation; we will find it pretty useful later on. It should also be mentioned that we are not confined to the use of the Euclidean metric employed here, and that more effective (in terms of computing effort) implementations than the one presented here are feasible. However, for the moment, we can introduce one application of the distance transform, which is related to a morphological operation called *thinning*. Morphological operations are introduced in Section 6.6. We can make the result of Example 5.4.10 a little bit more impressive by computing the distance transform of Figure 5.47. After applying a distance transform we can apply a thresholding technique which we already encountered in Example 5.4.10, and which we will deal with in detail in Section 6.3. A more significant result is the effort of such an operation, which can be found in Figure 5.49.

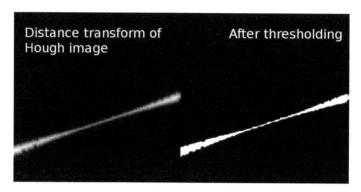

FIGURE 5.49: The distance transformation of Figure 5.47 and a binary version of that image after intensity thresholding. The centerline of Figure 5.47 is now emphasized.

Additional Tasks

Can you modify `DistanceMap_5.m` in such a manner that it produces something similar to Figure 5.49?

5.5 SUMMARY AND FURTHER REFERENCES

Filters and transformations are, as we have seen, two closely linked subjects. I admit that this chapter contains a lot of math, although I have only tried to motivate the use of separable transforms, namely the Fourier transform, in the complex domain. By no means can this short overview replace a solid background in applied and numerical mathematics. However, the importance of filtering operations justifies the effort since filtering is usually a vital component for other methods like segmentation, registration, and tomographic reconstruction. In this chapter, we have seen that the convolution operation, either in k-space or in the spatial domain can be arbitrarily combined in a linear manner to design more complex kernels. It is preferable to apply the convolution of more complex kernels in the Fourier-domain, and by means of the Fourier transform, we are also able to suppress periodic noise. Furthermore, we have learned about the PSF as a general tool for characterization of signal transmission in general, and how it is linked to the MTF. Finally, we made acquaintance with the Hough-transform, which allows to identify structures that are given in a parametric form.

Literature

R. C. Gonzalez, R. E. Woods: Digital Image Processing, Prentice-Hall, (2007)

M. Sonka, V. Hlavac, R. Boyle: Image Processing, Analysis, and Machine Vision, CL-Engineering, (2007).

W. Burger, M. J. Burge: Digital Image Processing – An Algorithmic Introduction using Java, Springer, (2008), `http://www.imagingbook.com`

CHAPTER 6

Segmentation

Wolfgang Birkfellner

CONTENTS

6.1 The segmentation problem 177
6.2 ROI definition and centroids 178
6.3 Thresholding 178
6.4 Region growing 181
6.5 More sophisticated segmentation methods 183
    6.5.1 ITK SNAP – a powerful implementation of a segmentation algorithm at work 185
6.6 Morphological operations 185
6.7 Evaluation of segmentation results 188
6.8 Practical lessons 190
    6.8.1 Count rate evaluation by ROI selection 190
    6.8.2 Region definition by global thresholding 192
    6.8.3 Region growing 192
    6.8.4 Region growing in 3D 195
    6.8.5 A very simple snake-type example 199
    6.8.6 Erosion and dilation 203
    6.8.7 Hausdorff-distances and Dice-coefficients 205
    6.8.8 Improving segmentation results by filtering 206
        6.8.8.1 Better thresholding 206
        6.8.8.2 Preprocessing and active contours 209
6.9 Summary and further references 212

6.1 THE SEGMENTATION PROBLEM

We have already learned that medical images map certain physical properties of tissue and store the resulting discrete mathematical function as an image. It is a straightforward and understandable desire that anyone who uses medical images wants to identify certain anatomical structures for further examination; identifying organs or other anatomical structures is an inevitable prerequisite for many operations that retrieve quantitative data from images as well as many visualization tasks.

Unfortunately, physical properties of tissue as recorded by a medical imaging device do usually not correlate completely with the anatomic boundaries of certain organs. That is a very fundamental problem since most organs do not consist of one type of tissue. Segmentation is therefore always a rather complex, specialized procedure often requiring considerable manual interaction, which renders image processing methods requiring segmentation to be quite unattractive. The need for highly specialized solutions is also documented by the plethora of research papers, which usually present rather specialized techniques for a certain type of application. The following chapter introduces the most basic segmentation methods, which usually are the basis for more complex approaches.

6.2   ROI DEFINITION AND CENTROIDS

The easiest way to identify a region on an image is to draw an area that defines the region-of-interest (ROI) and to evaluate gray values ρ only within that ROI. This method is by no means automatic, but does nevertheless play an important role for many practical applications. The selection of the rectangular signal-free area for Example 3.7.5 is a classical example for a ROI. An automatic registration algorithm delineating a certain area or volume within an image does also provide a ROI. Usually, it is planned that the ROI coincides with the anatomical region of interest as a result of the segmentation procedure. However, in certain imaging modalities, a ROI can also consist of a more general bounding box, where the remainder of the segmentation can be done by selecting intensities. A typical example is ROI selection in nuclear medicine, where absolute count rates, giving a measure of metabolic activity, may be of greater interest than anatomical detail connected to that region of the body. Section 6.8.1 gives a very simple example of such a procedure.

Connected to any ROI is also the centroid of this very region. The centroid of a ROI is usually defined as a central point that gives a reference position for that ROI. Throughout this book, we will encounter the centroid in several occasions, for instance if a precise figure for the position of an extended structure such as a spherical marker is required, or if a reference position for decoupling rotation and translation of point clouds is required. More on this topic can be found in Section 9. In general, a centroid is computed as the average vector of all vectors of the ROI-boundary:

$$\vec{r}_{\text{centroid}} = \frac{1}{N} \sum_{i=1}^{N} \vec{r}_i \qquad (6.1)$$

For a symmetrical ROI like a segmented fiducial marker of spherical shape, this centroid is also the most accurate estimate for the marker's position. However, if the ROI is not given by a boundary, but by an intensity region, the vectors pointing at the pixels which are part of the ROI are to be weighted with their actual gray value before they are summed up.

6.3   THRESHOLDING

The tedious process of drawing ROIs in images – especially if they are given in 3D – can be simplified by algorithms. Here, the ROI is defined by the segmentation algorithm. While the outcome of an image is usually a binary mask that delineates a ROI, we should be aware that such a mask can of course be used to remove unwanted parts outside the ROI of a grayscale image. If the ROI is given in a binary manner, a component-wise multiplication (see also Section 3.1.1) of the ROI mask (consisting of values 0 and 1) achieves this. In Figure 6.15, you can see such an image containing the grayscale information inside the ROI only.

The most basic approach is to divide the image in areas that contain interesting information vs. areas that are not interesting by making a binary classification based on gray levels. One knows, for instance from Table 4.1, that bone usually exhibits an image density ρ above 50 HU. A very basic approach towards segmentation is to get rid of all voxels which have a density ρ below that value. This process is called *thresholding*. When performing a thresholding operation, a binary model of voxels is built. Figure 6.1 shows a segmentation result for an axial slice from a multislice CT scan of a heart. The volume was acquired at an early phase after injection of contrast agent. The left ventricle, the atrium, and the aorta show excellent contrast.

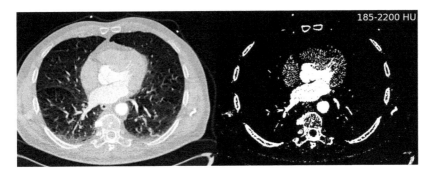

FIGURE 6.1: A segmentation example on a CT slice of the human heart. By defining an appropriate threshold, a binary image is created. The binary image contains, besides the bone and the contrast enhanced part of the heart, also parts of some large vessels in the lung and parts of the patient table. A full segmentation of the heart (or of parts of it containing contrast agent) without these additional structures is not possible by thresholding. Image data courtesy of the Dept. of Radiology, Medical University Vienna.

Usually, all gray scale information is lost and replaced by binary values, which automatically define a ROI. Another example is given in Figure 6.2, where a CT-scan of a patient's abdomen is thresholded, and subsequently, a rendering (a photo realistic visualization from the thresholded CT volume – see Chapter 8) of the thresholded volume was made using Analyze AVW.

In Figure 6.2, we see a lot of information, but none of these visualizations is very convincing. At no point in time do we see a particular part of the organs completely exposed. At lower thresholds, a mixture of soft tissue, contrast agent, and bone is visible. At higher thresholds, the bone with lesser density disappears, revealing quite ugly holes in the volume. A straightforward approach would be to apply an intensity transform that emphasizes the structure of interest, and to apply thresholding afterwards. Unfortunately, the diversity in man is so great that this only works to a very limited extent. Keep in mind that we are imaging physical properties of tissue, we are not taking images of organs. Therefore it cannot be excluded that two types of tissue have the same density. It is also a matter of fact that a certain type of tissue does not have one and only one type of radioopacity, but rather than that, a range in densities is covered. Things do even become more complicated when modalities with excellent soft tissue contrast such as MR are used. Here, a naive thresholding approach is bound to fail by nature.

A possibility to make thresholding a more sophisticated method is *local thresholding*; instead of defining a global threshold, which determines whether a pixel (or voxel) belongs to a given structure, one can also define a window around the local average gray value within a defined area. In short, a local thresholding algorithm consists of

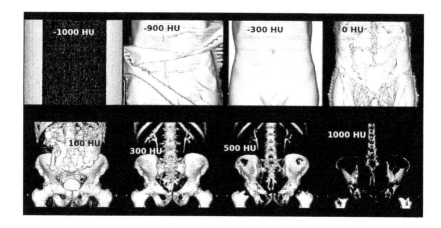

FIGURE 6.2: Eight rendered images of an abdominal CT-scan which underwent thresholding at different levels of the minimum image intensity. The first rendering was taken from the volume when setting the threshold to -1000 HU. The renderer displays the surface of the binary volume. Here, this is the shape of a cylinder. The threshold is so low that the air surrounding the patient in the CT was not removed. At a threshold of -900 HU, we see the blanket covering the patient. -300 HU is obviously a sufficient threshold to remove the blanket so that the skin of the patient becomes visible. The last image in the upper row was made at a threshold of 0 HU - the radioopacity of water. Part of the skin is now removed, and part of the musculoskeletal system becomes available. At 100 HU, large parts of the musculature are removed. The bladder containing contrast agent becomes visible, and so does part of the digestive system. At 300 HU, the bladder no longer gives sufficient contrast, but the renal system and the bones do. At 500 HU, we still see the renal system. Bone with lesser density is also removed. At 1000 HU, only the cortical bone remains. Image data courtesy of the Dept. of Radiation Oncology, Medical University Vienna.

the definition of a typical area (typically a circle with given radius, or a rectangle), in which the average gray value $\bar{\rho}$ is calculated.

the definition of a local threshold (or a pair consisting of an upper and lower threshold) which is defined as a percentage of $\bar{\rho}$.

the segmentation process itself, where the decision whether an image element belongs to the group to be segmented is based on the local threshold instead of the global threshold; this operation is confined to the previously defined area.

Local thresholding is rather successful in some situations, for instance when the image contains a gradient due to changing light – a classical example would be the photograph of a chessboard from an oblique angle. When using a global threshold, the change in image brightness may cause the rear part of the chessboard to vanish. A local threshold is likely to be successful in such a case. However, real life examples for such a situation in medical imaging are scarce, with the exception of video sequences from an endoscope.

Despite all of these problems, thresholding is an important step; it can be used to remove unwanted low-level noise outside the patient, for instance in SPECT or PET imaging, and it forms the base for more sophisticated algorithms like region growing and morphological operations, which we will explore in the next section.

6.4 REGION GROWING

The most straightforward measure to confine the thresholding process is to define a single image element, which belongs to the structure to be segmented. Such an element is called a *seed*. If a certain range of gray values is said to belong to a specific structure or organ, the region growing algorithm selects all image elements which are

within the defined threshold levels and

which are *connected* to the seed; connectedness is defined in such a manner that the image element must be in the vicinity of the seed, either by sharing a side, or by sharing at least one corner. You may recall Figure 5.9, where an illustration of connectedness is given. If an image element is connected to a seed, it becomes a seed by itself, and the whole process is repeated.

As you may recall from Chapter 5, two types of connectedness are possible in the 2D case – 4-connectedness and 8-connectedness. In the first case, only the four next neighbors of a seed are considered to be connected. These are the ones that share a common side. If one considers the neighbors that share a corner with the seed also as connected, we end up with eight nearest neighbors. In 3D, the equivalents are called 6-connectedness and 26-connectedness. An example of the region growing algorithm is the wand-tool in programs like Photoshop or GIMP (Figure 6.3 gives an illustration).

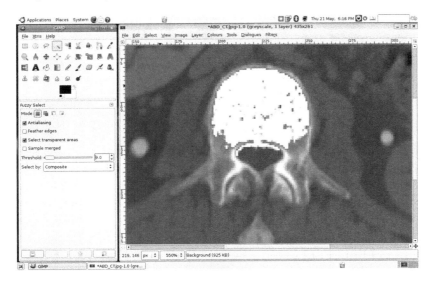

FIGURE 6.3: An effort to segment a vertebral body from the `ABD_CT.jpg` image from the lesson data using the wand-tool of GIMP. The cortical bones give a nice clear border; clicking in the interior spongeous bone of the vertebral body and selecting a window width of 9 gray values around the actual gray value at the location of a seed results in segmentation which is shown in white here. Selecting a larger window causes too large an area to be segmented; a smaller threshold results in a tiny spot around the seed; since GIMP is freely available, you are encouraged to try segmenting by changing the parameters of the wand tool. Image data courtesy of the Dept. of Radiology, Medical University Vienna.

While region growing is a huge leap compared to thresholding since it *localizes* segmentation information, it is also stricken with problems; playing around with the wand-tool of GIMP (or the equivalent tool in the Photoshop) gives an illustration of these problems. First of all, the choice of the upper and lower threshold is very tricky. Too small a threshold results in a cluttered segmented area, which is too small; a threshold window too wide causes an overflow of the segmented area. The wand is also not very powerful since the upper and lower threshold cannot be defined separately.

A segmentation effort of a contrast-filled compartment of the heart from a multislice CT-exam is given in Figure 6.4. The original image data are the same as in Figure 6.1. Here again, AnalyzeAVW was used. The three segmentation efforts should give the left ventricle, the atrium, and the aorta. Since the CT was taken at an early phase after injection of the contrast agent, these three parts of the organ give excellent contrast; by using a seed within the area of the aortic valve, it is to be expected that the method gives better results compared to simple thresholding as used in Figure 6.1, but still the algorithm is highly dependent on the internal parameters such as initial seed location and threshold window width. Furthermore, it is important to have a strong contrast in the initial image so that the anatomical region to be segmented can be clearly identified. Nonlinear intensity transforms and appropriate windowing as introduced in Chapter 4 are therefore also inevitable for a good segmentation result.

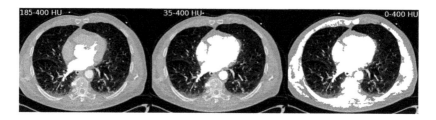

FIGURE 6.4: Three segmentation efforts of the contrast-filled phase of the heart CT-scan also shown in Figure 6.1. Different levels of minimum and maximum thresholds result in different ROIs to be segmented. The left image (with a threshold range of 185 – 400 HU) shows parts of the atrium, the left ventricle, and the aortic valve. Choosing a wider threshold of 35 – 400 HU also segments the parenchyma of the heart, and a small bridge also causes segmentation of the descending part of the aorta. When using a window of 0 – 400 HU, too many image elements are connected to the original seed, and large parts of muscle tissue and the skeleton are segmented as well. Image data courtesy of the Dept. of Radiology, Medical University Vienna.

Another problem with region growing in real life is the fact that anatomical regions do usually not show a sharp and continuous border to surrounding tissue. As the threshold window width grows, small "whiskers" usually appear in the segmented mask, which finally lead to a flooding of the whole image. These small structures are usually referred to as bridges; the straightforward way to deal with those is to manually introduce borderlines which must not be crossed by the region growing algorithm. In Example 6.8.3, you can experiment with implementing such a borderline. In real life, these bridges appear pretty often and require additional manual interaction, which is certainly not desirable. The middle and right part of Figure 6.4 show several bridges.

Having said all that, the most important problem is given by the fact that in medical imaging we often deal with 3D images, which are given as series of slices. While it is simple to apply global operations such as intensity transforms and thresholding, region growing in its raw form is pretty unsuitable for segmenting 3D volumes. In addition to adequate parameters for selecting the neighbors that belong to the structure to be segmented, we also need a method to propagate the seed through the volume, which is usually segmented slice-wise. If one naively transfers the seed to the next slice, the algorithm is bound to fail. The reason is the fact that structures which are connected in 3D may appear as separate structures in a single slice. A classical example is the aorta. If one looks at a contrast-enhanced CT scan of the heart like in Figure 6.4 it is evident that the aortic valve, the atrium and parts of the left ventricle are well saturated with contrast agent. The aorta, which leaves the heart in a caudal direction and makes a 180° turn (the aortic arch) to go down the spine, may appear as two circular structures on a single slice. Figure 6.5 illustrates this problem. Apparently it can be a difficult task to segment this structure using a slice-wise 2D region growing algorithm without additional knowledge of 3D anatomy. This 3D knowledge can be introduced by other methods such as statistical shape models or by level set methods, which will be introduced later on, but by itself, 2D-region growing cannot cope with such a problem.

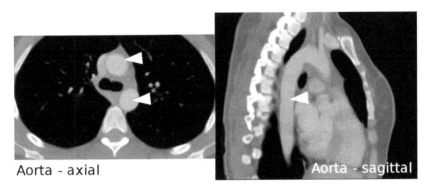

FIGURE 6.5: An illustration of typical problems encountered when dealing with 3D segmentation problems. The aorta in these CT images (indicated by white arrows) appears as a single structure in the right slice, which is reformatted in a sagittal orientation, whereas it shows up as two circles in the left axial slice. Image data courtesy of the Dept. of Radiology, Medical University Vienna.

6.5 MORE SOPHISTICATED SEGMENTATION METHODS

As pointed out before, segmentation of 3D structures can become intrinsically more delicate. In the following practical lessons, you will find two examples in Section 6.8.4, which give an illustration. Here, we demonstrate the effects of intelligent seed propagation in 3D. In general, all segmentation methods try somehow to define a ROI by following contours; they are, indeed, always based on propagating some kind of reference position towards a significant structure. In general, it might therefore be a good idea to apply some of the intensity transforms already encountered in Chapter 4. Furthermore, it might also prove useful to emphasize ridge lines that might correlate with anatomical structures using some of the methods from Chapter 5. The general problem of segmentation, however, stays the same – there is no simple solution to tell whether the intensities in an image give a good measure if an image element belongs to an anatomic structure or not. Therefore, the number of sophisticated algorithms published is considerable and goes beyond the scope of this book. For the sake of completeness, I will nevertheless try to give an outline of the common segmentation approaches.

Snakes or *active contours*: In general, snake-type algorithms are a special case of deformable models applied to volume data in a slice-wise manner. One may start with a general contour model, which adopts itself to a given contour by optimizing some sort of energy function. You may recall from Chapter 3 that an image is a mathematical function, which maps gray values ρ to pixel or voxel coordinates. ρ can be considered the height of a landscape – the valleys are, for instance, black, and the mountaintops are white. We know from basic physics that we can store *potential energy* when bringing a massive body to a mountaintop. If the points of our contour model are considered massive bodies, we may be able to find a contour by maximizing the potential energy. Example 6.8.5 gives a very simple illustration of this concept. Again, things are not as simple as they may sound – one has to define further boundary conditions. One of them may be that the adjacent points should stay close to each other, or more mathematically speaking, that the contour is steady and smooth. Or we may assume that the gain in potential energy of our mass points is diminished if they have to travel a very long way – in other words, it may be better to position your contour point on the nearest local peak of the ridge, rather than looking for the highest of all peaks. Finally, snakes are implicitly two dimensional. This is somewhat straightforward in medical imaging, where volume data are usually presented as slices. Still this is not very useful for many cases. Remember the example of the aorta in Section 6.4. A single anatomic entity such as the aorta may appear divided when looking at some of the slices. Therefore, the simple 2D way of looking at volumes is very often not optimal for segmentation tasks.

Live wire segmentation: A somewhat similar algorithm is the live wire algorithm, which takes a few edge points and fills the gaps to a contour; the merit function to be optimized for the image mainly operates on a gradient image, which can be derived by using edge detection methods such as those presented in Chapter 5.

Watershed transform: Another segmentation method for contours or contours derived from differentiated images is the watershed transform. Again, the contour of an image is considered a ridge line of a mountain range. When attaching buoys on each point of the ridge with a long rope, all you need is to wait for a diluvian and the line of buoys gives you the watershed transform of the mountain range. In other words, the valleys in the image are flooded, and while the water masses merge, they somewhat remember that they rose from different parts of the image.

Shape models: A technique to utilize a-priori knowledge of the organ to be segmented is the use of statistical shape models. Here, a gross average model of the organ to be segmented is generated from a large population of segmented 3D regions. Certain basis vectors for these shapes are computed by means of a *principal component analysis* (PCA). More details on the PCA and those basis vectors can be found in Chapter 7. In general, these shape models can be represented by a number of methods. The most simple way is to use the nodes of a surface mesh. Once a shape model is generated, it can be deformed by a linear combination of basis vectors. Intensity information, however, remains the main objective; the algorithm that selects the coefficients for the linear combination still relies on thresholding, region growing, or similar basic algorithms. However, by adopting the shape model, one also gets additional boundaries which mimic the organ to be segmented. The major advantage of shape-model type algorithms lies in the fact that it is 3D by nature and is not constrained by proceeding through slices, and that it takes more information than just the gray values of the image into account. Its disadvantage lies in the fact that the generation of the model requires a large number of representative samples, which all have to be segmented from clinical data. Furthermore, the use of a model constrains the algorithm's flexibility. One may generate, for instance a brain model. If this model is applied to a patient who underwent a neurosurgical procedure where part of the brain was removed, the algorithm is bound to fail. Unfortunately, we often encounter sick patients.

Level set segmentation: This is another method that utilizes some knowledge from beyond the intensity domain. Segmentation of a 2D image using level sets takes place by intersecting the 2D image with a surface model from 3D; in an iterative process, the higher-dimensional surface model given by a partial differential equation (PDE) may change its appearance until the intersection of the 3D surface with the 2D image yields the desired contours. It is of course also possible to intersect a 4D surface with a 3D volume, therefore the method is also an intrinsic 3D segmentation method. The adaptation of the higher-dimensional surface takes place by means of a so-called speed function, which is of course again coupled to image intensities. Active contours do offer the possibility to define the speed function.[1]

6.5.1 ITK SNAP – a powerful implementation of a segmentation algorithm at work

A beautiful implementation of a more sophisticated segmentation algorithm can be found if one searches for a program called *ITK SNAP*[2]. Figs. 6.6, 6.7 and 6.8 show the workflow of a typical segmentation progress, here again of a heart.

In short, ITK-SNAP utilizes an active contour model, which evolves based on the level set method. Intensity information from the image, together with an initial thresholding step are used for the definition of a primary model (called a *bubble* in ITK-SNAP) which evolves iteratively. The evolution is defined by a partial differential equation that also defines the shape of the higher-dimensional surface for the level set method. For the simple MATLAB-scripts used throughout this introductory course, the method is already too complex for a sample implementation. However, the reader is encouraged to download ITK-SNAP and to experiment with its capabilities.

6.6 MORPHOLOGICAL OPERATIONS

After a gross overview of the basic principles of segmentation, we also have to introduce a class of operations that are referred to as morphological operations. Once a model was segmented more or less successfully, one may encounter some residual debris, which may stem from intensity bridges – which is quite often the case when using region growing methods. Another source of stray image elements that are not connected to the actual segmented ROI may be image noise; when segmenting image data from nuclear medicine, this is actually pretty common since the main ROI can usually be segmented by thresholding.

---

[1] An introduction to the level set method with MATLAB® can be found in O. Demirkaya, M. H. Asyali, P. K. Sahoo: Image Processing with MATLAB: Applications in Medicine and Biology, CRC Press, 2008.

[2] A description can be found in PA Yushkevich, J Piven, HC Hazlett, RG Smith, J Ho, JC Gee, G Gerig: User-guided 3D active contour segmentation of anatomical structures: significantly improved efficiency and reliability, Neuroimage 31(3) 1116-1128, (2006)

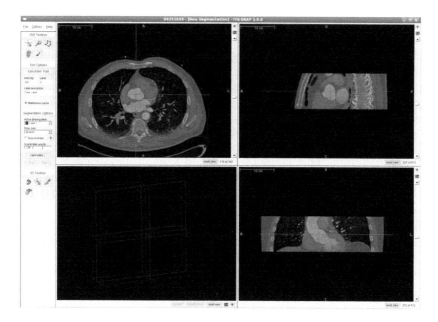

FIGURE 6.6: A screenshot of ITKSnap in its initial stage. Again, the heart CT scan already familiar from Figure 6.4 is used. The user can place a cross hair at an axial, sagittal and coronal slice; this is the 3D seed for the algorithm. Here, it is placed at the approximate location of the aortic valve. Image data courtesy of the Dept. of Radiology, Medical University Vienna.

A method to get rid of such segmented image elements that are either loosely connected or completely unconnected is a process called *erosion*. Erosion is the digital equivalent to sandblasting. When one wishes to clean a rusty piece of machinery, the method to clean such a piece of metal is to use an abrasive that is blown with high pressure onto the workpiece. The abrasive removes the surface layer of loose material and produces a ground surface. But as long as one does not use too much pressure or blasts onto one position for hours, the general structure of the workpiece is maintained. Erosion does the same thing to our segmented model. A kernel of defined shape wanders through the image; whenever the center of the kernel encounters an image element that is not zero (remember that the segmented model is usually binary), it checks whether its neighbors are non-zero as well; if the kernel is not completely contained within the segmented shape, the pixel at the center is removed. Mathematically speaking, the result of the erosion operation is the intersection of the original shape and the kernel. One may also remember the convolution operation introduced in Chapter 5, where a kernel is – figuratively spoken – intermixed with the image. The erosion operation is something similar, although it is non-linear by nature.

The opposite of erosion is *dilation*. Here, the union of the kernel and the shape is formed. If the center of the kernel lies within the segmented structure, it appends its neighbors to the shape. As a mechanical example, dilation can be compared to the coating of the shape with some sort of filler. Small defects in the shape, which might also stem from noise, can be closed by such an operation. In order to illustrate this operation, a rectangle with a small additional structure was drawn using the GIMP, and both erosion and dilation were applied. The result can be found in Figure 6.9.

The two operations can also be used together; if one applies an erosion followed by a

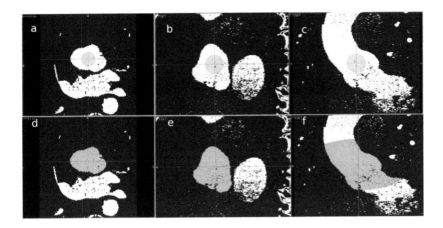

FIGURE 6.7: ITKSnap in progress. **a**, **b** and **c** show the initial bubble in the thresholded volume in axial, sagittal and coronal view. This is the *zero level* of the level set method. An appropriate global intensity threshold was also already applied to the image. As the algorithm iterates, it shows a constant growth in three dimensions, which reflects the change in the shape of the higher-dimensional manifold. This shape is bound by the borders indicated by the threshold. Note that the bubble does not penetrate every single gap in the pre-segmented image – it has a certain surface tension that keeps it from limitless growth. **d**, **e** and **f** show an intermediate stage of the segmentation process. Image data courtesy of the Dept. of Radiology, Medical University Vienna.

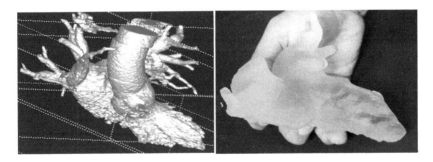

FIGURE 6.8: The result of the segmentation using ITKSnap after rendering (image on the left). The contrast agent's distribution mirrors the disease of the patient; he suffers from severe heart insufficiency, which causes little transport of the arterial blood and the contrast agent. Therefore, venous structures are also partially segmented. This 3D surface model can be "cleaned up" and smoothed using morphological operations, and transformed to a surface model – these techniques will be introduced in a later chapter. Once a triangulated surface model is available, the model can be printed using a 3D stereo lithographic printer. This tangible 3D model is shown in the photograph on the right.

dilation operation, the process is called *opening*; single image elements are removed by the erosion, and therefore cannot be dilated afterwards. Non-zero image elements enclosed by the segmented structure are widened and therefore are more likely not to be filled completely by the dilation process. The opposite operation – dilation followed by erosion – is called *closing*.

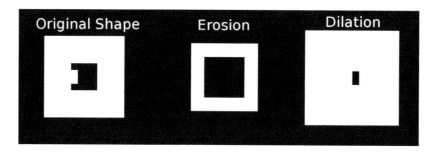

FIGURE 6.9: The effect of erosion and dilation using GIMP on a very simple shape (left image). After erosion, the rectangle is somewhat slimmer, and the internal additional structure is removed. Dilation causes the opposite effect; the internal structure was fused with the rectangle, and the whole rectangle got wider. Example 6.8.6 allows you to play with this image of 20 × 20 pixels. The shaping element is an eight-connected kernel of 3 × 3 pixel size.

Here, small black image elements within the segmented region are filled before the erosion process can open them up again. The advantage of both combined operations lies in the fact that they leave the surface and the shape of the segmented region somewhat invariant. Erosion by itself results in a thinner shape with less area than the original segmented shape. The dilation process compensates for this.

Given the fact that the generalization of erosion and dilation to 3D is pretty straightforward, it is evident that both operations can be extremely helpful when it comes to simplification and smoothing of segmented 3D models. Figure 6.8 gives a good illustration. The segmented 3D model of the left ventricle, the atrium, and the aorta was smoothed using an erosion process, which removed both loose residual 3D voxels and fine filaments connected to the pulmonary veins. In the fused deposition modelling process that generated the model shown in the left part of Figure 6.8, these fine structures would have caused considerable additional cost since the process deposits a fine powder in layers, which is cured by ultraviolet light. Each single stray voxel therefore requires a considerable deposit of so-called support material, which is necessary to keep the (completely useless) structure in position during the generation of the model.

6.7   EVALUATION OF SEGMENTATION RESULTS

Finally, we introduce two measures on the evaluation of segmentation results. If a model is segmented by an algorithm, it should be possible to compare this result to a gold standard segmentation. The first measure to evaluate the match of two contours is the *Hausdorff-distance* of two graphs. The Hausdorff-distance gives the *maximum distance* between to surfaces or contours. As a matter of fact, it is easier to program a Hausdorff-distance than to explain it. Let's consider two sets of contour points, S_1 and S_2. Each point s_i of contour S_1 has a set of distances $\{d_i\}$ to all other points of contour S_2. If we select the smallest of these distances in this set $\{d_i\}_{S_1 \to S_2}$ (this is the *infimum*) and proceed to the next point of S_1, we end up with a set of minimal distances for each point in S_1 to all other points in S_2. The maximum of this set is called the *supremum*. It is clear that if we perform the same operation for all points in S_2, the result can be different because the smallest distance of a point in S_2 to S_1 can be completely different from all the distances in $\{d_i\}_{S_1 \to S_2}$. Figure

6.11 illustrates this. The Hausdorff-distance is defined as

$$H\left(S_1, S_2\right) = \max \left\{ \sup_{s_2 \in S_2} \inf_{s_1 \in S_1} d\left(s_1, s_2\right), \sup_{s_1 \in S_1} \inf_{s_2 \in S_2} d\left(s_1, s_2\right) \right\}. \qquad (6.2)$$

Besides being a tool for evaluation, the Hausdorff-distance does of course also allow to construct a segmentation criterion, for instance in an active contour model.

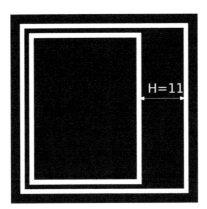

FIGURE 6.10: Two very simple shapes; the original image is used in Example 6.8.8.1 and is 40×40 pixel large. The Hausdorff distance is 11 pixels and is drawn into the image. There are of course larger distances from points on the inner rectangle to the outer square. But the one shown here is the *largest* of the possible *shortest* distances for points on the two shapes.

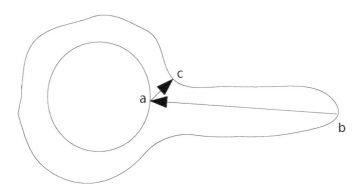

FIGURE 6.11: An illustration of the asymmetric nature of the Hausdorff distance. The minimum distance from point **a** to the outer shape leads to point **c**, whereas the shortest distance from point **b** on the outer shape leads to point **a**.

The other measure is a little bit easier to understand; it is the Dice-coefficient, defined by the overlap of two pixel sets A_1 and A_2. It is given as

$$D = \frac{2\left|A_1 \cap A_2\right|}{\left|A_1\right| + \left|A_2\right|} \qquad (6.3)$$

$|A_1 \cap A_2|$ is the absolute number of intersecting pixels (the pixels that share the same area) and $|A_i|$ is the sum of pixels in each area. Example 6.8.8.1 illustrates both concepts.

6.8 PRACTICAL LESSONS

6.8.1 Count rate evaluation by ROI selection

ROIExample_6.m implements the evaluation of activity in a given ROI, a common procedure from nuclear medicine. Here, we have a very simple series of images. It is a Petri–dish filled with a radioisotope, placed on a γ-camera. In the folder ROI in the LessonData, you find eight DICOM files alongside with the corresponding JPG images. Figure 6.12 shows a part of two of those images. A typical task in nuclear medicine is the monitoring of clearance rates of a tracer. For this purpose, one usually defines a ROI and measures the intensity as detected by the γ-camera or another modality for nuclear medicine. In this example, the ROI is the whole image since we only see the Petri dish. We therefore have to open the eight images, sum up the intensity in the ROI, and compare the results of this time series.

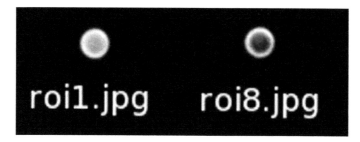

FIGURE 6.12: Two out of the eight images used for this example. We see the image of a Petri–dish filled with a radioisotope taken with a γ-camera. The bottom of the dish features a rim; according to the inverse-square law, the rim is brighter than the bottom of the dish, which is slightly elevated over the scintillator. The right image was taken at a later point in time, therefore the intensity in the image is lower. Image data courtesy of the Dept. of Nuclear Medicine, Medical University Vienna.

First, we have to change the working directory to the ROI directory by using the cd ROI command, and we have to find out about the DICOM-header sizes of the eight files in the ROI directory; I have already computed those header sizes. These are stored in a vector called headersize:

```
1:> cd ROI;
2:> headersize=zeros(8,1);
3:> headersize(1,1)=5710;
4:> headersize(2,1)=5712;
5:> headersize(3,1)=5682;
6:> headersize(4,1)=5696;
7:> headersize(5,1)=5702;
8:> headersize(6,1)=5700;
9:> headersize(7,1)=5704;
10:> headersize(8,1)=5698;
```

Next, we will allocate the matrix for the 256×256 image of 16 bit depth, and the vector for the cumulative image intensities. A text file storing the data will also be created:

```
11:> img = zeros(256,256);
12:> intens=double(zeros(8,1));
13:> ifp=fopen('Intensities.txt','w');
```

In the next few steps, we will open all eight DICOM files, skip their headers (whose size is stored in the **headersize** vector), and sum up the pixel intensities of the images. These are stored in a text file and plotted.

```
14:> for ind=1:8
15:> message=sprintf('Reading file #%d\n',ind);
16:> fname=sprintf('roi%d',ind);
17:> fp=fopen(fname, 'r');
18:> fseek(fp,headersize(ind,1),'bof');
19:> img(:)=fread(fp,(256*256),'short');
20:> fclose(fp);
21:> intsum = 0;
22:> for j=1:256
23:> for k=1:256
24:> rho = double(img(j,k));
25:> intsum = intsum + rho;
26:> end
27:> end
28:> intens(ind,1)=floor(intsum);
29:> fprintf(ifp,'%d\n',intens(ind,1));
30:> end
31:> fclose(ifp);
32:> plot(intens)
33:> cd ..
```

All of this you have seen before, and the example so far is trivial. It can even be made more simple if you use the **dicomread** functionality available in MATLAB's image processing toolbox. So here is the part that requires some work on your side:

Additional Tasks

Which isotope was used?

Repeat the procedure with **roi....jpg** images in the **ROI** folder; the corresponding file **ROIExampleWithJPGs_6.m** is also in the **LessonData**-folder. What is the result for the radioisotope, and why is it wrong?

In order to answer the first question, you have to find out about the half-life of the isotope. For this purpose, one has to find out about the time between the images. This can be done by checking the DICOM-header. Tag (0008|0032) gives you the acquisition time as a text string as hour, minute and second. You can write the acquisition times in a spreadsheet and plot the content of the **Intensities.txt** file with the appropriate time intervals. What you see then is the reduction of cumulative image intensity caused by the decay of the isotope. The recorded image intensity is proportional to the radioactive nuclei available, and their number follows the *law of radioactive decay*:

$$N(t) = N(t_0) * e^{-\lambda t} \tag{6.4}$$

$N(t)$ is the number of nuclei at time t, and $N(t_0)$ is the number of nuclei when the measurement starts. λ is the so called decay constant. The half-life $T_{\frac{1}{2}}$ is given as $T_{\frac{1}{2}} = \frac{\ln 2}{\lambda}$. As long as the detector of the γ camera takes its measurements in a more or less linear part of its dynamic range (see Figure 4.2), the cumulative image intensity at time t is proportional to $N(t)$. Therefore, half-life can be computed from the data in the `Intensities.txt` file. As a further hint, I can assure you that the isotope used here is a pretty common one in nuclear medicine.

The second question is a more philosophical one. The answer lies in the fact that *medical images are not just pretty pictures*. Most common image formats like JPG store grayscale images at 8 bit depth, and this is fine if you don't want to do anything but to look at them. For analytical use, this compression in intensity space is not permissible since the cumulative intensities are no longer proportional to the measured count rate of the γ-camera, which is by itself proportional to the number of nuclei. Remember – we are dealing with mathematical functions showing the physical properties of tissue, we are not just taking photographs. For the same reason, we have used DICOM images in Example 3.7.5 for the computation of SNR values.

6.8.2 Region definition by global thresholding

Here is a simple one; we try a global threshold on the `ABD_CT.jpg` image provided with the example. The threshold is set to 150. You should try different thresholds and interpret the image. The script is called `Threshold_6.m`:

```
1:> img = imread('ABD_CT.jpg');
2:> segimg = zeros(261,435);
3:> thresh = 150;
4:> for i=1:261
5:> for j=1:435
6:> if img(i,j) >= thresh
7:> segimg(i,j)=64;
8:> end
9:> end
10:> end
11:> colormap(gray)
12:> image(segimg)
```

Additional Tasks

The result of `Threshold_6.m` is a binary image with pixel intensities of 0 and 64; by using image algebra techniques such as the ones introduced in Section 3.1.1 and Example 3.7.1, it is possible to generate a greyscale image of the segmented ROI. Modify `Threshold_6.m` accordingly.

6.8.3 Region growing

First, we will implement region growing using a very simple 2D image, which is shown before and after segmentation by region growing in Figure 6.13. This is, again, not a very clinical image; however, it is usually a good idea to test algorithms on very simple images before proceeding to the more complex material encountered in real life.

So here we go with a very simple implementation of region growing; the script is found

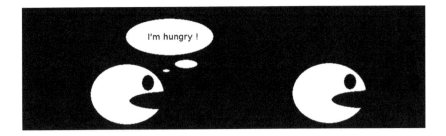

FIGURE 6.13: The left image is the original phantom image, which will be used for our example in the first place. After choosing a seed within the head of this little character and an appropriate threshold range, applying a region growing algorithm using four-connected neighbors results in the right image.

in the `LessonData` folder, and it is named `RegionGrowing_FourConnected_6.m`. As usual, we open the image first, and we cast it by force to the data type `uint8`. A second matrix named `seedmask` is openend, and an initial seed is placed at the pixel coordinate (130, 210). This seed assumes the value 64 as opposed to the remainder of the matrix. The intensity of the pixel at the location of the seed is retrieved:

```
1:> img = uint8(imread('PACMAN_THINKS.jpg'));
2:> seedmask=zeros(261,435);
3:> seedmask(130,210)=64;
4:> seedintensity=img(130,210);
```

Next, we define a range of possible pixel intensities around the intensity of the seed; here, we define a range of ± 10 gray values around the intensity of the seed. If these intensity limits are beyond the image range, they are truncated to the upper and lower bound of the image range. Strictly speaking, this is not necessary since too large a range will not affect the outcome. But it is good manners to take care of things like that:

```
5:> seedrangemin=seedintensity-10;
6:> if seedrangemin < 0
7:> seedrangemin = 0;
8:> end
9:> seedrangemax=seedintensity+10;
10:> if seedrangemax > 255
11:> seedrangemax = 255;
12:> end
```

Now, an iterative process is started; we initialize two counter variables, `oldseeds` and `newseeds`, which hold the number of seeds during each iteration. After that, we enter a `while`-loop, which terminates when no new seeds are found in the next iteration – the operator ~=, which is "not equal" in MATLAB, is introduced here. In each iteration, the `newseeds` found in the previous run become the `oldseeds` of the current run. Next, we inspect every pixel of the image `seedmask` containing the seeds; only the pixels on the very edge of the image are not taken into account since this simplifies life when looking for neighboring pixels (otherwise we would need a special check whether we are still inside the image while looking for neighbors). If a seed is encountered, the algorithm looks whether the image intensity `intens` of its four-connected neighbors is within the intensity range; if this is the case, these neighbors also become seeds. The `while` loop terminates if the number of seeds becomes constant. Finally, the segmented area, stored in `seedmask` is displayed. The results should resemble the right image in Figure 6.13. However, the image is a 1 bit image, which simplifies the segmentation task considerably.

```
13:> oldseeds = 1;
14:> newseeds = 0;
15:> while newseeds ~= oldseeds
16:> oldseeds = newseeds;
17:> newseeds = 0;
18:> for i = 2:260
19:> for j = 2:434
20:> if seedmask(i,j) > 0
21:> intens=img((i-1),j);
22:> if (intens >= seedrangemin) &
(intens <= seedrangemax)
23:> newseeds = newseeds + 1;
24:> seedmask((i-1),j) = 64;
25:> end
26:> intens=img((i+1),j);
27:> if (intens >= seedrangemin) &
(intens <= seedrangemax)
28:> newseeds = newseeds + 1;
29:> seedmask((i+1),j) = 64;
30:> end
31:> intens=img(i,(j-1));
32:> if (intens >= seedrangemin) &
(intens <= seedrangemax)
33:> newseeds = newseeds + 1;
34:> seedmask(i,(j-1)) = 64;
35:> end
36:> intens=img(i,(j+1));
37:> if (intens >= seedrangemin) &
(intens <= seedrangemax)
38:> newseeds = newseeds + 1;
39:> seedmask(i,(j+1)) = 64;
40:> end
41:> end
42:> end
43:> end
44:> end;
45:> colormap(gray)
46:> image(seedmask)
```

Additional Tasks

Another image, `PACMAN_THINKS_WITH_A_BRIDGE.jpg`, features an artifact. A thin line connects the head of the character with another structure. If you try to segment this image, you will end up with a larger segmented image, containing unwanted areas.

You can suppress this by adding an additional border, which can, for instance, be a straight line from pixel coordinates (110,240) to (110,270). In the algorithm, this line should represent a taboo, where no new seeds are accepted. Implement such a border in the `RegionGrowing_FourConnected_6.m` script so that the original image as in Figure 6.13 is segmented again.

Try to use the algorithm on the `ABD_CT.jpg` image provided, and segment the vertebral body from the image. The seed can remain on the same location, but you should experiment with the intensity range. Initially, the result is found in Figure 6.14. It may also be useful to manipulate overall image contrast, for instance by applying the algorithms presented in Example 4.5.4. Figure 6.15 shows two more segmentation efforts using region growing that were made using the AnalyzeAVW software; it is evident that the seed location and the intensity window obviously play a crucial role.

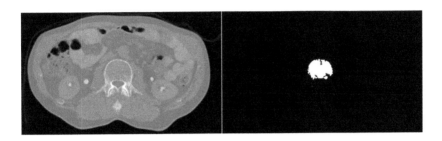

FIGURE 6.14: The result when using the `RegionGrowing_FourConnected_6.m` script on the `ABD_CT.jpg` image. The vertebral body is not fully segmented. Changing the image intensities and the intensity range for the segmentation algorithm may improve the result. However, this segmentation can be directly compared to Figure 6.3. Image data courtesy of the Dept. of Radiology, Medical University Vienna.

6.8.4 Region growing in 3D

In this example, we will show some principles of 3D segmentation. For this purpose, we will again design a simple theoretical phantom. The volume consists of a 3D matrix, where a tubular structure proceeds from slice # 1 to slice # 80. Figure 6.16 shows some of these slices.

So here is the variation of the `RegionGrowing_FourConnected_6.m` script that operates in 3D. First, a volume named `vol` with $100 \times 100 \times 70$ voxels is generated. In the following `for ...` loop, each slice – the z-component of the 3D matrix `vol` – is visited, and a circle of 19 pixels diameter is drawn. The center of the circle follows the 3D diagonal of the data cube. The `if ...` statements make sure that only the pixels within a circular shape are drawn into the slices, and that the circles remain within the boundaries of the slices. The script is called `RegionGrowing_WanderingStaticSeed_6.m`.

```
1:> vol = zeros(100,100,70);
2:> for i=1:70
3:> sl=sqrt(2*i*i);
4:> for x=-9:9
5:> for y=-9:9
6:> if (x*x+y*y < 100)
```

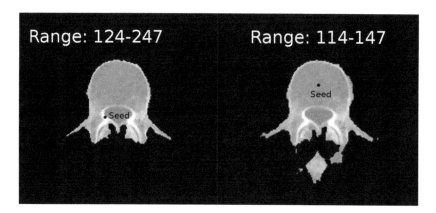

FIGURE 6.15: Two more segmentations of the vertebral body from the `ABD_CT.jpg` image. These results were achieved using the Analyze AVW software. As we can see, both seeds are located within the vertebral body; despite the fact that the range for finding connected pixels was adopted, the result varies significantly. As a conclusion, we see that the region growing algorithm is highly dependent on internal parameters. Image data courtesy of the Dept. of Radiology, Medical University Vienna.

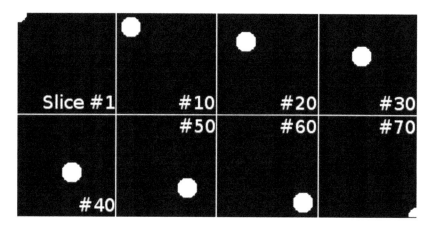

FIGURE 6.16: Some of the slices in the simple tube phantom volume generated by the `RegionGrowing_WanderingStaticSeed_6.m` script. The tube starts at the bottom of the volume in the upper left corner and proceeds along the 3D diagonal of the volume to the lower right corner in the last slice.

```
7:> sx=floor(sl+x);
8:> sy=floor(sl+y);
9:> if (sx > 0) & (sx < 100)
10:> if (sy > 0) & (sy < 100)
11:> vol(sx,sy,i)=255;
12:> end
13:> end
14:> end
```

```
15:> end
16:> end
17:> end
```

In the next part of the script, we proceed through the volume slice by slice again. For this purpose, again a `for` ... loop is used, and the slices are copied from the `vol` datacube to a 2D slice image `img`.

```
18:> for slice=1:70
19:> img = zeros(100,100);
20:> for i=1:100
21:> for j=1:100
22:> img(i,j)=vol(i,j,slice);
23:> end
24:> end
```

What follows is mostly a copy of code from the already well-known `RegionGrowing_FourConnected_6.m` script. The only difference is the location of the seed, which is given at a static position $\mathbf{x} = (2, 2, \# \text{ of slice})^T$; its intensity is also fixed to $\rho = 255$, and all four connected neighbors within an intensity range of $\rho \in \{245 \ldots 255\}$ are segmented.

```
25:> seedmask=zeros(100,100);
26:> seedmask(2,2)=255;
27:> seedintensity=255;
28:> seedrangemin=seedintensity-10;
29:> if seedrangemin < 0
30:> seedrangemin = 0;
31:> end
32:> seedrangemax=seedintensity+10;
33:> if seedrangemax > 255
34:> seedrangemax = 255;
35:> end
36:> oldseeds = 1;
37:> newseeds = 0;
38:> while oldseeds ~= newseeds
39:> oldseeds = newseeds;
40:> newseeds = 0;
41:> for i = 2:99
42:> for j = 2:99
43:> if seedmask(i,j) > 0
44:> intens=img((i-1),j);
45:> if (intens >= seedrangemin) &
(intens <= seedrangemax)
46:> newseeds = newseeds + 1;
47:> seedmask((i-1),j) = 255;
48:> end
49:> intens=img((i+1),j);
50:> if (intens >= seedrangemin) &
(intens <= seedrangemax)
51:> newseeds = newseeds + 1;
52:> seedmask((i+1),j) = 64;
```

```
53:> end
54:> intens=img(i,(j-1));
55:> if (intens >= seedrangemin) &
(intens <= seedrangemax)
56:> newseeds = newseeds + 1;
57:> seedmask(i,(j-1)) = 64;
58:> end
59:> intens=img(i,(j+1));
60:> if (intens >= seedrangemin) &
(intens <= seedrangemax)
61:> newseeds = newseeds + 1;
62:> seedmask(i,(j+1)) = 64;
63:> end
64:> end
65:> end
66:> end
67:> end
```

After each slice, the result is shown; after a few iterations, nothing but the seed itself remains in the image. At that point in time, you may terminate the script by pressing `Ctrl-C`. The `Press RETURN to proceed` ... statement halts the script in a very old fashioned way.

```
68:> colormap(gray)
69:> image(seedmask)
70:> foo=input('Press RETURN to proceed ...');
71:> end
```

Additional Tasks Since it is obvious that this naive approach does not work in 3D, you should find a method to change the seed position in such a manner that the whole tube is being segmented. Two methods of migrating the seed appear straightforward.

> Instead of just pushing the seed up one slice, you can compute the centroid of your segmented ROI according to Equation 6.1, and use this position as your new seed after propagating it to the next slice. As long as the tube does not get too thin (which is not the case here), you should be able to succeed.

> You may also push your seed to the next slice and initiate a search within a finite radius which looks for pixels in the desired intensity range. As soon as a pixel is found, it becomes the new seed. If no pixel is found, you may terminate the script.

In order to make the whole thing a little bit less tedious to watch, you may add an `if` clause at the end of the script which only shows every tenth segmented image:

```
...:> if mod((slice-1),10) == 0
...:> image(seedmask)
...:> foo=input('Press RETURN to proceed ...');
...:> end
...:> end
```

In this example, we have introduced an important principle of advanced segmentation algorithm, which may be described as *adaptive* – the seed (or, in more complex algorithms, the boundary) of the segmented ROI adopts itself to a new situation using prior knowledge.

6.8.5 A very simple snake-type example

SimpleSnakeSeeds_6.m is another example where we try to segment the vertebral body from the ABD_CT.jpg image. Spoken in a highly simplified manner, snakes are graphs that adopt themselves to border lines of strongly varying intensity in an image. In our example, we will initiate such a graph by drawing a circle around the vertebral body. Figure 6.17 shows the initial phase and the result of the SimpleSnakeSeeds_6.m script. The seeds search for the brightest pixel in a nearby area, and we hope that these correspond to the structure we want to segment.

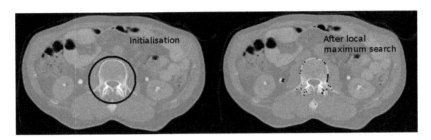

FIGURE 6.17: The initialization phase and the outcome of the SimpleSnakeSeeds_6.m script. First, seeds are defined around the vertebral body by placing them on a circle of 50 pixels radius. Then, the brightest pixel within a range of 20 pixels is determined. The seed migrates to that position. As we can see, the result shows some outliers where the seeds migrated to the contrast-filled leg arteries. Also, the subtle structure of the dorsal part of the vertebral body is not covered very well. Image data courtesy of the Dept. of Radiology, Medical University Vienna.

So here is the code of the SimpleSnakeSeeds_6.m:

```
1:> img = imread('ABD_CT.jpg');
2:> img=transpose(img);
3:> edgepoints=zeros(400,2);
4:> numberOfValidEdgepoints=0;
5:> for x=-50:50
6:> for y= -50:50
7:> if ((x*x+y*y) > 2401) & ((x*x+y*y) < 2601)
8:> numberOfValidEdgepoints =
numberOfValidEdgepoints+1;
9:> edgepoints(numberOfValidEdgepoints,1) = 210 + x;
10:> edgepoints(numberOfValidEdgepoints,2) = 145 + y;
11:> end
12:> end
13:> end
```

So far, we have read the well-known ABD_CT.jpg image, and switched the rows and columns of the resulting matrix. A 400×2 matrix edgepoints is allocated, which should hold a number of seeds. None of these edgepoints is allocated so far, therefore the counter numberOfValidEdgepoints is set to zero. Next, we define the coordinates of a circle of radius 50 around pixel $\vec{x} = (210, 145)^T$ using the well known parametric representation of a circle $x^2 + y^2 = r^2$ where x and y are the Cartesian coordinates of the diameter of the circle, and r is its radius. In order to avoid round-off errors from our discrete coordinates, every coordinate where $\sqrt{x^2 + y^2}$ is within the range of $\{49 \ldots 51\}$ is accepted. The result can be found in the left half of Figure 6.17. Next, we will instantiate a search for the brightest pixel in a neighborhood of radius `searchradius = 20` pixels.

```
14:> searchrad=20;
15:> for ei=1:numberOfValidEdgepoints
16:> ximax = edgepoints(ei,1);
17:> yimax = edgepoints(ei,2);
18:> imax=img(ximax,yimax);
19:> for x=-searchrad:searchrad
20:> for y=-searchrad:searchrad
21:> if ((x*x+y*y) < (searchrad*searchrad))
22:> xs=edgepoints(ei,1)+x;
23:> ys=edgepoints(ei,2)+y;
24:> if img(xs,ys) > imax;
25:> imax=img(xs,ys);
26:> ximax=xs;
27:> yimax=ys;
28:> end
29:> end
30:> end
31:> end
32:> edgepoints(ei,1)=ximax;
33:> edgepoints(ei,2)=yimax;
34:> end
```

All pixels within the `edgepoints`-matrix are visited, and using the already known parametric representation of a circle, the brightest pixel within `searchradius` is sought after. We also remember the coordinates of this brightest pixel using the variables `ximax` and `yimax`. After the search, the coordinates of an `edgepoint` are reset to the coordinates of this brightest pixel. All we have to do now is mark this position of the new `edgepoints` by drawing a small black cross at this position, and furthermore, the result is displayed using `image`. The result can also be found in the right part of Figure 6.17.

```
35:> for ei=1:numberOfValidEdgepoints
36:> img(edgepoints(ei,1)+1,edgepoints(ei,2)) = 0;
37:> img(edgepoints(ei,1),edgepoints(ei,2)) = 0;
38:> img(edgepoints(ei,1)-1,edgepoints(ei,2)) = 0;
39:> img(edgepoints(ei,1),edgepoints(ei,2)+1) = 0;
40:> img(edgepoints(ei,1),edgepoints(ei,2)-1) = 0;
41:> end
42:> img=transpose(img);
43:> maximg=double(max(max(img)))/64.0;
44:> img=img/maximg;
45:> colormap(gray)
46:> image(img)
```

The result is, admittedly, not very convincing. A few `edgepoints` migrated towards intense structures such as the femoral artery, and many converged to the same location, resulting in a very sparse outline. However, some of them did somehow find the cortex of the vertebral body.

The problem here lies in the fact that the energy of the single `edgepoint` – remember the introduction of the snake-algorithm in Section 6.5 – is defined in a very trivial way. We simply search for the highest peak within the search radius `searchrad`. A more intelligent version of our algorithm should consist of additional boundary conditions that define the energetic optimum. For instance, we can add a term that diminishes the potential energy if we try to place our `edgepoint` at a position that is already occupied by another `edgepoint`. The easiest way to achieve this is to set the intensity of a peak in the ridge of intensities to zero. A subsequent `edgepoint` will therefore find this position to be ineligible for an edge point, and will search for another maximum within `searchrad`. A modified script, `BetterSnakeSeeds_6.m`, does exactly this. The assignment

```
...:> edgepoints(ei,1)=ximax;
...:> edgepoints(ei,2)=yimax;
```

from `SimpleSnakeSeeds_6.m` is augmented by another assignment in `BetterSnakeSeeds.m`:

```
...:> edgepoints(ei,1)=ximax;
...:> edgepoints(ei,2)=yimax;
...:> img(ximax,yimax)=0;
```

The result is found in Figure 6.18. Compared to Figure 6.17, we see an improvement, although we still face the problems that some of our contour points still migrate to other structures of high intensity.

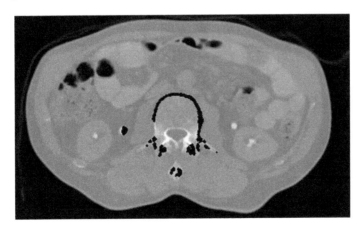

FIGURE 6.18: The result of the `BetterSnakeSeeds_6.m` script. Here, seeds cannot select the same position as an intensity maximum. Still, some seeds wander off to other structures since we have not yet introduced a criterion of contour smoothness. Image data courtesy of the Dept. of Radiology, Medical University Vienna.

Additional Tasks

In this oversimplified example, we were at least able to define parts of the cortex of the vertebral body. Still we are far from a satisfying result. Therefore, it would be interesting to take a few more measures. The one measure that might really help in this endeavor, however, would be a smoothness constraint on the contour; in a very simple manner, this can be introduced by taking care that neighboring contour points stay close together when migrating from the initial shape to the most intense pixel available. A simple way to achieve this in `BetterSnakeSeeds_6.m` is to move each point to the position of its predecessor before starting a search for a maximum pixel. The only problem here is a rather technical one. We have to take care that all the starting positions are sorted, so that two neighboring `edgepoints` are also indexed next to each other. This was done in a third script `BetterSnakeSeedsConstrained_6.m`. The result of `BetterSnakeSeedsConstrained_6.m` can be found in Figure 6.19. Compared to the earlier efforts from Figs. 6.17 and 6.18, the result is more encouraging – at least all the `edgepoints` finally migrated to the vertebral body, although the contour is still not well defined. Your task with this script is to inspect the code from `BetterSnakeSeedsConstrained.m` and find out what actually happens. Sorting the `edgepoints` is, by the way, achieved with the nasty old trick from Example 3.7.5. Why is this sorting necessary? Finally, you might also try to use some of the windowing and edge-enhancement operations from Chapters 4 and 5 to further improve the result.

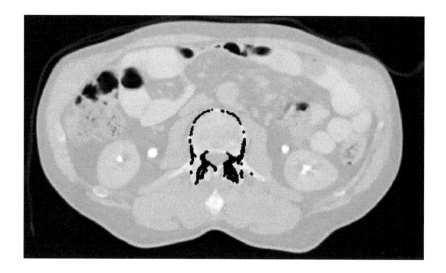

FIGURE 6.19: The result of the `BetterSnakeSeedsConstrained_6.m` script. By taking a few additional measures, smoothness of the contour was introduced in such a manner that each of the `edgepoints` searches for a maximum intensity in the immediate vicinity of its predecessor, who has already found a maximum. By this, it is made sure that the single `edgepoints` stay together. On the other hand, a full contouring of the cortex of the vertebral body has not been achieved. Image data courtesy of the Dept. of Radiology, Medical University Vienna.

We stop further efforts to refine the result of our contour-based segmentation algorithm, which is, in its simplicity, more a mixture of ideas from various segmentation methods. One possibility would be, for instance, adding the Hausdorff-distance as a further constraint. By subsequently adding constraints, we were able to refine the result – first, we were just pushing contour points towards the maximum pixel intensity ρ available. Second, we added the constraint that contour points must not occupy the same position, therefore the contour cannot contract to a single point. Finally, we told the contour points to stay close to each other. Figure 6.20 illustrates our approach. If we would continue our efforts, we might even be able to get a full segmentation of the vertebral body, but the effort to achieve this would make a rather extensive script necessary. Furthermore, we could also let our `edgepoints` propagate similar to the seed in Example 6.8.4 in order to get a three dimensional segmentation. In the case of region growing, we learned that the algorithm is highly dependent on internal parameters such as the intensity range defining the region, and initial seed location. We conclude from this example that this dependence on a proper choice of parameters also holds true for other algorithms such as contour models.

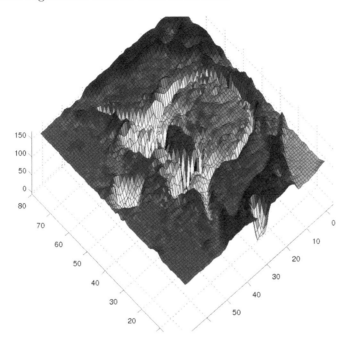

FIGURE 6.20: A surface plot of the vertebral body from `ABD_CT.jpg` illustrates our measures taken in the snake-type segmentation example. The image was inverted, and the contour of the vertebral body to be segmented now appears as a deep ridge in this plot. In the first example, we arranged a ring of marbles around the cortex of the vertebral body, and most of them fell into this groove, but they were infinitely small – therefore, several marbles could take the same place. In the next refinement, only one marble could take a position at the bottom of the groove. In the third step, we made magnetic marbles. The contour points stick to each other, and therefore they take positions at the bottom of this surface next to each other. In Example 6.8.8.2, we will deepen the groove using filtering techniques.

6.8.6 Erosion and dilation

`MorphologicalOps_6.m` is a script that implements erosion on the very simple shape from Figure 6.9. Let's take a look at it:

```
1:> img = imread('MorphologicalSquare.jpg');
2:> modimg = zeros(20,20);
```

So far, nothing new. We have opened an image, and allocated the memory for another image of the same size, which will contain the result of the operation. Next, we will visit every pixel besides those on the very edge of the image; if we encounter a non-black pixel, we will copy this pixel to the new image `modimg`. If we see that there is a neighbor that is zero, this pixel is deleted. The kernel hides in the `if` statement – the operator `||` is a logical OR, by the way.

```
3:> for i=2:19
4:> for j=2:19
5:> if img(i,j) > 0
6:> modimg(i,j)=1;
7:> if (img(i-1,j) == 0) || (img(i+1,j) == 0) ||
(img(i,j-1) == 0) || (img(i,j+1) == 0)
8:> modimg(i,j) = 0;
9:> end
10:> end
11:> end
12:> end
13:> colormap(gray)
14:> image(64*modimg)
```

Finally, the image is displayed. Figure 6.21 shows the result.

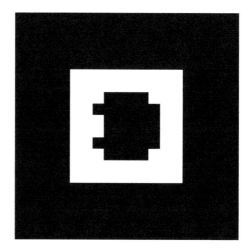

FIGURE 6.21: A shape, generated by erosion in `MorphologicalOps_6.m` from the shape `MorphologicalSquare.jpg`, which can be found in the `LessonData` folder and Figure 6.9. Denote the difference in this shape and the middle image in Figure 6.9, which was generated by using the erosion operator in the GIMP.

Additional Tasks

Modify the erosion kernel in such a manner that `MorphologicalOps_6.m` produces the same eroded shape as GIMP in Figure 6.9.

Modify `MorphologicalOps_6.m` in such manner that it performs a dilation, an opening, and a closing operation.

Threshold `ABD_CT.jpg` and perform some morphological operations on the result.

6.8.7 Hausdorff-distances and Dice-coefficients

`Hausdorff_6.m` implements a Hausdorff-distance on Figure 6.10. We have two images `Hausdorff1.jpg` and `Hausdorff2.jpg`, which can be combined to Figure 6.10. Let's take a look at the script; we read the two images, and we allocate a vector for the two Hausdorff-distances as well as a vector d which holds all possible distances for a point. `ind` is a counter variable:

```
1:> imgOuter = imread('Hausdorff1.jpg');
2:> imgInner = imread('Hausdorff2.jpg');
3:> dmax=zeros(2,1);
4:> d=zeros(1600,1);
5:> ind=1;
```

Next, we enter `imgInner` and if we encounter a non-zero pixel, we start computing its distance `dd` to all non-zero pixels in `imgOuter`. If `dd` is smaller than the smallest distance `dist` encountered so far, it is declared to be the smallest distance. `dist` is initialized to the diagonal of the 40×40 images, and by this, we compute the infimum of all distances. When all pixels in `imgOuter` were visited, this infimum of distances is stored in the vector d. If we are done with all pixels in `imgInner`, we determine the supremum of all distances as the maximum member of d and store it in the vector `dmax`. The same procedure is repeated with `imgInner` and `imgOuter` permuted, but this part of the code is not printed here. The Hausdorff-distance is the maximum of the two values in `dmax`. In this case, the two Hausdorff-distances are the same due to the geometric shape of the sample.

```
6:> for i=1:40
7:> for j=1:40
8:> if imgInner(i,j) > 0
9:> dist=57;
10:> for k=1:40
11:> for l=1:40
12:> if imgOuter(k,l) > 0
13:> dd=sqrt((i-k)^2+(j-l)^2);
14:> if dd < dist
15:> dist=dd;
16:> end
17:> end
18:> end
19:> end
20:> d(ind,1) = dist;
21:> ind=ind+1;
22:> end
23:> end
24:> end
25:> dmax(1,1)= max(d);
...
...:> HausdorffDistance=round(max(dmax))
```

`Dice_6.m` is comparatively simple. It implements Equation 6.3. The images `Dice1.jpg` and `Dice2.jpg` are the same as in the Hausdorff-example, but the contours are filled with white pixels. We read the images and compute the area of intersection as well as the areas of the single segmented areas. The resulting Dice-coefficient is 0.73. In an optimum case, it should be 1.

Additional Tasks

In the `LessonData` folder, you will find the outline of the two segmentation results from Figure 6.15. These are named `RGOutline1.jpg` and `RGOutline2.jpg`. Compute the Hausdorff-distance, and compare the two values in `dmax`.

6.8.8 Improving segmentation results by filtering

In the `LessonData/6_Segmentation`, you will find a subfolder named `ComplexExamples`. It contains examples on improving segmentation outcome by filtering and other operations.

6.8.8.1 Better thresholding

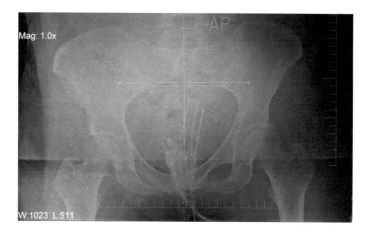

FIGURE 6.22: An x-ray image taken during a brachytherapy session. The localization of small radioactive pellets in hollow needles is monitored. Therefore, this image is a multi-exposure taken during the dwell times of the pellets, which are retracted by a flexible wire during the irradiation. Our target here is to segment the cross-shaped positioning aid by thresholding. Image data courtesy of the Dept. of Radiation Oncology, Medical University Vienna.

In this example, to be found in the subfolder `BrachyExample`, we have an x-ray taken during a brachytherapy session for treatment of cervical cancer (Figure 6.22). The patient receives a high local dose from small radioactive pellets inserted in the body through hollow needles. This is a multi-exposure x-ray, where the path of the brachytherapy-pellets (seen as bright spots on the image) is monitored while the pellets are retreated. Our (somewhat academic) task is to segment the positioning aid, that shows up as a cross in the image. In a further step, it would be possible to remove this structure from the image by local image interpolation. The x-ray shows a local gradient from right to left, which is most likely caused by the Heel effect.[3] One is encouraged to segment the structure from the image, for instance by using GIMP. The original image, already optimized for optimum gray scale representation by using methods similar to those presented in Chapter 4, can be found as

---

[3]The fact that some x-ray photons are trapped inside the anode cause this effect since the photons are generated in a region below the anode surface. Given the fact that the anode is sloped, a gradient in the resulting image is not uncommon.

image **a** in Figure 6.24. Thresholding this eight bit image with varying thresholds using GIMP yielded the following results:

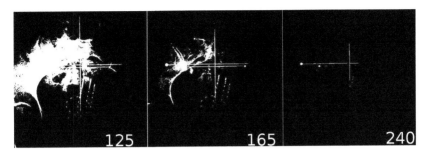

FIGURE 6.23: The x-ray image from Figure 6.24 after thresholding. The target structure is the cross-shaped positioning aid. Full segmentation of this image structure is not possible by thresholding. Image data courtesy of the Dept. of Radiation Oncology, Medical University Vienna.

In order to improve the segmentation, we can apply various operations which we already know from Chapter 5. First, the image is enhanced using an unsharp masking operation, similar to the operation we have introduced in Example 5.4.4. Next, a Sobel-filter (as it can be found in the examples from Chapter 5) is applied. The result undergoes thresholding and dilation – two operations we know from this chapter. The single preprocessing steps, carried out with GIMP, can be found in Figure 6.24.

Now, we will use some of our own scripts to go further. We could have done all this by ourselves as well, but the result would be the same. Since the cross-shaped structure consists of straight lines, we can apply a Hough-transform. The script from Chapter 5 was changed slightly; it is now named `StepOne_Hough_6.m`. It produces an image named `brachyhough.pgm`. In order to compensate for roundoff errors, this image is dilated using a script named `StepTwo_DilateHough_6.m`, which was derived from the script `MorphologicalOps.m` described in Example 6.8.6. The result is an image `brachydilate.pgm`. The third script, `StepThree_Threshold_6.m`, applies a threshold of 170 to the original image and stores the result as `brachythreshold.pgm`.

These three scripts are carried out by a fourth script, which is the only script one has to execute if you want to run the sample. It is called `BrachyCleanup_6.m`. First, it executes the three aforementioned scripts and clears the MATLAB workspace:

```
1:> StepOne_Hough_6;
2:> StepTwo_DilateHough_6;
3:> StepThree_Threshold_6;
4:> clear;
```

Next, we read the dilated retransform of the Hough-operation, and we load the thresholded image. Both images are scaled to an intensity range of $\rho \in \{0 \ldots 1\}$.

```
5:> dilimg=imread('brachydilate.pgm');
6:> dilimg=round(dilimg/255.0);
7:> thimg=imread('brachythreshold.pgm');
8:> thimg=round(thimg/255.0);
```

Now, we allocate memory for a new image, `mask`, and we perform a pixelwise multiplication of the thresholded image `thimg` and the dilated Hough-retransform `dilimg`. The result

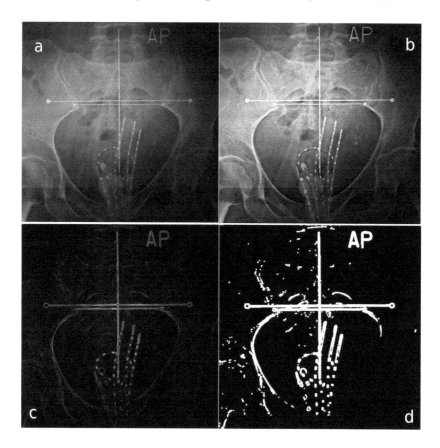

FIGURE 6.24: **a** shows the original x-ray, after optimization of image contrast. In order to improve the segmentation of the target structure, several preprocessing steps were carried out. **b** shows the image after enhancement by unsharp masking. In **c**, a Sobel filter was applied. This image was thresholded and dilated. The result, which will undergo further processing, can be found in **d**. Image data courtesy of the Dept. of Radiation Oncology, Medical University Vienna.

is a logical AND operation – only if both pixels are non-zero, the pixel in `mask` is non-zero as well. The results can be found in Figure 6.25. Finally, the result is saved as `Cross.pgm` and displayed using the `image` command.

```
9:> mask=zeros(512,512);
10:> mask=thimg.*dilimg*255;
...:>
```

I admit that this example is a little bit academic, but it illustrates two important aspects of segmentation; first, appropriate preprocessing of the image does help. And second, using a-priori knowledge (in this case the fact that our target structures are straight lines) can be incorporated for better segmentation results. The preprocessing steps shown in Figure 6.24 are also very effective when trying region growing. Figure 6.26 shows the outcome of segmenting the cross structure using the region growing algorithm of AnalyzeAVW.

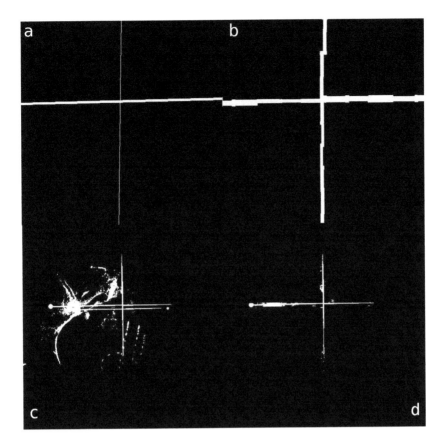

FIGURE 6.25: The single steps carried out by the `BrachyCleanup_6.m` script. Image **d** from Figure 6.24 undergoes a Hough-transform (**a**). The result is dilated (**b**) and undergoes a logical AND operation with the binary result of thresholding at a threshold of 165 (**c**), which results in the segmented structure **d**. You are encouraged to compare the result with Figure 6.23, namely illustration **b**, which was also segmented using the same threshold. Image data courtesy of the Dept. of Radiation Oncology, Medical University Vienna.

Additional Tasks

Compute the Dice-coefficient and the Hausdorff-distance for the images `brachyRegionGrowing.jpg` (Figure 6.26) and `Cross.jpg`, which is the output of the `BrachyCleanup_6.m` script. Both images can be found in the `LessonData` folder.

6.8.8.2 Preprocessing and active contours

The same principle of enhancing prominent structures can also be applied to our simple active contour example. The results from Example 6.8.5 were, in the end, already quite good. Still our snake also tends to converge to the inner cortex – this could be solved by modifying our initial shape to a torus – and it tends to neglect the processus transversus. We will try to apply some preprocessing to improve this outcome in the example given in the subfolder `ComplexExamples/SnakeWithPreprocessing`. Therefore, a few initial steps were applied using GIMP. First, contrast was optimized using a non-linear intensity transform,

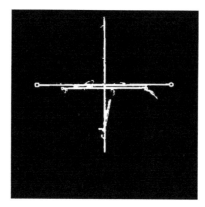

FIGURE 6.26: The effect of region growing on the preprocessed x-ray image shown in Figure 6.24 **d**. Image data courtesy of the Dept. of Radiation Oncology, Medical University Vienna.

similar to the Sigmoid-shaped intensity transform from Example 4.5.4. Next, we apply a Sobel-filter; the result undergoes thresholding. The steps are shown in Figure 6.27.

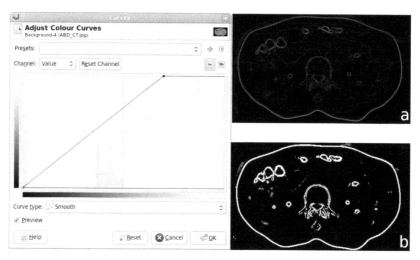

FIGURE 6.27: The preprocessing steps carried out using GIMP prior to applying a modified version of the `BetterSnakeSeedsConstrained_6.m` script. First, non-linear intensity transform is carried out in order to optimize the contrast of the image. Second, a Sobel-filter is applied. The resulting image is thresholded. Image data courtesy of the Dept. of Radiology, Medical University Vienna.

Next, one could apply the `BetterSnakeSeedsConstrained_6.m` directly to the thresholded Sobel-image from Figure 6.27. That is, however, not a brilliant idea since there is absolutely no gradient information in that image. Instead of this simple approach, we invest a little bit more effort in the image to be segmented. A small script named `Preprocessing_6.m` does all the work; first, it loads the original image `ABD_CT.jpg` and the image modified using GIMP called `ABD_CTSobeledThresh.jpg`:

```
1:> img=imread('ABD_CT.jpg');
```

```
2:> dimg=imread('ABD _CTSobeledThresh.jpg');
```

Next, it scales `dimg` to an intensity range $\rho \in \{0 \dots 1\}$, and the intensity range is shifted by one so that black is 1 and white is 2. Next, we avoid problems with the eight bit datatype of our images by scaling the original image `img` to a range $\rho \in \{0 \dots 127\}$, and we carry out a piecewise multiplication of `img` and `dimg`. As a result, the edges of the image are enhanced, and the result is saved as `ABD_CT_ENHANCED.jpg`.[4] The outcome of our operation is a gray scale image with strongly emphasized edges; it can be found in Figure 6.28. The operation we carried out was not very subtle since we have to avoid datatype-related problems for the sake of simplicity, but it serves the purpose.

```
3:> maxint=max(max(dimg));
4:> dimg=(dimg/maxint)+1;
5:> newimg=zeros(261,435);
6:> newimg=0.5*img.*dimg;
7:> imwrite(newimg,'ABD_CT_ENHANCED.jpg','JPG');
```

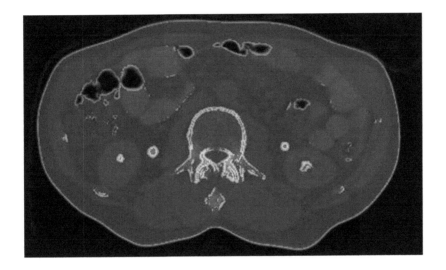

FIGURE 6.28: The result of the `Preprocessing_6.m` script. It loads the thresholded Sobel image from Figure 6.27, scales the intensities of the original `ABD_CT.jpg` image appropriately and enhances the edges in the image by a pixelwise binary multiplication. The result is not very beautiful – a more sophisticated operation would require some manipulations in image depth – but the result serves our purpose. Image data courtesy of the Dept. of Radiology, Medical University Vienna.

The second script we already know – it is a slightly modified version of `BetterSnakeSeedsConstrained_6.m` named `BetterSnakeSeedsConstrainedTwo_6.m`. This modified script

carries out `Preprocessing_6.m`.

operates on the result `ABD_CT_ENHANCED.jpg` (see Figure 6.28).

has a reduced radius of local search `searchrad` of 15 instead of 20 pixels.

---

[4]If you encounter problems with `imwrite` in Octave, you may as well save the image as a PGM file.

plots the `edgepoints` into the original image.

The result can be found in Figure 6.29. Now, at least the processi are also part of the contour, which was not the case in the original script. A further refinement would be possible by changing our initial shape – a circle – to the topologically correct model of a torus. Still, preprocessing by filtering has enhanced the result. In this case, region growing on the differentiated and thresholded image does not yield a satisfying result as it did in Example 6.8.8.1 since the contour cannot be segmented as clearly on the differentiated image.

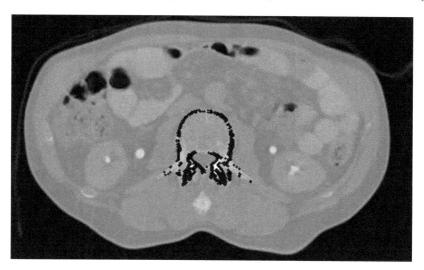

FIGURE 6.29: The result of `BetterSnakeSeedsConstrainedTwo_6.m`; one may compare the outcome with Figure 6.19. The edge-enhancement operation has led to a better approximation of the vertebral body shape – at least the transverse process is now also part of the contour, which may be refined by using less initial points and a second adaption step which uses interpolated points between those seeds. Image data courtesy of the Dept. of Radiology, Medical University Vienna.

6.9 SUMMARY AND FURTHER REFERENCES

Segmentation is certainly one of the more difficult areas in medical image processing. The large body of highly complex and innovative current research work documents this. However, the basic problem is that image intensities map physical properties of tissue, but not the tissue in its entirety. Unfortunately, the more sophisticated the imaging device, the bigger the segmentation problem may become. Segmenting muscle tissue in CT may be cumbersome, but it can be done. An MR image of the same area, which excels in soft tissue contrast, might be even the bigger problem, just because of that very good contrast. However – a large arsenal of segmentation methods exists and the skillful use of these methods should usually solve many problems. Still, manual interaction remains a necessity in many cases. In general, we can categorize the algorithms presented as follows:

Segmentation based on intensity values (thresholding).

Segmentation based on intensity values and one point being part of the ROI (region growing).

Segmentation based on intensity values and a topologically equivalent ROI boundary (snakes and similar algorithms).

Segmentation based on intensity values and a morphologically similar ROI boundary (statisitical shape models).

Sometimes it is also possible to avoid segmentation by using intensity based methods as we will learn in Chapters 9 and 8. In this chapter, only the most basic concepts were introduced: thresholding, region growing, and simple contour based algorithms. An important point also has to be emphasized: segmentation in medical imaging is, in many cases, a 3D problem. A slice-wise approach will not succeed in many cases. Therefore it is necessary to propagate seeds or edge points in an intelligent manner in 3D space.

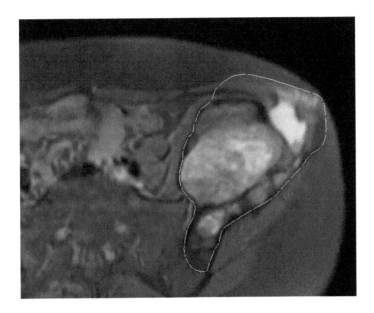

FIGURE 6.30: An illustration of the difficulties associated with segmentation. This axial MR slice shows a malignant orthopedic tumor in the hip. The manually drawn border shows the extent of this tumor as drawn by an expert. On image data like this, an automatic segmentation effort will always fail due to the considerable contrast detail of the malignant tissue and the complex and random shape of the lesion. Alternatively, the same lesion shows virtually no detail on other imaging modalities like CT. Image data courtesy of the Dept. of Radiology, Medical University Vienna.

Literature

T. S. Yoo: Insight into Images: Principles and Practice for Segmentation, Registration, and Image Analysis, A. K. Peters, (2004)

J. M. Fitzpatrick, M. Sonka: Handbook of Medical Imaging, Volume 2. Medical Image Processing and Analysis, SPIE Press, (2009)

E. R. Dougherty, R. A. Lotufo: Hands-on Morphological Image Processing, SPIE Press, (2003)

R. Baldock, J. Graham: Image Processing and Analysis: A Practical Approach, Oxford University Press, (2000)

CHAPTER 7

Spatial Transforms

Wolfgang Birkfellner

CONTENTS

7.1   Discretization – resolution and artifacts 215
7.2   Interpolation and volume regularization 216
7.3   Translation and rotation 219
    7.3.1   Rotation in 2D – some properties of the rotation matrix 219
    7.3.2   Rotation and translation in 3D 222
    7.3.3   A special case – the principal axis transform 224
    7.3.4   The quaternion representation of rotations 226
7.4   Reformatting 228
7.5   Tracking and image-guided therapy 229
7.6   Practical lessons 233
    7.6.1   Spatial image transforms in 2D 233
    7.6.2   Two simple interpolation examples 236
    7.6.3   A special case – the PCA on binary images 240
    7.6.4   A geometric reformatting example – conic sections 242
    7.6.5   A reformatting example on a small volume data set 245
    7.6.6   Convolution revisited 247
7.7   Summary and further references 249

7.1 DISCRETIZATION – RESOLUTION AND ARTIFACTS

Ever since Chapter 3, we are aware that images consist of 2D or 3D image elements. These elements are, by their nature, discrete. A change in image size therefore introduces artifacts, which may be considered rounding errors. Figure 7.1 gives an illustration. The original image is a PET-scan with 128×128 pixels in-plane resolution of a gynecological tumor located in the pelvis. The left part of the image was resized without interpolation – the single pixels appear blocky and enlarged. If we apply an interpolation procedure, which distributes the pixel intensities in a more sophisticated manner, we get the result on the right hand side. In short, enlarging the image consists of putting a finer mesh of image elements on the image data. If we don't distribute the image intensities in a smooth manner, a blocky appearance is inevitable. It is to be emphasized that interpolation does not add image information, but improves visualization of image data.

Another interpolation problem is illustrated in Figs. 7.12 and 7.17. Here, a rotation operation does not transfer all gray values from the original image to the rotated image due

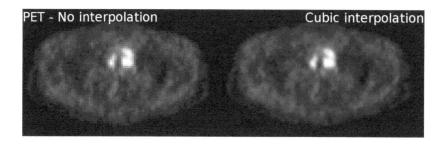

FIGURE 7.1: The effects of interpolation. The original image is an [18]FDG PET slice of a tumor located in the lower abdomen. The sub-image of the slice shown here was resampled from 84×50 pixels to 638×398 pixels, without and with interpolation. The left image fills the new pixels by the values from the nearest neighbor in the old image, whereas the right image distributes gray values ρ using a bicubic interpolation model. While there is no new information in the right image, visualization and interpretation is improved. Image data courtesy of the Dept. of Nuclear Medicine, Medical University Vienna.

to discretization artifacts. Figure 7.14 illustrates that, in such a case, even nearest neighbor interpolation can yield an improved result. Before we proceed to the more complex problem of rotation and translation in 2D and 3D, we will take a look at the interpolation problem and scaling.

7.2 INTERPOLATION AND VOLUME REGULARIZATION

Let's take a look at interpolation; the easiest way to interpolate between two discrete data pairs $(x_i, \rho_i)^T$ and $(x_j, \rho_j)^T$ is to draw a straight line. We know that the general shape of a linear function is $\rho = \rho_0 + ax$ where ρ_0 is the value that is connected to the doublet $(0, \rho_0)^T$ – this is the position on the ordinate where the straight line intersects it. a is the gradient of the function. If we interpolate, we can rewrite this function as

$$\rho = \rho_0 + \frac{\rho_1 - \rho_0}{x_1 - x_0}(x - x_0) \tag{7.1}$$

The term *bilinear interpolation* refers to the generalization of this method to a function in two variables. Here, a linear interpolation is carried out in one direction, and then the other direction follows. We can estimate the function values on the grid as shown in Figure 7.2 as follows:

$$\rho_{x,y_0} = \frac{x_1 - x}{x_1 - x_0}\rho_{00} + \frac{x - x_0}{x_1 - x_0}\rho_{10} \tag{7.2}$$

$$\rho_{x,y_1} = \frac{x_1 - x}{x_1 - x_0}\rho_{01} + \frac{x - x_0}{x_1 - x_0}\rho_{11} \tag{7.3}$$

$$\rho_{x,y} = \frac{y_1 - y}{y_1 - y_0}\rho_{x,y_0} + \frac{y - y_0}{y_1 - y_0}\rho_{x,y_1} \tag{7.4}$$

A closer look at Eqs. 7.2, 7.3 and 7.4 shows that we interpolate first in the x-direction, starting from coordinates y_0 and y_1. The final value is given by an interpolation in y-direction between the previously interpolated values. Just as we did in Section 5.1.2, we can

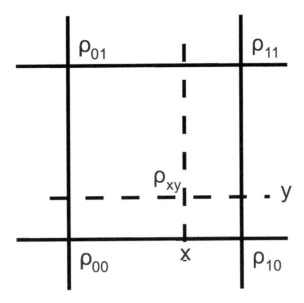

FIGURE 7.2: The basic principle of bilinear interpolation on a regular grid. Four nodes with known function values $\rho_{00} \ldots \rho_{11}$ are given. The function value ρ_{xy} on an arbitrary position $(x, y)^T$ is estimated by performing a linear interpolation in both directions.

simplify the whole thing by assuming the difference between pixel positions $x_1 - x_0$ and $y_1 - y_0$ to be one. Equation 7.4 therefore simplifies to

$$\rho_{x,y} = (y_1 - y)((x_1 - x)\rho_{00} + (x - x_0)\rho_{10}) + \\ (y - y_0)((x_1 - x)\rho_{01} + (x - x_0)\rho_{11}). \qquad (7.5)$$

Equation 7.5 can be written as a product of vectors and matrices (the subject of matrix multiplication will be reviewed in more detail in Section 7.3.1) if we assume x_0 and y_0 to be zero and x_1 and y_1 to be one:

$$\rho_{xy} = \begin{pmatrix} 1-y \\ y \end{pmatrix}^T \begin{pmatrix} \rho_{00} & \rho_{10} \\ \rho_{01} & \rho_{11} \end{pmatrix} \begin{pmatrix} 1-x \\ x \end{pmatrix}. \qquad (7.6)$$

The application of Equation 7.6 to image interpolation is obvious; we subdivide the original pixel into smaller units, and the gray value of these smaller pixels is computed from the four gray values $\rho_{00} \ldots \rho_{11}$. We can of course expand the bilinear interpolation to the 3D-domain. In such a case, the interpolated values for ρ_{xyz_0} and ρ_{xyz_1} are computed for the corresponding interpolated in-slice pixels for neighboring slices. Finally, a linear interpolation in the intra-slice z-direction is carried out. Unfortunately, an elegant formulation of trilinear interpolation requires the introduction of matrices with three indices (so-called tensors). This is beyond the scope of this book, therefore we will refrain ourselves to the following formula:

$$\rho_{xyz} \; = \; \begin{pmatrix} (1-x)(1-y)(1-z) \\ (1-x)(1-y)z \\ (1-x)y(1-z) \\ (1-x)yz \\ x(1-y)(1-z) \\ xy(1-z) \\ x(1-y)z \\ xyz \end{pmatrix}^{T} \begin{pmatrix} \rho_{000} \\ \rho_{001} \\ \rho_{010} \\ \rho_{011} \\ \rho_{100} \\ \rho_{110} \\ \rho_{101} \\ \rho_{111} \end{pmatrix}. \qquad (7.7)$$

The position of the eight gray values $\rho_{000} \dots \rho_{111}$ can be found in Figure 7.3.

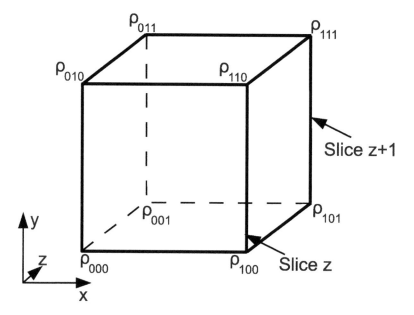

FIGURE 7.3: The conventions for performing a trilinear interpolation according to Equation 7.7.

More sophisticated interpolation methods, based on more complex functions that are usually modeled as differentiable numerical models (so-called splines), are available as well; however, for most applications, bi- and trilinear interpolation work just fine if we do not enlarge the image to a huge extent. Figure 7.4 shows a few examples of different interpolation techniques on the PET-image from Figure 7.1.

A special case of interpolation is the regularization of volumes. As pointed out in Section 3.1, voxels in medical imaging do not usually have a cubic shape. Therefore, it is a good idea to apply an interpolation procedure that assigns isotropic voxel dimensions to the volume before applying further image processing routines. This is a common problem in 3D US, where a number of images is taken. Depending on the imaging geometry of the 3D US scanhead, the slices can be positioned in a fan-shaped geometry relative to each other. In such a case, the spatial resolution may vary depending on the location of the voxels.

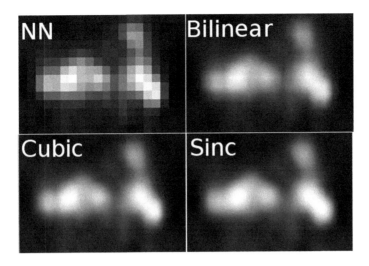

FIGURE 7.4: Different interpolation techniques, presented on a subimage from the PET image in Figure 7.1. The image was magnified fifteen times; at such a magnification, differences in interpolation models are evident. The image on the outer left was not interpolated; what follows are images that underwent bilinear interpolation, cubic interpolation, and interpolation using a sinc-function. All images were generated using GIMP. The image of the bilinear interpolation also shows an important property of this method: despite its name, bilinear interpolation is not a linear operation – it is the product of two linear operations. Therefore it is only linear in the direction of the coordinate axes; this results in the star-shape artifacts visible in the example. Image data courtesy of the Dept. of Nuclear Medicine, Medical University Vienna.

7.3 TRANSLATION AND ROTATION

7.3.1 Rotation in 2D – some properties of the rotation matrix

When rotating a single point given by $\vec{x} = (x, y)^T$, it is a useful approach to use a matrix R which is applied to this vector – the result is a new vector $\vec{x}'$. Such a matrix, which rotates a point in 2D by an angle ϕ is given by

$$R = \begin{pmatrix} \cos(\phi) & -\sin(\phi) \\ \sin(\phi) & \cos(\phi) \end{pmatrix} \tag{7.8}$$

The transformation of our 2D-point $\vec{x}$ can now be written as

$$\vec{x}' = R\vec{x} \tag{7.9}$$

As you may have read in the foreword, working in this book requires only little mathematics, but even a basic course in image processing cannot be mastered without some basics; some of them were already encountered in Chapter 5. Multiplication of matrices is another one of those basics; in order to multiply a matrix such as R from Equation 7.8 with a vector $\vec{x}$, we have to form the inner products of the matrix rows with the vector, and each of those inner products gives a component of the resulting vector. Inner products, however, are already well known from Chapter 5. As we know, the inner product can be computed as a sum of products of the corresponding vector elements. If we perform the matrix multiplication in

Equation 7.9, we get

$$\vec{x}' = \begin{pmatrix} \cos(\phi)x - \sin(\phi)y \\ \sin(\phi)x + \cos(\phi)y \end{pmatrix} \qquad (7.10)$$

That is the only time we will fully write down the transform of a position $\vec{x}$ to another position. When dealing with more complicated spatial transformations, we would drown in chaos if we would continue to deal with sines and cosines. However, a few more important words on matrix multiplication are necessary:

When multiplying two matrices, the number of matrix columns has to match the rows of the other matrix – otherwise, the matrix product cannot be computed. The components of the resulting matrix are given as the inner products of the respective rows and columns of the matrices; when computing the product of two matrices A and B, the components c_{ij} of the resulting matrix C are given as the inner product of the row number i of matrix A and column number j of matrix B.

Matrix multiplication is *not commutative*; let's consider two matrices A and B. The result of the matrix multiplication depends on the order of the multiplication: $AB \neq BA$. Furthermore, the transposition operation – the exchange of rows and columns – is connected to this behavior: $(AB)^T = B^T A^T$.

Matrix multiplication is, however, *associative*. The identity $A(BC) = (AB)C$ is true.

The inverse operation of multiplication with a matrix A is the multiplication with the inverse A^{-1} of the matrix. In MATLAB®, the inverse is computed by calling the command `inv`. The inverse only exists if A is not *singular*. A matrix is singular if its *determinant* is zero. In MATLAB, the determinant is computed using the command `det`. For a 2×2 matrix A, the determinant is given as

$$\det A = a_{11}a_{22} - a_{12}a_{21}. \qquad (7.11)$$

For a 3×3 matrix, a roughly similar scheme named the *Rule of Sarrus* can be used. The product of a matrix and its inverse is the identity matrix, where all components are zero besides those on the diagonal axis, which are one. An identity matrix has the same number of rows and columns. In MATLAB, an $N \times N$ identity matrix is generated by calling `eye(N)`.

Multiplication in MATLAB or Octave is always matrix multiplication. For single numbers (called scalars), this does not matter. A scalar is, however, a 1×1 matrix. If one wishes to multiply each element of a matrix with the corresponding element of the other matrix – which is not matrix multiplication and, more strictly speaking, not a multiplication in a mathematical sense – one should use the operator `.*` instead of `*`. This operation is also already known from Chapter 5. It requires that the matrices are of the same size.

For rotation matrices, we will use radians as the unit of choice for specifying angles; remember that an angle in radians is given as the fraction of the diameter of a circle with radius 1. Ninety degrees correspond to $\frac{\pi}{2}$.

Rotation matrices have two special properties. First, a rotation transformation does not change the length of a vector. Therefore, its *determinant* is always 1. If it is -1, the matrix introduces also a reflection. If you end up with a determinant of -1 after some transformations using rotation matrices, you have usually made a mistake.

Another possibility, for instance when registering two volume image datasets, is the fact that not all scanners necessarily produce images in a frame of reference of the same handedness; usually, the z-direction has to be flipped in order to get a useful result. The other property of the rotation matrix is that it can easily be inverted. The inverse of a rotation matrix is its transpose: $R^{-1} = R^T$. These two properties give the group of rotation matrices the name SO(2) (for 2D rotations) and SO(3) (for 3D rotations). Rotation matrices form the *special* and *orthogonal* group. A matrix A is special if its determinant is 1, and it is orthogonal if $A^{-1} = A^T$.

We usually carry out matrix multiplication from left to right. When generating the product of a matrix and a vector, we write this operation down as $A\vec{x} = \vec{x}'$. Those of you who work with OpenGL, a widespread API for visualization of 3D surface data, will notice that OpenGL uses a different convention. Vectors in OpenGL are given as a single row, whereas in our widespread convention, a vector is given by a single column. Therefore the same operation reads $\vec{x}^T A^T = \vec{x}'^T$ in OpenGL.

If we want to rotate an image by an angle ϕ, all we have to do is apply Equation 7.9 to every single pixel position $\vec{x}$, and to store its gray value ρ at the new position $\vec{x}\prime$. Example 7.6.1 illustrates this, and the result of this very simple operation can be found in Figure 7.12. However, the result of such an operation is usually not an integer, and therefore rounding artifacts may be inevitable.

After talking about rotation, we also have to take into account the second operation which allows for changing the location of pixels in an image – translation. Compared to rotation, translation – the shifting of image content by a constant vector $\vec{\Delta r} = (\Delta x \; \Delta y)^T$ is simple. We just add this vector to every pixel location $\vec{x}$ by adding $\vec{\Delta r}$. In Section 7.3.2 we will learn how to combine rotation and translation in matrix notation. However, the problem lies in the fact that translation and rotation do not commute either. Applying a translation before applying the rotation gives a different result compared to translation followed by rotation. Figure 7.5 illustrates this problem.

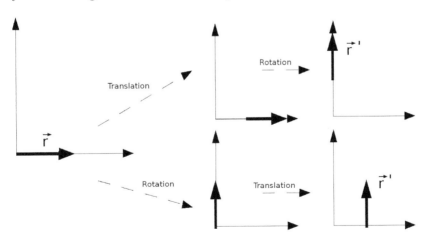

FIGURE 7.5: The effects of a combined rotation and translation on a simple vector $\vec{r}$ located on the abscissa of a Cartesian coordinate system. If translation by one unit is applied prior to rotation by 90°counterclockwise, the upper position for the transformed vector $\vec{r}'$ is the outcome. Otherwise, the lower situation is the result. Translation and rotation do therefore not commute.

Figure 7.5 shows something else; while we have to take care which operation to handle first, we can also choose the center of rotation by a translation; when rotating an image, Example 7.6.1 shows us that we move the image content out of the image domain quickly. Instead of making the image domain larger, we can as well

> Move the center of the image (or the centroid of a ROI as given in Equation 6.1) to the origin of the coordinate system; if the image dimensions are width W and height H, this translation vector is given as $\vec{\Delta c} = - \left(\frac{W}{2}, \frac{H}{2} \right)^T$.

> Next, the shifted coordinates are rotated.

> Finally, the rotated coordinates are shifted back to the image domain by a translation $-\vec{\Delta c}$. This is actually the inverse transform of shifting the pixel coordinates to the image origin.

In an additional task in Example 7.6.1, you have to carry out this operation. By applying both rotation and translation, we do now have all the degrees-of-freedom (dof) of rigid motion in 2D available.

7.3.2 Rotation and translation in 3D

However, medical imaging is three dimensional in many cases. All of a sudden, we have three dof in rotation and three dof in translation; apparently, life gets more complicated if you add more dof. However, we will see that the handling of rotations is not that much different from the 2D case. First, we have three so-called Euler angles which act as parameters for the rotation around the axes of a 3D Cartesian coordinate system. The rotation matrix that rotates a point in space around the x-axis looks like this:

$$R_x = \begin{pmatrix} 1 & 0 & 0 \\ 0 & \cos(\phi_x) & -\sin(\phi_x) \\ 0 & \sin(\phi_x) & \cos(\phi_x) \end{pmatrix} \tag{7.12}$$

As one can see, the whole thing looks pretty similar to the matrix R from Equation 7.8. Before we proceed, we should take a closer look at this matrix. As we have learned in Chapter 5, a Gaussian stays a Gaussian when applying the Fourier transform. It changes its width, but not its shape. In special cases, it is even an eigenfunction. A matrix is a transformation applied to a vector with a finite number of elements. The *eigenvector* retains its direction, but it may be stretched by a factor λ that represents the *eigenvalue*. If we want to find the eigenvectors and eigenvalues of a matrix, we have to solve the following linear system of equations: $R_x \vec{x} = \lambda \vec{x}$. We can make sure by computing the transpose and the determinant of R_x that it is a rotation indeed. Therefore, the eigenvalue λ has to be one since a rotation cannot change a vector's length. Without further math, we can easily verify that every vector $\vec{x} = (x_i, 0, 0)^T$ – that is, all vectors collinear to the x-axis – is an eigenvector of R_x. The corresponding matrices for rotation around the y- and z- axis are:

$$R_y = \begin{pmatrix} \cos(\phi_y) & 0 & -\sin(\phi_y) \\ 0 & 1 & 0 \\ \sin(\phi_y) & 0 & \cos(\phi_y) \end{pmatrix} \tag{7.13}$$

and

$$R_z = \begin{pmatrix} \cos(\phi_z) & -\sin(\phi_z) & 0 \\ \sin(\phi_z) & \cos(\phi_z) & 0 \\ 0 & 0 & 1 \end{pmatrix}. \tag{7.14}$$

By using R_x, R_y, and R_z, we can now compose rotations in 3D by successively applying these three matrices. An arbitrary rotation of a point in 3D - space with coordinates $\vec{x}$ is simply given as $\vec{x}' = R\vec{x}$, where R is a combination of the three matrices R_i. The only problem lies in the fact that matrix multiplication is not commutative, therefore the product $R_{xyz} = R_x R_y R_z$ gives a completely different rotation than $R_{zyx} = R_z R_y R_x$. If we provide Euler-angles as parameters for 3D rotation, we also have to define a convention on the order of applying these angles. Euler angles are handy since they can be easily interpreted, but they can cause terrible chaos when handling them. In short, we will be acquainted with a different parameter set that is not very demonstrative but extremely powerful.

If we handle rotation by a combination of 3D rotation matrices, it is only straightforward to do the same thing for translations. Until now, we have not dealt with a translation matrix, but it would be very handy to combine the matrix notation of rotations with a similar method for translations. Let's take a look at the translation problem; shifting positions by a vector $\vec{\Delta s}$ using a translation matrix T should look like this:

$$T\vec{x} = (x_1 + \Delta s_1,\ x_2 + \Delta s_2,\ x_3 + \Delta s_3)^T .$$

If we try to guess the shape of such a 3×3 matrix, we realize that it would look rather cumbersome. A little trick does indeed yield a way more simple solution. We can *augment* the 3×3 matrix T to a 4×4 matrix by adding a row and a column; the same is done with the vector $\vec{x}$. the fourth element of $\vec{x}$ is said to be one, and the added row and column of the augmented matrix T contains zeros besides the main diagonal element t_{44}, which is also set to 1. The translation operation now looks like this:

$$T\vec{x} = \begin{pmatrix} 1 & 0 & 0 & \Delta s_1 \\ 0 & 1 & 0 & \Delta s_2 \\ 0 & 0 & 1 & \Delta s_3 \\ 0 & 0 & 0 & 1 \end{pmatrix} \begin{pmatrix} x \\ y \\ z \\ 1 \end{pmatrix} = \begin{pmatrix} x + \Delta s_1 \\ y + \Delta s_2 \\ z + \Delta s_3 \\ 1 \end{pmatrix}. \tag{7.15}$$

Equation 7.15 actually does what we expect it to do; at the cost of augmenting the translation operator T, we do have a matrix that gives us a translation if we only look at the first three components of the resulting vector. Next, it would be interesting to merge this formalism with the already known matrix formulation of rotations. Of course, we also have to augment the rotation matrices. We therefore get

$$R_x = \begin{pmatrix} 1 & 0 & 0 & 0 \\ 0 & \cos(\phi_x) & -\sin(\phi_x) & 0 \\ 0 & \sin(\phi_x) & \cos(\phi_x) & 0 \\ 0 & 0 & 0 & 1 \end{pmatrix}$$

and similar matrices R_y and R_z; again, all we did was an augmentation by adding an additional row and column with all elements besides the diagonal element equal zero. A little problem, however, arises; if we add additional matrices like a perspective projection operator (which we will encounter in Chapter 8), the fourth element of the resulting transformed position will usually not be 1. In such a case, we have to *renormalize* the result of our operation by multiplying all four elements of the resulting 4×1 vector with the inverse of the fourth element.

This representation of the spatial transforms is called *homogeneous coordinates*. The reader who is ready to suffer may try to express an arbitrary transform of three translations and three rotations by carrying out the matrix multiplications and inspect all the sines and cosines that will pop up; therefore we refrain from the explicit transformation as given in

Equation 7.10. It is noteworthy that another important operation can also be carried out using homogeneous coordinates – scaling of coordinates, which is especially important for medical imaging since we usually encounter volumes where the in-plane resolution differs from the slice spacing. If we want to scale voxel positions, we can use the *scaling matrix S*:

$$S = \begin{pmatrix} \sigma_x & 0 & 0 & 0 \\ 0 & \sigma_y & 0 & 0 \\ 0 & 0 & \sigma_z & 0 \\ 0 & 0 & 0 & 1 \end{pmatrix}$$

where σ_i gives the scaling factor in each dimension. However, I personally have never made use of the scaling matrix in my work – I rescale the volume prior to any operation in order to avoid further confusion. In all operations using homogeneous coordinates, we still have to be aware that also the matrices T and S do not commute with the rotation matrices R_i – the order in which the transformation is carried out is still crucial.

We conclude that we can use a product of matrices for all rigid-body transformations in 3D – that is, all transformations that map each voxel position in the same manner. These are also called *affine transformations*. This matrix, which we may call *volume transformation matrix* V can be composed as $V = T R_x R_y R_z S$ or $V = R_z R_y R_x T S$, or in another sequence. If one chooses to scale the coordinates using a scaling matrix S, this one should always be carried out first, otherwise the whole operation would be completely pointless. It is also noteworthy that both S and T have a non-zero determinant, therefore they are invertible. The inverse matrices S^{-1} and T^{-1} are given as:

$$S^{-1} = \begin{pmatrix} \frac{1}{\sigma_x} & 0 & 0 & 0 \\ 0 & \frac{1}{\sigma_y} & 0 & 0 \\ 0 & 0 & \frac{1}{\sigma_z} & 0 \\ 0 & 0 & 0 & 1 \end{pmatrix} \text{ and } T^{-1} = \begin{pmatrix} 1 & 0 & 0 & -\Delta s_1 \\ 0 & 1 & 0 & -\Delta s_2 \\ 0 & 0 & 1 & -\Delta s_3 \\ 0 & 0 & 0 & 1 \end{pmatrix}$$

When inverting a volume transformation matrix V, one also has to keep in mind that the inverse of a product of two matrices A and B is given as $(AB)^{-1} = B^{-1}A^{-1}$. The inverse of a transformation $V = TRS$ is therefore given as $V^{-1} = S^{-1}R^T T^{-1}$. Finally, the centering of the rotation operation as shown in Example 7.6.1 can be written as $T^{-1}RT$. Its inverse is $T^{-1}R^T T$. The true power of the use of matrices lies in the fact that we can combine transformations – the matrices are not commutative, but they are associative. A series of transformations can be written down as a product of matrices. The resulting matrix can be computed and applied to the 3D coordinates in a given application.

7.3.3 A special case – the principal axis transform

A special case of a 2D transformation, which incorporates a more general concept from statistics name *principal component analysis* (PCA), is the principal axis transform. In a PCA procedure, a set of random variable pairs x_i and y_i, which may be correlated, is transformed to a subset of uncorrelated variables. Basically, correlated variables are connected by a *correlation coefficient*, which we will encounter in Chapter 9 again. If we plot all values of x_i and y_i in a so-called scatterplot, we may get something that looks like Figure 7.6. The grade of dependency between values of x_i and y_i can be defined by *Pearson's correlation coefficient* r, which is defined as

$$r = \frac{\overbrace{\sum_{i=1}^{N} (x_i - \bar{x})(y_i - \bar{y})}^{\text{Covariance of x and y}}}{\underbrace{\sqrt{\sum_{i=1}^{N} (x_i - \bar{x})^2}}_{\text{Standard deviation of x}} \underbrace{\sqrt{\sum_{i=1}^{N} (y_i - \bar{y})^2}}_{\text{Standard deviation of y}}}. \tag{7.16}$$

Pearson's correlation coefficient $r \in \{-1 \ldots 1\}$ gives the amount of *linear dependency* of two independently measured variables x_i and y_i. If $r = 1$, a high value x_i causes a high value of y_i, and the dependence of the two is strictly linear. The standard deviation of x_i and y_i, usually called σ_x or σ_y is a measure of the variability of single values versus the expectation value $\bar{x}$ or $\bar{y}$. It is also known as the width of a Gaussian if the values of x_i or y_i follow a normal distribution – therefore, approximately 68% of all values x_i can be found in an interval $\bar{x} \pm \sigma$. The expectation value $\bar{x}$ in a normal distribution is, of course, the average value of x_i. The *covariance* is something new – it measures to what extent a large deviation of a single value x_i from $\bar{x}$ causes a large deviation of the corresponding value y_i from $\bar{y}$. The correlation coefficient is tightly connected to *linear regression analysis*, where the straight line that describes the linear dependency of the variable pairs x_i and y_i is defined as the optimum model for the functional correspondence of the variables. The gradient a of the regression line $y = ax + b$ is given as:

$$a = r\frac{\sigma_y}{\sigma_x}.$$

One may ask why this is of any importance in the context of medical image processing. It is in many contexts, but within our current subject – spatial transformations – it is of special interest. One may guess from Figure 7.6 that the PCA-transform is indeed a rotation and a translation in the coordinate system spanned by the values of x and y. The PCA is carried out as follows.

Compute the average vector $\vec{E}$ from all vectors containing the paired values $(x_i, y_i)^T$.

The *covariance matrix* C is given as the averaged sum of the matrix product

$$C(x,y) = \frac{1}{N} \sum_{i=1}^{N} \begin{pmatrix} x_i \\ y_i \end{pmatrix} (x_i, y_i) - \vec{E}\vec{E}^T. \tag{7.17}$$

The eigenvectors and eigenvalues of $C(x,y)$ are computed, and the eigenvectors are sorted in a descending manner according to their eigenvalues. A matrix R is formed where the columns represent the eigenvectors.

The PCA transformation is carried out by computing $R\left((x_i, y_i)^T - \vec{E}\right)$.

Example 7.6.3 implements a PCA on a binary image; the non-zero pixels are considered correlated variable pairs. Figure 7.16 shows the initial image; after carrying out the PCA, the image is aligned alongside the main axis where most image information is found (Figure 7.17).

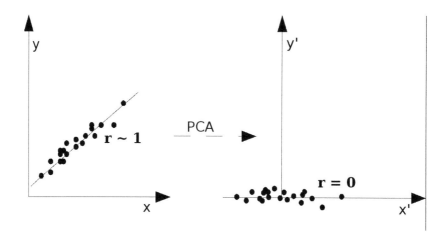

FIGURE 7.6: The principle of the PCA transform. Pairs of variables x_i and y_i are plotted in so-called scatterplot. If a linear functional correspondence between x_i and y_i exists, the correlation coefficient r is either close to 1 or -1, depending on the gradient of the functional correspondence. This is the situation on the left hand side. The goal of the PCA is to transform the variables (x_i, y_i) in such a manner that the correlation coefficient becomes minimal. In this new frame of reference, the variables are uncorrelated to the largest extent possible. For uncorrelated variables, the correlation coefficient is zero. Since r is closely connected to the slope of the regression line, this slope becomes zero as well (see also the right hand side of the illustration).

7.3.4 The quaternion representation of rotations

By now, we have mastered the most important tool for 3D visualization and processing of tomographic images. We now know how to manipulate images in the spatial domain, we are aware of its pitfalls, and with the formalism of matrix transformations, we have a comprehensive and simple tool at hand – those of you who don't believe this are encouraged again to carry out a multiplication of three rotation matrices and take a look at the result. Still, there is a major blemish: the order in which rotations are carried out is not arbitrary since the single rotation matrices do not commute. In aviation, where the rotation around the x-axis is called roll, the rotation around the y-axis is the pitch, and the z-axis rotation is called yaw, this is even regulated by an official norm (otherwise, aviation control would yield catastrophic results in five out of six cases). This parametrization in Euler-angles gives rise to even more problems since in a certain position, one of the Euler-angles becomes arbitrary. This is the so-called Gimbal lock problem. And finally, it is extremely cumbersome to interpolate rotation motion from angles.

Therefore, a more convenient parametrization of the group of rotations in 3D space would be helpful; it should be unambiguous, and it should allow for some sort of commutative math in order to allow for adaptive filtering. Such a parametrization was introduced in the middle of the nineteenth century, and the parameters are called *unit quaternions*.

In order to give a tangible interpretation of unit quaternions, it is useful to introduce another possible way of giving rotation parameters – the *eigenvector* of the rotation matrix R and the angle of rotation around this single vector. The eigenvector $\vec{u}$ of length 1 is the one axis defined by all points that do not change their position when carrying out the rotation. The only remaining degree of freedom is the one angle ϕ that gives the amount of the clockwise rotation around $\vec{u}$. A quadruple q derived from $\vec{u}$ and ϕ can be represented as

$$q = (q_0, q_1, q_2, q_3)^T = \left(\cos\left(\frac{\phi}{2}\right), \vec{u}^T \sin\left(\frac{\phi}{2}\right)\right)^T. \tag{7.18}$$

This representation is extremely useful if one wants to find out about projection properties since it allows for an easy check. Furthermore, one can use this property to interpolate rotations. In Section 9.7.1, we will encounter a very useful application for this set of parameters q, the *unit quaternion*. Unit quaternions fulfill the identity $q_0^2 + q_1^2 + q_2^2 + q_3^2 = 1$.

You may recall that in Chapter 5, I announced the return of complex numbers. Here they are. Quaternions are a quadruple of one scalar and three complex numbers. The imaginary unit $\mathbf{i}$ now has two more brothers, usually named $\mathbf{j}$ and $\mathbf{k}$. For all of those, the identity $i^2 = j^2 = k^2 = -1$ is true. A quaternion q is given as $q = q_0 + \mathbf{i}q_1 + \mathbf{j}q_2 + \mathbf{k}q_3$ and can therefore be expressed as $q = (q_0, q_1, q_2, q_3)^T$, analog to a complex number. The multiplication of two unit quaternions is not commutative, but it is anti-commutative; the multiplication of two quaternions u and v yields the following result: $uv = w$ or $vu = -w$. Compared to the behavior of rotation matrices, this is a huge simplification.

In medical image processing, namely in image-guided therapy and registration, quaternions play an important role. First, almost all tracking systems (see also Section 7.5) give their output as quaternions. Second, one can easily determine the eigenvector of rotation and the associated eigenvalue of an arbitrary complex transform in 3D space. And finally, one can interpolate the angulations in a complex 3D trajectory, for instance in biomechanics.

Therefore, we need to know how a quadruple of unit quaternions q can be expressed as a rotation matrix. This is done by carrying out the following calculation:

$$R = \begin{pmatrix} 1 - 2\left(q_2^2 + q_3^2\right) & 2\left(q_1q_2 - q_0q_3\right) & 2\left(q_0q_2 + q_1q_3\right) \\ 2\left(q_0q_3\right) & 1 - 2\left(q_1^2 + q_3^2\right) & 2\left(q_2q_3 - q_0q_1\right) \\ 2\left(q_1q_3 - q_0q_2\right) & 2\left(q_0q_1 + q_2q_3\right) & 1 - 2\left(q_1^2 + q_2^2\right) \end{pmatrix}. \tag{7.19}$$

The inverse operation is, of course, also possible:

Compute the trace of the rotation matrix: $\operatorname{tr}R = \sum_{i=1}^{3} R_{ii}$.

Compute four values $p_0 \ldots p_3$ as follows:

$$\begin{aligned} p_0 &= 1 + \operatorname{tr}R \\ p_1 &= 1 + 2R_{11} - \operatorname{tr}R \\ p_2 &= 1 + 2R_{22} - \operatorname{tr}R \\ p_3 &= 1 + 2R_{33} - \operatorname{tr}R \end{aligned} \tag{7.20}$$

Determine the maximum $p_{\max}$ of $\{p_0 \ldots p_3\}$.

Compute $p_s = \sqrt{p_{\max}}$.

The index s of $p_{\max}$ determines which of the four following computations has to be carried out:

$$\begin{aligned} s = 0: \quad q_0 &= \frac{1}{2}p_0 \\ q_1 &= \frac{1}{2p_0}\left(R_{32} - R_{23}\right) \\ q_2 &= \frac{1}{2p_0}\left(R_{12} - R_{21}\right) \\ q_3 &= \frac{1}{2p_0}\left(R_{21} - R_{12}\right) \end{aligned} \tag{7.21}$$

$$s = 1 : \quad q_0 = \frac{1}{2p_1}(R_{32} - R_{23})$$

$$q_1 = \frac{1}{2}p_1$$

$$q_2 = \frac{1}{2p_1}(R_{21} + R_{12})$$

$$q_3 = \frac{1}{2p_1}(R_{13} + R_{31}) \tag{7.22}$$

$$s = 2 : \quad q_0 = \frac{1}{2p_2}(R_{13} - R_{31})$$

$$q_1 = \frac{1}{2p_2}(R_{21} + R_{12})$$

$$q_2 = \frac{1}{2}p_2$$

$$q_3 = \frac{1}{2p_2}(R_{32} + R_{23}) \tag{7.23}$$

$$s = 3 : \quad q_0 = \frac{1}{2p_3}(R_{21} - R_{12})$$

$$q_1 = \frac{1}{2p_3}(R_{13} + R_{31})$$

$$q_2 = \frac{1}{2p_3}(R_{32} + R_{23})$$

$$q_3 = \frac{1}{2}p_3 \tag{7.24}$$

If q_0 is negative, all values $q_0 \ldots q_3$ should be multiplied with -1.

Check if the result is still a unit quaternion.

As said before, the unit quaternion is a representation of the eigenvector of an arbitrary rotation matrix R as given by an arbitrary product of Eqs. 7.12, 7.13 and 7.14. The inverse operation given above is therefore an algorithm that derives the eigenvector and the angle of rotation of R.

7.4 REFORMATTING

Now that we are able to master spatial transformations in 3D, we can turn to the most important visualization method for 3D volume image data. As already said before, tomographic images must not be considered stacks or collections of single images; they are, indeed, images defined on a 3D domain. The fact that 3D images are acquired in a slicewise manner in many imaging systems, does, however, not simplify this model. However, CBCT and SPECT, for instance, do not work in such a manner. Rather than that, they acquire projection data, and the volume is reconstructed from a multitude of these projections. More about this will come in Chapter 10. MR machines do acquire data as slices, but the position of the imaging plane is determined using the MR machine parameters and can be chosen arbitrarily.

The other problem lies in the fact that visualization of a function $I(x, y, z) = \rho$ is not as trivial as in the case of 2D images. A possibility to visualize the 3D datasets is to compute new slices. Another possibility is the use of visualization techniques such as rendering, which we will encounter in Chapter 8. However, the generation of new slices is the most important visualization technique. It is referred to as reformatting. We can distinguish between *orthogonal reformatting* – this is the derivation of new slices from the volume alongside the main anatomical directions – axial/transversal, sagittal and coronal. However, the exactness of this definition is limited. If a patient lies in the scanner at a slightly tilted position (a CT machine, for instance, can tilt the whole unit with an angle of up to 15°), the axial direction is not coincident with the orientation of the body stem. Reformatting of slices in arbitrary orientations is called *oblique reformatting*. And finally, we can define an arbitrary 2D manifold, which intersects the volume image. This is generally referred to as *curved reformatting*. Figure 7.7 shows such an image; this is a so-called pantomographic reformatting from dental radiology, where a CT of the mandible was reformatted in such a manner that the reformatting plane follows the arc of the jaw, thus producing an image similar to panoramic x-ray.

The derivation of orthogonal and oblique sections is actually rather simple. We have our data volume, built up from voxels and defined in a Cartesian coordinate system. We may consider the x-y plane to be the initial cutting plane. All we have to do is rotate and translate this plane to the desired position, and to transfer the gray values ρ from a voxel at the position $(x, y, z)^T$ that intersects a pixel in the cutting plane to exactly this pixel in the 2D image. Interpolation of an appropriate gray value from the surrounding voxels is usually a necessity. Examples 7.6.4 and 7.6.5 illustrate reformatting, which from now on allows us to visualize 3D data at arbitrary orientations.

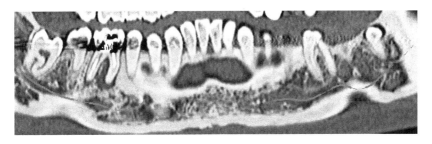

FIGURE 7.7: A curved reformatting from dentistry. Here, a standard CT of the mandible was acquired, and a curved reformatting plane matching the arc of the jaw is defined. Therefore, a slice image of the whole jaw is provided, similar to the well-known panoramic x-ray used in dentistry for more than 80 years. Image courtesy of A. Gahleitner, Dental School, Medical University Vienna.

7.5 TRACKING AND IMAGE-GUIDED THERAPY

With the tools to handle spatial transforms at hand, we can proceed to an application field where diagnostics and therapeutic measures are joined – image-guided therapy, often also referred to as stereotactic surgery, frameless stereotaxy, neuronavigation, or computer-aided surgery. Here, we use three components to guide the physician during an intervention or a surgical procedure:

Tracking of patient position and 3D pose of instruments.

Registration of the patient coordinate system to the reference frame of an image dataset.

Visualization of the actual situation by generating views from the registered image data.

We will deal with registration in Chapter 9. Visualization techniques beyond reformatting will be introduced in Chapter 8. What is left for now in the context of this chapter is tracking. Tracking in general refers to the real-time measurement of six degrees of freedom of several rigid bodies. Several techniques for tracking exist.

Optical Tracking: Several calibrated cameras (see Section 9.6) acquire an image of active or reflective optical beacons of known geometry (see also Figure 7.11). By reconstructing the 3D position of at least two (for 5 dof) or three beacons (for 6 dof), one can derive the volume transformation V of the rigid body carrying the beacons relative to the camera coordinate system; an algorithm for deriving an affine transformation from known position pairs in two coordinate systems is presented in Section 9.7.1. It is possible to track multiple rigid bodies (usually referred to as *tools*) since these are either connected by cable to the control unit of the camera, or they feature a unique configuration of markers in the case of wireless systems (see Figure 7.10). In the latter case, the beacon consists of a reflective sphere. Optical tracking systems are the most widespread tracking technology, with typical accuracy in the range of 0.3 mm; their main disadvantage lies in the fact that a free line-of-sight between the tool and the camera is necessary. Figure 7.8 shows a typical camera bar of an optical tracker. Another type of optical tracking system that is not very widespread in medicine sweeps the digitizer volume with laser fans; the beacons on tools are replaced by photoresistors in these systems.

Electromagnetic Tracking: Another widespread technology is electromagnetic tracking, where the field strength or the magnetic flux of a specially designed electromagnetic field is measured by small sensors like search coils or flux-gate sensors. The electromagnetic field permeates soft tissue and does therefore not require a free line-of-sight. Furthermore, the sensors can be built with an extremely small form factor that allows for the use of electromagnetic trackers within flexible instruments such as endoscopes. A drawback of electromagnetic trackers, however, is the fact that the reference field may be distorted by conductive or ferromagnetic materials, which depreciates the accuracy achievable with these devices. Still, these systems provide the technology of choice in current image – guided therapy systems if flexible instruments are to be tracked within the body. Figure 7.9 shows an image of a current electromagnetic tracker.

Mechanical Tracking: The earliest systems for computer-aided neurosurgery consisted of a single passive arm with encoders on each joint. Since the relative position of the joints relative to each other is known, the position of the instrument tip at the end of the device can be determined from the kinematic chain. In neurosurgery, the patient's calvaria is fixed by means of a so-called Mayfield clamp,[1] therefore one tracked tool is sufficient. These systems are very accurate, but bulky, difficult to sterilize, and were more or less replaced by optical trackers. Nevertheless, position information from decoders still plays an important role in medical robotics.

---

[1] I would prefer to call it a vise.

Ultrasonic Tracking: A system similar to optical trackers can be built using ultrasound-emitters and microphones. The ultrasound emitter acts like an optical beacon, and an array of microphones takes the position of the camera in an optical tracker. However, the ultrasound tracker suffers from the same problem as the optical tracker, which is the requirement for a free line-of-sight between the emitter and the detector. Furthermore, changes in air humidity and temperature affect the speed of sound, which also affects tracker accuracy. Therefore, ultrasonic tracking systems have not found widespread usage in image-guided therapy despite the fact that cost-effective systems are available.

Passive HF-Tracking: An interesting approach consists of small passive transponders which emit a signal when being exposed to an electromagnetic field of high frequency. These transponders, contained in small glass capsules, can be implanted near a tumor in healthy tissue. By monitoring the position of the beacon during radiotherapy, internal organ motion can be monitored to spare healthy tissue. The positioning of the emitter is somewhat delicate, therefore tracking applications for a large range of motion appear difficult and were not yet realized.

Inertial Tracking: One can derive position from a known starting point by integrating acceleration twice in the time domain. The same holds true for angulation, where an integration of angular velocity yields a change in rotation. Acceleration and angular velocity can be measured by special sensors. However, the time integration step yields an inevitable drift over a longer period of time. Therefore, such inertial trackers were only used as supporting systems in augmented or virtual reality application, where they provide input for adaptive filtering of position data.

Image-based Tracking: Finally, it is possible to retrieve motion directly from medical images if the imaging modality is located within the operating room. By applying registration techniques presented in Chapter 9, 3D motion can, for instance, be derived from 2D projective data. In the case of x-ray imaging, this may cause considerable additional dose. But also monitoring of interventional progress by US- and MR-imaging is used in clinical routine.

Common to all tracking systems is the fact that their output is usually in quaternions, which have to be converted to rotation matrices R using Equation 7.19. The clinical application fields of image-guided therapy range from neurosurgery, ear-, nose-, and throat surgery, craniomaxillofacial surgery, orthopedics, plastic and trauma surgery to interventional radiology, radiotherapy, and surgical training.

An example for an image-guided therapy system was developed by the author;[2] it uses an optical tracking system to report the position of a surgical drill relative to the patient. After preoperative planning (in this case, it was implant sites for oral and extraoral dental implants in cranio- and maxillofacial surgery), the patient was registered to the CT with planning data using a point-to-point registration technique, and by continuous reading of tracker measurements, the actual drill position was displayed both on three obliquely reformatted slices and volume renderings (see also Figure 7.11).

---

[2]A more detailed description of this system can be found in W. Birkfellner, K. Huber, A. Larson, D. Hanson, M. Diemling, P. Homolka, H. Bergmann: A modular software system for computer-aided surgery and its first application in oral implantology, IEEE Trans Med Imaging 19(6):616-20, (2000).

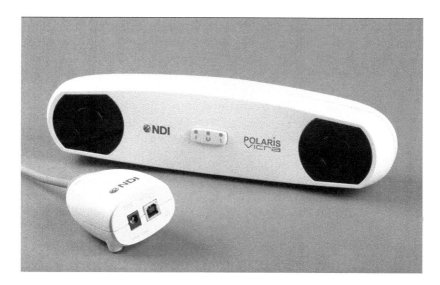

FIGURE 7.8: An image of a camera bar of an optical tracking system, the Polaris Vicra by Northern Digital Inc. (Ontario, Can). This is a system featuring two planar cameras with a filter that blocks visible light. The digitizer volume is flooded with infrared light from an array of light-emitting diodes surrounding the camera. Reflective spheres on the tool show up in the camera images. By knowing the relative configuration of the beacons and the projection geometry of the camera system, one can derive an affine transformation in six dof. Image courtesy of Northern Digital Inc.

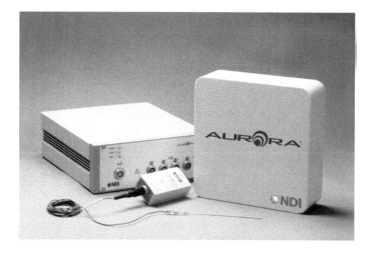

FIGURE 7.9: An electromagnetic tracking system, the Aurora, also from Northern Digital Inc. (Ontario, Can). The field emitter generating the electromagnetic reference field can be found in the right half of the image. A needle containing a small position sensor located at the needle tip is shown in front of the control hardware which processes the raw sensor data and interfaces to a computer. Image courtesy of Northern Digital Inc.

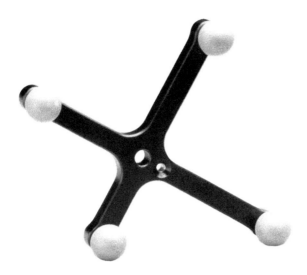

FIGURE 7.10: A passive optical tracking probe. The tracking system flushes the digitizing volume with infrared light, which is reflected by the four spheres. Due to the known unique configuration of the beacons on the tool, the tracker can distinguish between several tools. Since the system is passive, no additional wiring is necessary. Image courtesy of Northern Digital Inc.

7.6   PRACTICAL LESSONS

7.6.1   Spatial image transforms in 2D

The `Simple2DRotation_7.m` script rotates an T1-weighted MR-slice of a pig, which we have already encountered in Examples 3.7.2 and 4.5.1. This time, another slice in coronal orientation is given. First, we load the image `PorkyPig.jpg`, and we scale it to 6 bit depth. Next, we allocate some memory for the rotated image `rotimg`, and we define the angle of rotation. Here, we have chosen -20°. Finally, we define a rotation matrix `rotmat` according to Equation 7.8.

```
1:> img=imread('PorkyPig.jpg');
2:> img=round(img/4.0);
3:> rotimg=zeros(350,350);
4:> angle=-20;
5:> rotmat=zeros(2,2);
6:> rotmat(1,1)=cos(angle*pi/180);
7:> rotmat(1,2)=-sin(angle*pi/180);
8:> rotmat(2,1)=sin(angle*pi/180);
9:> rotmat(2,2)=cos(angle*pi/180);
```

Next, we can check whether `rotmat` is really a rotation matrix; therefore we compute the determinant of the matrix `rotmat` (which should be one for a true rotation matrix), and we compute the product of the matrix `rotmat` and its transpose. The result should be the unity matrix since the transpose gives the inverse of a rotation matrix.

```
10:> DeterminantOfMatrix=det(rotmat)
```

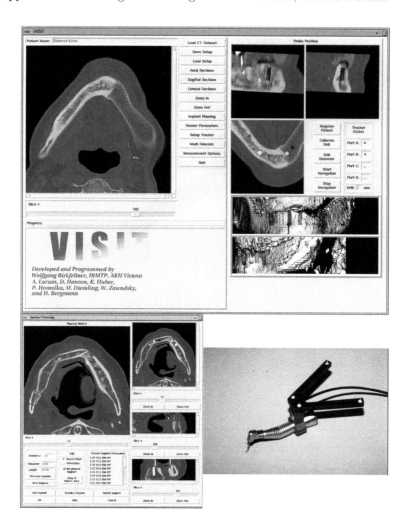

FIGURE 7.11: Some screenshots of VISIT, a system for image-guided cranio- and maxillo-facial surgery developed by the author. The top screenshot shows the main screen of the program, where a dental CT scan can be browsed, and planned sites for dental implants are shown in dependence of surgical drill position on oblique reformatted slices and volume renderings. After preoperative planning (lower left screenshot) of implant channels on the CT, the patient was registered using a point-to-point registration technique. The position of the surgical drill (lower right image) is reported by an optical tracking system; the tool for the optical tracker is rigidly attached to the drill.

```
11:> foo=input('This is the determinant of the
rotation matrix - Press RETURN...');
12:> invrotmat=transpose(rotmat);
13:> ProductOfMatrixAndInverse=rotmat*invrotmat
14:> foo=input('This is the product of the
rotation matrix and its transpose - Press RETURN...');
```

Now, we apply the rotation transform from Equation 7.9 to every pixel in the image;

the rotated image `rotimg` is slightly larger than the original image `img`. Of course we have to take care that the transformed pixel remains within the domain of the image. Since `img` was already scaled to 6 bit and we have done nothing to the image intensities here, we can simply display the result, which is found alongside the original image in Figure 7.12.

```
15:> oldpix=zeros(2,1);
16:> newpix=zeros(2,1);
17:> for i=1:300
18:> for j=1:300
19:> oldpix(1,1)=i;
20:> oldpix(2,1)=j;
21:> rho=img(i,j);
22:> newpix=round(rotmat*oldpix);
23:> if (newpix(1,1) > 0) & (newpix(1,1) < 350) &
(newpix(2,1) > 0) & (newpix(2,1) < 350)
24:> rotimg(newpix(1,1),newpix(2,1))=rho;
25:> end
26:> end
27:> end
28:> colormap(gray)
29:> image(rotimg)
```

Additional Tasks

Modify this script by applying a translation of the image content to the center of the image, carry out the rotation, and shift the image back again. The result should look like Figure 7.13.

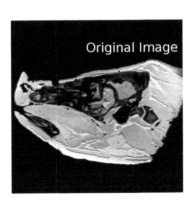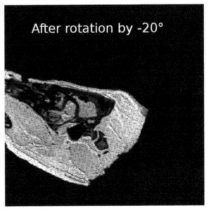

FIGURE 7.12: The result of our initial image rotation effort; the original image `PorkyPig.jpg`, which can be seen on the left hand side, was rotated by -20° around the origin of the image, which lies in the upper left corner. Discretization artifacts, which stem from rounding the transformed pixel coordinates are clearly visible on the rotated image (right side). Furthermore, the location of the origin causes the image content to move out of the image domain.

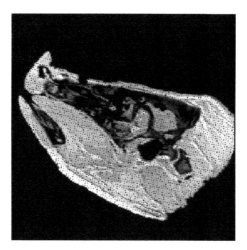

FIGURE 7.13: When shifting the pixel locations to the centroid reference system of the picture, we can avoid moving the image content out of the image domain such as in Figure 7.12. Your modification of `Simple2DRotation_7.m` should yield this result. The ugly artifacts from rounding errors remain but will be tackled in the next example.

7.6.2   Two simple interpolation examples

In `NNInterpolation_7.m`, we will use a nearest-neighbor interpolation model to beautify the rotated MR image of the pig head without the ugly black spots in the image; the script is derived from `Simple2DRotation_7.m`. The first few lines are identical:

```
1:> img=imread('PorkyPig.jpg');
2:> img=round(img/4.0);
3:> rotimg=zeros(300,300);
4:> angle=-20;
5:> rotmat=zeros(2,2);
6:> rotmat(1,1)=cos(angle*pi/180);
7:> rotmat(1,2)=-sin(angle*pi/180);
8:> rotmat(2,1)=sin(angle*pi/180);
9:> rotmat(2,2)=cos(angle*pi/180);
```

Now, we introduce the special trick which allows us to cover all pixels in `rotimg`. Instead of transforming the gray values ρ from `img` to `rotimg`, we invert the transformation, so that pixels in `rotimg` are mapped to `img`. Therefore we have to invert the matrix `rotmat`. By doing so, we can cover all pixels in `rotimg` – the annoying black dots, which stem from roundoff-errors, are therefore avoided. Next, a few vectors are initialized, and a variable `rho` is defined, which holds the gray value ρ from the pixel position in the original image `img`.

```
10:> rotmat=transpose(rotmat);
11:> oldpix=zeros(2,1);
12:> newpix=zeros(2,1);
13:> shift=zeros(2,1);
14:> shift(1,1)= 150;
15:> shift(2,1)= 150;
16:> rho=0;
```

Now, we visit each pixel in `rotimg`, apply the inverse transformation to these pixel coordinates, and store the gray value `rho` for each pixel in `img`. One may take a closer look at the vector `shift` and its role in the transformation. If the transformed pixel position `oldpix` in `img` lies within the domain of `img`, `rho` is stored in `newimg` at the position `newpix`. The result is displayed and can be found in Figure 7.14.

```
17:> for i=1:300
18:> for j=1:300
19:> newpix(1,1)=i;
20:> newpix(2,1)=j;
21:> oldpix=round(rotmat*(newpix-shift)+shift);
22:> if (oldpix(1,1) > 0) & (oldpix(1,1) < 300) &
(oldpix(2,1) > 0) & (oldpix(2,1) < 300)
23:> rho=img(oldpix(1,1),oldpix(2,1));
24:> end
25:> rotimg(i,j)=rho;
26:> end
27:> end
28:> colormap(gray)
29:> image(rotimg)
```

We use a nearest neighbor interpolation in an implicit manner. We round the transformed pixel coordinates and acquire the corresponding gray value ρ in the original image.

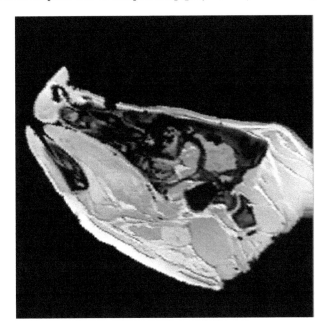

FIGURE 7.14: The result of `NNInterpolation_7.m`; a nearest-neighbor interpolation, introduced in an implicit manner by using the inverse transform from the target image to the original is used to remove the rounding errors that can be seen in Figure 7.13.

The script `BiLinearInterpolation_7.m` implements a bilinear interpolation to a PET image. The output can be directly compared to Figure 7.4. The script directly implements

Equation 7.6. First, we read the image `PET_Sample.jpg`, scale its intensity to six bit, and display it; furthermore, memory for a larger image `newimg` is allocated:

```
1:> img=(imread('PET_Sample.jpg'))/4.0;
2:> newimg=zeros(512,512);
3:> colormap(gray)
4:> image(img)
5:> foo=input('The original image at 64 x 64 pixel
resolution - press RETURN...');
```

Next, we scale the image to `newimg` using a nearest neighbor interpolation; the interpolation is implemented by rounding the new intermediate pixels to the nearest pixel position in the original image:

```
6:> for i=1:512
7:> for j=1:512
8:> si=round(i/8.0);
9:> sj=round(j/8.0);
10:> if si > 0 & si < 65 & sj > 0 & sj < 65
11:> rho=img(si,sj);
12:> newimg(i,j)=rho;
13:> end
14:> end
15:> end
16:> colormap(gray)
17:> image(newimg)
18:> foo=input('The scaled image at 512 x 512 pixel
resolution, nearest neighbor interpolation -
press RETURN...');
```

So far, nothing mysterious happened. Next, we proceed to bilinear interpolation. A matrix `rhoMat` for holding the four gray values ρ from Equation 7.6 is allocated, and the pixel which is located in the lower left corner of the interpolation grid (see also Figure 7.2) is found at `pivot00i` and `pivot00j`. After checking that we are still in the domain of the original image, we retrieve the four gray values `rho00` ... `rho11`. Next, we define the two vectors $((1 - y), y)$ and $((1 - x), x)^T$ from Equation 7.6 and assign the gray values to the matrix `rhoMat`. The matrix multiplication is carried out, and the interpolated gray value is assigned in the bigger image `newimg`. Figure 7.15 shows the three results provided by the script.

```
19:> rhoMat=zeros(2,2);
20:> for i=1:512
21:> for j=1:512
22:> pivot00i=floor(i/(512/64));
23:> pivot00j=floor(j/(512/64));
24:> if pivot00i > 1 & pivot00i < 64 & pivot00j > 1 & pivot00j < 64
25:> rho00=img(pivot00i,pivot00j);
26:> rho01=img(pivot00i,(pivot00j+1));
27:> rho10=img((pivot00i+1),pivot00j);
28:> rho11=img((pivot00i+1),(pivot00j+1));
```

Next, we compute the modulus of the operation 512/64 – that is the remainder of the integer division. The modulus in MATLAB is given by the function `mod`.

```
29:> denx=mod(i,(512/64));
30:> deny=mod(j,(512/64));
31:> leftVect=([(1-deny/(512/64)),(deny/(512/64))]);
32:> rhoMat(1,1)=rho00;
33:> rhoMat(1,2)=rho10;
34:> rhoMat(2,1)=rho01;
35:> rhoMat(2,2)=rho11;
36:> rightVect=transpose([(1-denx/(512/64)),...
(denx/(512/64))]);
37:> newimg(i,j)=leftVect*rhoMat*rightVect;
38:> end
39:> end
40:> end
41:> colormap(gray)
42:> image(newimg)
```

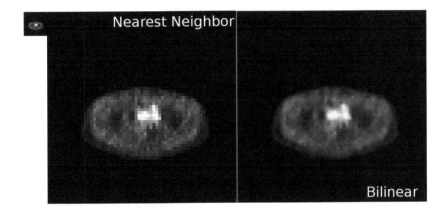

FIGURE 7.15: The output of the `BiLinearInterpolation_7.m` script. The small image in the upper left corner is the original image, drawn to scale compared to the middle and the right image. The middle image shows the result of scaling `PET_Sample.jpg` to 512×512 pixels using nearest neighbor interpolation. The right image shows the result of our bilinear interpolation effort. Image data courtesy of the Dept. of Nuclear Medicine, Medical University Vienna.

Additional Tasks

Compose the transform in homogeneous coordinates, and invert the resulting transform using the MATLAB command `inv` instead of carrying out the transformation steps one by one in `NNInterpolation_7.m`.

Apply a bilinear interpolation in `NNInterpolation_7.m` instead of a nearest neighbor interpolation.

Scale `PET_Sample.jpg` to 150×150 pixels using `BiLinearInterpolation_7.m`.

7.6.3 A special case – the PCA on binary images

In `BinaryPCA_7.m`, we will perform a principal component analysis (PCA) on a binary image. The mouse-topogram that was already heavily misused in Chapter 5 returns here (see Figure 7.16). It was rotated and segmented to a binary image using a simple thresholding operation which we have already encountered in Chapter 6. The example was placed in this chapter since it is actually a spatial transformation in this context, although the PCA is a much more general concept from statistics. Here, we handle the x and y components of all non-zero pixels as independent variables in a scatterplot. Using the PCA on the pixel coordinates results in the main axes of the image. The result of the PCA is a rotation matrix that aligns the image in the direction where most of the pixels lie.

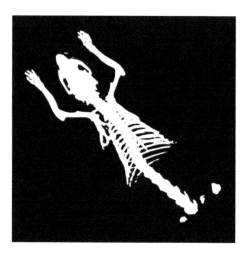

FIGURE 7.16: The initial image used for a demonstration of the PCA on binary images. The topogram of a mouse, already encountered in Chapter 5 for a number of times, was segmented using a simple thresholding operation, and rotated. The PCA on the coordinates of non-zero pixels yields a spatial transform in 2D that aligns the principal axis – that is, the axis that contains the most pixels. Image data courtesy of C. Kuntner, AIT Seibersdorf, Austria.

So let's take a look at `BinaryPCA_7.m`. First, the binary mouse image is read; we also make sure that it is absolutely binary, although this is not necessary:

```
1:> img = imread('BinMouseCT.jpg');
2:> maxint=max(max(img));
3:> img=round(img/maxint);
```

Next, we compute the expectation value for the coordinates occupied by a pixel. The expectation value is simply the average of the coordinates for all occupied pixels. You may recognize that this average vector `expVect` is in fact identical with the centroid as defined in Equation 6.1. So far, there is nothing mysterious going on:

```
4:> expVect=zeros(2,1);
5:> hit= 0;
6:> for i=1:400
7:> for j=1:400
```

```
8:> if img(i,j) > 0
9:> hit = hit+1;
10:> expVect(1,1) = expVect(1,1)+i;
11:> expVect(2,1) = expVect(2,1)+j;
12:> end
13:> end
14:> end
15:> expVect=expVect/hit;
```

Next, we allocate some memory for further vector and matrix operations:

```
16:> posVect=zeros(2,1);
17:> covarianceMatrix= zeros(2,2);
18:> expMatrix=expVect*(transpose(expVect));
```

The last line deserves a little bit of explanation; we may recall that the PCA consists of an eigenvector-decomposition of the $N \times N$ covariance matrix C, which is defined in Equation 7.17. The important thing here is the multiplication of vectors and transposed vectors. Remember that vectors are matrices as well, and the product $\vec{x}_n \vec{x}_n^T$ results in a matrix:

$$\vec{x}_n \vec{x}_n^T = \begin{pmatrix} x_{n_1} \\ x_{n_2} \end{pmatrix} (x_{n_1}\, x_{n_2}) = \begin{pmatrix} x_{n_1}^2 & x_{n_1} x_{n_2} \\ x_{n_1} x_{n_2} & x_{n_2}^2 \end{pmatrix}.$$

expMatrix as well as covarianceMatrix, which follows in the next paragraph, are therefore 2×2 matrices. In the following code, the covariance matrix covarianceMatrix is generated:

```
19:> for i=1:400
20:> for j=1:400
21:> if img(i,j) > 0
22:> posVect(1,1)=i;
23:> posVect(2,1)=j;
24:> covarianceMatrix=covarianceMatrix+(posVect*
(transpose(posVect)));
25:> end
26:> end
27:> end
28:> covarianceMatrix=covarianceMatrix/hit-expMatrix;
```

Next, we have to compute the eigenvectors of covarianceMatrix. We already know that an eigenvector of a matrix C, associated with eigenvalues, is a vector that does not change its shape when C is applied to it. A possibility to compute eigenvectors and eigenvalues of a matrix is called the *Jacobi-decomposition*. We elegantly avoid programming something like that by simply using the internal function eig of MATLAB®, which returns both the eigenvectors and eigenvalues. For programming languages like C++, similar commands are provided by mathematical libraries like the GSL.

```
29:> [eigenVectors,eigenValues]=
eig(covarianceMatrix);
30:> rotmatrix=zeros(2,2);
31:> rotmatrix(1,1)=eigenVectors(1,2);
32:> rotmatrix(1,2)=eigenVectors(1,1);
33:> rotmatrix(2,1)=eigenVectors(2,2);
34:> rotmatrix(2,2)=eigenVectors(2,1);
```

The matrix A for the PCA is composed by the eigenvectors of the covariance matrix C. However, the order of the vectors is defined by the magnitude of the associated eigenvalue. `eig`, unfortunately does not sort the eigenvectors. This results in a matrix of eigenvectors that has a determinant of -1– a reflection is introduced. We remove this blemish by re-ordering the `eigenVectors` in `rotmatrix`.

Now, we carry out the PCA on the vectors $\vec{x}_n$ of the occupied pixels; $\vec{x}'_n = A\,(\vec{x}_n - \vec{e})$. The centroid $\vec{e}$, which was called `expVect` in the script, is shifted to the origin of the coordinate system. Next, A (which is called `rotmatrix` in the script) is applied to the resulting shifted coordinates. By inserting the line `det(rotmatrix)` in the script, one can easily verify that A is a rotation, indeed. However, our image has the origin of the coordinate system in the upper left corner. Therefore we have to shift the rotated pixel coordinates back to the centroid. And we have to make sure that the pixels stick to the image domain; finally, the image is displayed. The result can be found in Figure 7.17.

```
35:> newPos=zeros(2,1);
36:> newimg=zeros(400,400);
37:> for i=1:400
38:> for j=1:400
39:> if img(i,j) > 0
40:> posVect(1,1)=i;
41:> posVect(2,1)=j;
42:> newPos=round((rotmatrix*(posVect-expVect))
+expVect);
43:> if (newPos(1,1) > 0 & newPos(1,1) < 400 &
newPos(2,1) > 0 & newPos(2,1) < 400)
44:> newimg(newPos(1,1),newPos(2,1))=64;
45:> end
46:> end
47:> end
48:> end
49:> colormap(gray)
50:> image(newimg)
```

Additional Tasks

Introduce a nearest neighbor interpolation in the script so that the annoying artifacts in Figure 7.17 disappear.

7.6.4 A geometric reformatting example – conic sections

For this example, we will leave the domain of medical images and introduce reformatting on something that is already well known for a few thousand years – conic sections. It was already known in ancient Greece that cutting a plane out of a cone results in curves which may be closed or open, depending on the angle at which the cutting plane intersects the cone. If the cutting plane is normal to the central axis of the cone, the resulting shape will be a circle. The diameter of the circle depends on the distance of the cutting plane from the cone tip. If the cutting plane is tilted relative to the central axis by an angle smaller than half the opening angle, the resulting shape will be an ellipse, which is deformed relative to a circle, but closed. If the angle of the cutting plane equals half the opening angle of the cone, an open curve will form – the parabola. A tilting angle beyond half the opening angle

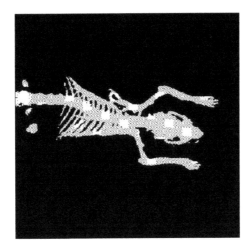

FIGURE 7.17: The segmented mouse after a principal axes transform in `BinaryPCA_7.m`. Discretization artifacts are, however, clearly noticeable. Image data courtesy of C. Kuntner, AIT Seibersdorf, Austria.

produces another open curve, the hyperbola. Quite a number of people have derived the various properties of the cone sections. We will simply take a look at them by reformatting a 3D volume of a cone's outer hull.

The script for this example is called `Conesects_7.m`. First of all, we have to generate a volume matrix in MATLAB which contains a cone. The cone is formed in such a manner that each slice in the volume contains a circle which fulfills the requirement $\sqrt{x^2 + y^2} = z/2$ which is the parametric definition of a circle of radius $z/2$. In other words – the circle gets bigger in diameter as we advance through the volume. Here we have a volume of $101 \times 101 \times 101$ voxels. The opening angle is 53.1 degrees:

```
1:> conevol=zeros(101,101,101);
2:> for vz=1:100
3:> for vx=-49:50
4:> for vy=-49:50
5:> zsqr=floor(vz/2);
6:> circlePos=floor(sqrt(vx*vx+vy*vy));
7:> if ((circlePos > (zsqr-1))&&(circlePos<(zsqr+1)))
8:> circlePixX=vx+50;
9:> circlePixY=vy+50;
10:> if (circlePixX > 0) && (circlePixY> 0)
11:> if (circlePixX <= 100) && (circlePixY <= 100)
12:> conevol(circlePixX,circlePixY,vz) = 64;
13:> end
14:end
15:> end
16:> end
17:> end
18:> end
```

What happens? First, the internal memory is cleared, and a three-dimensional matrix conevol is reserved (a little extra space is left here, as indexing problems may sometimes occur). Each voxel of coordinates $(x, y, z)^T$ is visited. The radius of a circle in plane z is given by the last coordinate, which is also the slice number. By rounding off the geometric mean of the pixel coordinates $(x, y)^T$ in a single slice and by taking care that the result is within a range of ± 1 pixel, the pixels forming the circle are found. Finally, the origin is shifted from $(0, 0)^T$ to $(50, 50)^T$, the center of the slice. Finally, it is taken care that the resulting circle is within the boundaries of the single slice, and the pixel is set to a value of 64. conevol is now a volume containing the hull of a cone with its origin at $(50, 50, 1)^T$ and its base of 100 pixels diameter at the last slice of the volume.

Next, we can do the reformatting. We define an image img of 100×150 pixels size so that reformatted images can have a length of $\sqrt{2} * 100$ pixels. Two 4×1 vectors pixPos and nPixPos are defined. The first one holds the pixel position in the reformatting plane prior to moving the reformatting plane, and the latter holds the transformed voxel position in homogeneous coordinates. In other words – prior to transforming the reformatting plane, it is coincident with the first slice of the conevol volume. After transformation, the adequate grayvalue ρ is taken from the volume and assigned to the coordinates given by the first two components of vector pixPos. Next, a rotation matrix around the x-axis Rx is defined. The tilt of the reformatting plane in degrees is defined as the parameter xangledegrees, which is subsequently converted to radians. The 4×4 rotation matrix around the x-axis as defined in Equation 7.12 can be found in the next few lines. After tilting the reformatting plane, it has to be shifted; this follows in the next few lines, where the 4×4 translation matrix is defined. Finally, the full spatial transform is computed as $V = TR_x$.

```
19:> img =zeros(100,150);
20:> pixPos=zeros(4,1);
21:> nPixPos=zeros(4,1);
22:> Rx=zeros(4,4);
23:> xangledegrees=0;
24:> xangle=xangledegrees*3.14159/180.0;
25:> Rx(1,1) = 1;
26:> Rx(2,2) = cos(xangle);
27:> Rx(2,3) = -sin(xangle);
28:> Rx(3,2) = sin(xangle);
29:> Rx(3,3) = cos(xangle);
30:> Rx(4,4) = 1;
31:> T=zeros(4,4);
32:> T(1,1)=1;
33:> T(2,2)=1;
34:> T(3,3)=1;
35:> T(4,4)=1;
36:> T(1,4)=0;
37:> T(2,4)=0;
38:> T(3,4)=50;
39:> V=zeros(4,4);
40:> V=T*Rx;
```

After generating the volume and defining the transformation of the reformatting plane, the actual reformatted slice can be computed.

```
41:> for rfx=1:100
```

```
42:> for rfy=1:150
43:> pixPos(1,1)=rfx;
44:> pixPos(2,1)=rfy;
45:> pixPos(3,1)=1;
46:> pixPos(4,1)=1;
47:> nPixPos=V*pixPos;
48:> nPixPos=floor(nPixPos);
49:> if ((nPixPos(1,1) > 0)&(nPixPos(1,1) <100)) &
((nPixPos(2,1)>0 )&(nPixPos(2,1)<100 )) &
((nPixPos(3,1)>0 )&(nPixPos(3,1)<100))
50:> img(rfx,rfy)=conevol(floor(nPixPos(1,1)),
floor(nPixPos(2,1)),floor(nPixPos(3,1)));
51:> end
52:> end
53:> end
54:> colormap(gray)
55:> image(img)
```

Here, every pixel in the untransformed imaging plane of img is visited, transformed to the position of the reformatting plane using V, and the result is rounded off to integer pixel values. The lengthy if-statement takes care that only voxels within the volume conevol are visited, and the gray value ρ at that voxel position is copied to the two dimensional pixel position in the image img. Finally, the image is displayed. Since Octave and MATLAB sometimes display images with a skewed width/height ratio, the result may also be saved as a PGM. Figure 7.18 shows a few results.

7.6.5 A reformatting example on a small volume data set

For this example introducing orthogonal reformatting, we have two scripts at hand; ReformattingSmall_7.m reads a CT from the already well-known pig dataset named pigSmall.img. The dataset features an isotropic resolution of 3mm^3 and is meant for those of you whose computer power is not that overwhelming. There is also a better dataset with 1.5mm^3 resolution named pigBig.img, which is read by a script named ReformattingBig_7.m. Both scripts do the same – they read the volume and produce a set of coronal slices. The volume was generated using AnalyzeAVW and saved in the Analyze 7.5 file format that was used by earlier releases of Analyze (see also Section 3.5); in this format, header information is stored separately from the image information, but the whole volume is stored as one chunk of data. We already scaled intensities down to 64 shades of gray to save disk and memory space. First, the file is opened and read into a 3D array of data named vol. We read the information byte by byte. In order to have some progress information, the actual z-coordinate is being displayed.

```
1:> vol=zeros(193,193,220);
2:> fp = fopen('pigBig.img','r');
3:> for z=1:220;
4:> z
5:> for i=1:193
6:> for j=1:193
7:> rho=fread(fp,1,'char');
8:> vol(i,j,z)=rho;
```

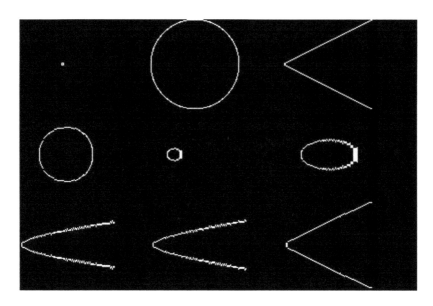

FIGURE 7.18: A few results of reformatting the 3D cone. The three slices in the first row give an impression of the cone shape. In the first two images, the reformatting plane was not tilted; a slice at position z=2 shows a small circle at the tip of the cone, and the second slice was taken at position z=98 at the base of the cone. Tilting the imaging plane by 90 degrees and shifting the tilted plane by 50 pixels in the y-direction resulted in the third image – a cross section of the cone, which is of course a triangle (and an extreme case of a hyperbola as well). The second row shows the effects of tilting and shifting the reformatting plane by an angle smaller than 63.45 degrees, which is the limit where an ellipse turns into a parabola. Tilting the reformatting plane by 10 degrees and shifting the tilted plane by 50 pixels towards the base of the cone gives the first figure, which is barely eccentric. Tilt angles of 30 and 50 degrees followed by a shift of 30 pixels in the y-direction results in the other two ellipses, which are more eccentric. One may also recognize the round-off errors at the right hand of the ellipses. We do not do any interpolation – intersection at a grazing angle results in these artifacts. The third row finally shows the result of tilting the image plane even further. If the tilting angle is parallel to a straight line on the cone, we get a parabola; tilting angle is 90 – 53.1/2 degrees, the plane is translated by 48 pixels in the y direction. The other two images show two hyperbolas which result if the tilting angle is further increased to 65 and 80 degrees while keeping the translation to 48 pixels in y-direction.

```
 9:> end
10:> end
11:> end
```

Next, we re-orientate the coordinates in a new image img so that the original axial orientation becomes a coronal orientation; every tenth slice is displayed, and the user is prompted to proceed. Figure 7.20 shows some output. In the additional tasks, you are prompted to visualize the axial and the sagittal view.

```
12:> img =zeros(220,220);
13:> for pos=1:19
```

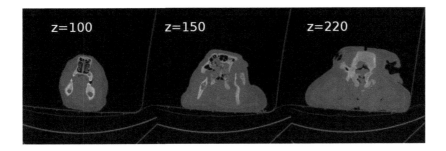

FIGURE 7.19: Three sample slices in original axial orientation from the CT-dataset used in this example. The volume we already know from Example 3.7.2. In this example, we read the full 3D volume. On the slices, we see the snout, the forehead, and the occipital region of the pig skull.

```
14:> for rfx=1:220
15:> for rfy=1:193
16:> img(rfx,rfy)=vol((pos*10),rfy,rfx);
17:> end
18:> end
19:> colormap(gray)
20:> image(img)
21:> foo=input('Press RETURN to proceed to the...
next slice ...');
22:> end
```

Additional tasks

Implement the axial and sagittal reformatting of the CT-dataset.

Based on Example 7.6.4, one should implement oblique reformatting; bear in mind that in Example 7.6.4, the cutting plane was tilted first, and then shifted. The sequence of transformations therefore was TR. Here, it would be a good idea to shift the center of the volume to the origin of the coordinate system, carry out the rotation, and then shift everything back just like we did in Example 7.6.1.

The eager among you may also implement a trilinear interpolation as given in Equation 7.7.

7.6.6 Convolution revisited

Two scripts named ThreeDConvolutionBig_7.m and ThreeDConvolutionSmall_7.m show a generalization of the convolution concept from Chapter 5. As said many times before, many concepts of 2D image processing generalize to 3D; we will now apply a simple edge detection kernel from Equation 5.8 to our CT-volume. With reformatting at hand, we have a simple way of visualizing our efforts. Again, we have a script for the less patient, and one with better resolution. First, we read the volume, just as we did in Example 7.6.5:

```
1:> vol=zeros(97,97,110);
```

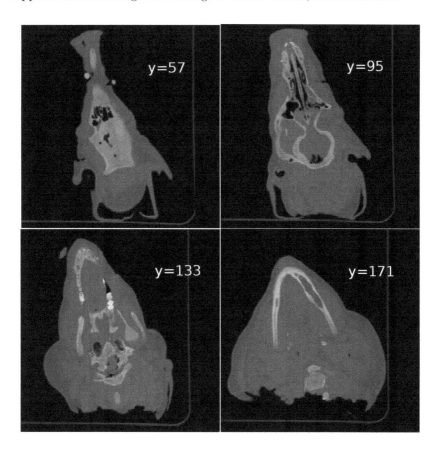

FIGURE 7.20: A set of orthogonally reformatted slices from the `pigBig.img` CT dataset. This is an output of the `ReformattingBig_7.m` script. Due to the different anatomy of a pig, it is hard to tell whether the sections are coronal or not. In a human, these slices would represent a coronal orientation.

```
2:> fp = fopen('pigSmall.img','r');
3:> for z=1:110;
4:> z
5:> for i=1:97
6:> for j=1:97
7:> rho=fread(fp,1,'char');
8:> vol(i,j,z)=rho;
9:> end
10:> end
11:> end
```

We assign a new volume named `diffvol`, and we apply a 3D version of the central difference kernel, resulting in three partial derivatives `dx`, `dy`, and `dz`. We compute the geometric mean of these partial derivatives to get the total differential, scale the volume back to 6 bit, and save the result using MATLAB's `fwrite` function. The script does not display an image.

```
12:> diffvol=zeros(97,97,110);
```

```
13:> for i=2:96
14:> for j=2:96
15:> for z=2:109
16:> dx = 0.5*(-vol((i-1),j,z) + vol((i+1),j,z));
17:> dy = 0.5*(-vol(i,(j-1),z) + vol(i,(j+1),z));
18:> dz = 0.5*(-vol(i,j,(z-1)) + vol(i,j,(z+1)));
19:> diffvol(i,j,z) = sqrt(dx*dx+dy*dy+dz*dz);
20:> end
21:> end
22:> end
23:> minint=min(min(min(diffvol)));
24:> diffvol=diffvol-minint;
25:> maxint=max(max(max(diffvol)));
26:> diffvol=diffvol/maxint*64;
27:> fp = fopen('pigSmallDiff.img','w');
28:> rho=fwrite(fp,diffvol);
```

We can use our efforts from Example 7.6.5 to visualize the resulting `pigSmallDiff.img` or `pigBigDiff.img`; as you may recognize, the oblique reformatting reveals that we are indeed dealing with a volume of edges at any orientation. For illustration purposes, a cutting plane was rotated by 45° in the x-, y- and z-axis subsequently; the result can be found in Figure 7.21.

7.7 SUMMARY AND FURTHER REFERENCES

A fairly verbose chapter has come to an end. But we were able to introduce interpolation, a very basic concept from image processing, and we spent a lot of effort in understanding spatial transforms. This is actually vital for medical image processing and 3D data visualization. Understanding the way position is given, and the ability to decompose it will keep us busy in the next section anyhow. The PCA, a very general technique in data processing, was also introduced in a manner that gives a very tangible result. And we have learned about reformatting, the most important technique for visualization of tomographic image data.

Literature

G. Strang: Introduction to Linear Algebra, Wellesley Cambridge Press, (2009)

T. S. Yoo: Insight into Images: Principles and Practice for Segmentation, Registration, and Image Analysis, A. K. Peters, (2004)

T. Peters, K. Cleary (Eds.): Image-Guided Interventions: Technology and Applications, Springer, (2008)

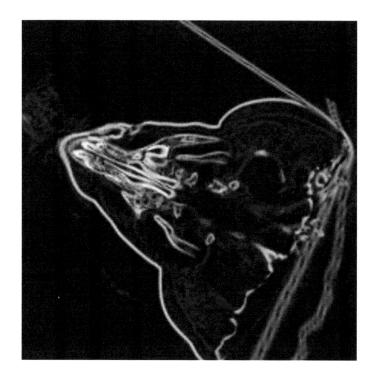

FIGURE 7.21: An oblique reformatting of the volume generated by `ThreeDConvolutionBig_7.m`; the reformatting plane was rotated by 45° around the x-, y- and z-axis. As one can see, the result of the 3D convolution is indeed a volume that contains edges in all arbitrary orientations.

CHAPTER 8

Rendering and Surface Models

Wolfgang Birkfellner

CONTENTS

8.1	Visualization	251
8.2	Orthogonal and perspective projection, and the viewpoint	252
8.3	Raycasting	252
	8.3.1 MIP, DRRs and volume rendering	253
	8.3.2 Other rendering techniques	258
8.4	Surface–based rendering	258
	8.4.1 Surface extraction, file formats for surfaces, shading and textures	261
	8.4.2 Shading models	266
	8.4.3 A special application – virtual endoscopy	266
8.5	Practical lessons	267
	8.5.1 A perspective example	267
	8.5.2 Simple orthogonal raycasting	269
	8.5.3 Viewpoint transforms and splat rendering	272
	8.5.4 Volume rendering using color coding	275
	8.5.5 A simple surface rendering – depth shading	280
	8.5.6 Rendering of voxel surfaces	283
	8.5.7 A rendering example using *3DSlicer*	286
	8.5.8 Extracting a surface using the cuberille algorithm	287
	8.5.9 A demonstration of shading effects	291
8.6	Summary and further references	295

8.1 VISUALIZATION

Visualization, generally speaking, is the art and science of conveying information to a human observer by means of an image; we already learned about the most important and widespread visualization techniques in medical imaging – *windowing*, which makes information hidden in the full intensity depth of the image visible, and *reformatting*, which allows for exploring a data cube or volume in arbitrary directions. However, when speaking about medical image processing, the beautiful and astonishing photorealistic images generated from volume data often come to mind. Rendering is the core technology for generating these visualizations. In this chapter, we will learn about the most important rendering paradigms.

8.2 ORTHOGONAL AND PERSPECTIVE PROJECTION, AND THE VIEWPOINT

The basic idea of rendering is to generate a 2D image from 3D data; every camera and every x-ray machine does this actually. It is therefore straightforward to mimic the behavior of these devices mathematically, and we will see again in Section 9.6 how we can derive the most important property of an imaging device – the distance of the viewpoint (or x-ray focus) from the 3D scene to be imaged.

However, for this purpose we need a matrix that gives us a projection, the projection operator P. If one assumes that the origin of all rays that project the 3D scene to the 2D imaging plane lies at infinity we get the following matrix:

$$P_\infty = \begin{pmatrix} 1 & 0 & 0 & 0 \\ 0 & 1 & 0 & 0 \\ 0 & 0 & 0 & 0 \\ 0 & 0 & 0 & 1 \end{pmatrix} \tag{8.1}$$

This projection images everything onto the x-y plane; the eyepoint is located at infinity in the direction of the z-axis. This is an orthogonal projection: all rays hitting the object are parallel. The term *infinite* only refers to the fact that the viewer is located at a large distance from the object. It therefore depends on the size of the object viewed. Example 8.5.1 illustrates this.

Orthogonal projection, which is computationally more efficient than perspective rendering, is the common geometry for rendering. We do, however, want to be able to look at our object from different viewpoints. In real life, we have two possibilities to look at something from a different point of view. We can change *our position*, or we can change the *position of the object*. When rendering an object, we can do the same. We can either apply a volume transform V on every voxel of our object and apply the projection $PV\vec{x}$ or we can apply another volume transform V' to the projection operator: $V'P\vec{x}$. The difference between the two will be demonstrated in Example 8.5.3.

One can also introduce perspective using the operator P; in this case the matrix has to be modified to

$$P = \begin{pmatrix} 1 & 0 & 0 & 0 \\ 0 & 1 & 0 & 0 \\ 0 & 0 & 0 & 0 \\ 0 & 0 & -\frac{1}{f} & 1 \end{pmatrix} \tag{8.2}$$

where f is the distance of the eyepoint located on the z-axis. Remember that in homogeneous coordinates, the fourth component of the vector $\vec{x} = (x, y, z, 1)^T$ always has to be one. This is not the case when applying P as given in Equation 8.2. Therefore, the resulting vector $\vec{x}' = P\vec{x}$ has to be *renormalized* by an operation $\vec{x}'_{\text{renormalized}} = \vec{x}' * \frac{1}{x'_4}$ so that the fourth element of $\vec{x}'$ becomes one again.

8.3 RAYCASTING

The projection operator is very helpful, but not very intuitive. Let's go back to the idea of simulating a camera, or an x-ray machine. Such a device records or emits rays of electromagnetic radiation (for instance light). The most straightforward approach is to simulate an x-ray. X-rays emerge from the anode of the x-ray tube and pass through matter. In dependence of the density and radioopacity of the object being imaged, the x-ray is attenuated. The remaining intensity produces a signal on the detector. *Raycasting*[1] can simulate this behavior if we sum up all gray values ρ in the path of the ray passing through a volume. This is, mathematically speaking, a line integral. If we want to simulate a camera, the situation is similar, but a different physical process takes place. Rather than penetrating the object, a ray of electromagnetic radiation is reflected. Therefore we have to simulate a ray that terminates when hitting a surface, and which is weakened and reflected; the amount of light hitting the image detector of a camera after reflection is defined by the object's surface properties. These properties are defined by *lighting models*, *shading* and *textures*. From these basic considerations, we can derive several properties of these rendering algorithms:

Volume rendering: A ray that passes an object and changes its initial intensity or color during this passage is defined by a *volume rendering* algorithm. Such an algorithm does not know about surfaces but draws all of its information from the gray values in the volume. It is an *intensity-based* algorithm.

Surface rendering: If we simulate a ray that terminates when hitting a surface, we are dealing with a *surface rendering* algorithm. The local gradient in the surrounding of the point where the ray hits the surface determines the shading of the corresponding pixel in the image plane. The drawback lies in the fact that a surface rendering algorithm requires segmentation, which can be, as we already learned in Chapter 6, cumbersome.

Raycasting is an image-driven technique – each pixel in the imaging plane is being assigned since it is the endpoint of a ray by definition. This is a huge advantage of raycasting since round-off artifacts as the ones we encountered in Example 7.6.1 cannot occur. Every pixel in the imaging plane has its own dedicated ray. If the voxels are large in comparison to the resolution of the image, discretization artifacts may nevertheless occur. In such a case, one can interpolate between voxels along the path of the ray by reducing the increment of the ray. Performance does, of course, suffer from this.

8.3.1 MIP, DRRs and volume rendering

Let's stick to volume rendering first; if we simulate an x-ray tube and simplify the attenuation model in such a manner that we just project the most intense voxel, we are dealing with *maximum intensity projection* (MIP). Figure 8.3 shows such a rendering. While the method sounds extremely simple, it is astonishingly efficient if we want to show high contrast detail in a volume. The appearance is somewhat similar to an x-ray with contrast agent.

Example 8.5.2 implements a very simple algorithm for MIP rendering; as usual in our sample scripts, the resolution of the volume to be used is coarse, but it shows the basic principle of raycasting. In this implementation, a straight line parallel to the z-axis is drawn from each pixel on the image plane to the boundary of the volume. The most intense pixel in the path of this straight line is finally saved on the image plane. Example 8.5.2 also introduces another important component of rendering, which is *intensity clipping*. In order to keep the image tidy from a gray film that stems, for instance, from non-zero pixels of air surrounding the object, it is recommendable to introduce a minimum rendering threshold – if a voxel does not show high intensity, it is omitted. Intensity clipping by introducing a

---

[1]A synonymous term is *raytracing*; we encountered this method earlier, in Chapter 5, where the imaging behavior of a spherical mirror was simulated using a raytracing software for optical design.

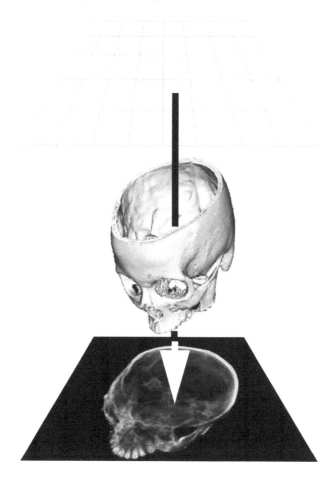

FIGURE 8.1: Orthogonal raycasting consists of projecting a beam emanating from a grid parallel to the image plane; the ray determines the appearance of the pixel it aims at on the imaging plane. If a volume rendering algorithm is implemented using raycasting, it integrates the voxel values using a defined transfer function. In the most simple case, this function is a simple max-function; only the most intense voxel is returned and conveyed to the pixel on the rendered image. This rendering technique is called *maximum intensity projection* (MIP). Image data courtesy of the Dept. of Radiology, Medical University Vienna.

rendering threshold must not be mistaken for the segmentation method named thresholding, where a binary volume is constructed by omitting voxels below or above a given threshold. Nevertheless, we have already seen the effects of introducing a rendering threshold in Figure 6.2, where the problems of segmentation based on thresholding were illustrated by using a rendering threshold.

If we simply *sum up* the voxels encountered by the ray, we end up with a render type that is called *summed voxel rendering*. It is the most simple type of a DRR which we already know from Section 9.7.2. Figure 8.4 shows such a summed voxel rendering; it is not exactly a simulation of an x-ray image since the exponential attenuation of the x-ray is not taken into account. It is nevertheless a very good approximation, and besides 2D/3D

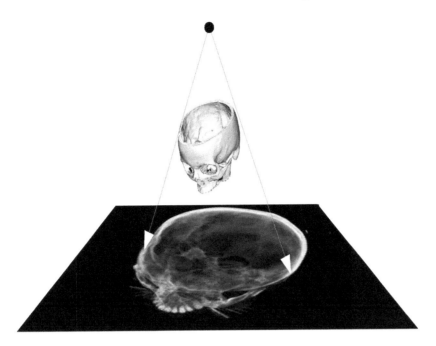

FIGURE 8.2: Raycasting can also be used for *perspective rendering*; here, all rays emanate from an eyepoint; the remaining steps are similar to orthogonal raycasting. Image data courtesy of the Dept. of Radiology, Medical University Vienna.

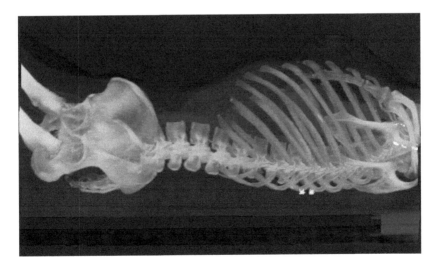

FIGURE 8.3: An orthogonal maximum intensity projection (MIP) from a whole-body CT, taken from a lateral viewpoint. In MIP, only the most intense voxel is projected to the imaging plane. MIP is the most primitive form of a volume rendering technique. Image data courtesy of the Dept. of Radiology, Medical University Vienna.

registration, DRRs are widely used in clinical radiation oncology for the computation of so called simulator images.

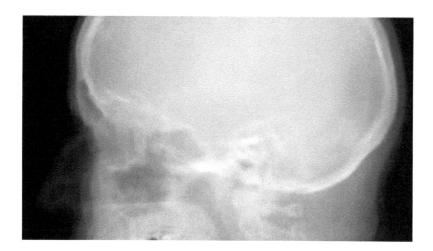

FIGURE 8.4: *Summed voxel rendering* is a simple sum of all voxel intensities in a ray's path. This is a simplified model of x-ray imaging, where the attenuation of the ray's energy is not taken into account. Being a volume rendering technique, summed voxel rendering also presents the simplest form of an algorithm for computing *digitally rendered radiographs* (DRRs). Image data courtesy of the Dept. of Radiology, Medical University Vienna.

The MIP and the DRR are simple volume rendering techniques; in volume rendering, a *transfer function* determines the final intensity of the rendered pixel. The two transfer functions we encountered so far are

$$\mathcal{T}_{\text{MIP}} = \max(\rho) \quad \forall \rho \in \{\vec{x}\} \tag{8.3}$$

$$\mathcal{T}_{\text{DRR}} = \sum \rho \quad \forall \rho \in \{\vec{x}\} \tag{8.4}$$

where ρ is the intensity of voxels located at positions $\{\vec{x}\}$, which is the set of all voxels within the *path of the ray*. The strength of volume rendering lies in the fact that segmentation is not necessary. However, a MIP or a DRR is usually not what one expects from a visualization algorithm for 3D data. If one wants to show, for instance, the surface of the body and some internal organs, more sophisticated volume rendering approaches are necessary. A transfer function that shows both high-intensity contrast from structures inside the body as well as the surface could look something like this:

Assign a high value of a given color to the first voxel above the rendering threshold encountered by the ray; one could also introduce some sort of shading here in such a manner that voxels with a greater distance to the origin of the ray appear darker. This very simple type of surface shading is called *depth shading* (see also Figure 8.7 and Example 8.5.5). More sophisticated shading methods will be introduced in the Section 8.4. However, the ray is not terminated (or *clipped*) here.

If the ray encounters a structure with a gray value within a defined section of the histogram, it may add an additional color and voxel opacity to the pixel to be rendered.

These more complex transfer functions can, of course, be refined and combined with surface shading techniques in order to improve visual appearance. However, it does not require segmentation in a strict sense. The definition of ROIs for rendering takes place by choosing

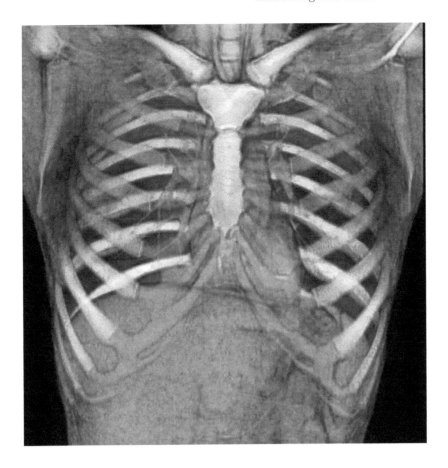

FIGURE 8.5: If one chooses a transfer function that assigns opacity and color to gray values, a more sophisticated type of summed voxel rendering is possible. A color version of this image rendered by volume compositing can be found in the JPGs folder on the accompanying CD. This image was created using AnalyzeAVW. The dialog showing the definition of the transfer function is found in Figure 8.6. Image data courtesy of the Dept. of Radiology, Medical University Vienna.

the area of the histogram that gets a color assigned. A sophisticated volume rendering algorithm creates beautiful images, similar to old anatomical glass models, and circumvents the problems of segmentation. An example of a rendering generated by such a *volume compositing* technique can be found in Figure 8.5; the associated transfer function is given in Figure 8.6. Example 8.5.4 shows how such a colorful rendering can be made.

Finally, we have to discuss the choice of the viewpoint in the rendering process. Changing the view of an object is easy; all we have to do is apply a spatial transform to the volume. Example 8.5.2 presents such a transform. The only problem here is the considerable confusion if the object leaves the rendering domain – it is hard to debug a code that is formally correct but renders nothing but a void volume. The more complex operation is the change of the viewpoint. If we transform the position of the observer, we also have to transform the imaging plane accordingly, otherwise the image will be skewed. Example 8.5.3 gives an illustration of viewpoint transforms.

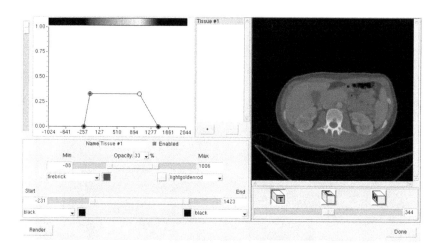

FIGURE 8.6: The dialog of AnalyzeAVW for defining a transfer function for the volume compositing process. Opacity and color assigned to voxel gray values are given by manipulating the transfer function. Image data courtesy of the Dept. of Radiology, Medical University Vienna.

8.3.2 Other rendering techniques

The main problem of raycasting lies in the fact that it is computationally expensive, especially when switching to a perspective view model. Various refinements to improve the performance of raycasting do exist, for instance *shear-warp rendering*. But we can also use our old pal, the projection operator P to render images. This method is called *splat rendering*. An example is given in Example 8.5.3. It is a *volume driven rendering*[2] method, and implementing a MIP or summed voxel rendering is pretty straightforward – all we have to do is apply the projection operator to the voxel positions and map the gray values to the appropriate pixel positions in the rendering plane. The quality of such a rendering is inferior to a raycasting, but since we usually use a rendering threshold, another huge advantage pops up – we don't have to keep or visit all voxels in a volume since the spatial context of the voxels does not play a role. Look at Figure 8.7, where we only render the bony part of a volume that has approximately $4.5 * 10^7$ voxels. Approximately 15% belong to bony tissue. It is therefore a considerable waste to employ a raycasting technique here.

8.4 SURFACE–BASED RENDERING

In Figure 8.7, we make a step from volume rendering to surface rendering. The main difference of surface rendering compared to volume rendering methods lies in the fact that we do not use the gray values in the image to assign a gray value or a color to the rendered pixel, but we encode the *properties of a surface element to the gray value*. An example already mentioned is *depth shading* – the distance of a voxel to the imaging plane determines its gray value. An example can be found in Figure 8.7. The transfer function for depth shading is given as

$$\mathcal{T}_{\mathrm{DS}} = \max \|\vec{x} - \vec{x}_{\mathrm{Render\ Plane}}\| \quad \forall \{\vec{x}\}. \tag{8.5}$$

---

[2]This refers to the fact that the location of the voxel determines the position of a pixel in the rendering. It must not be confused with *volume rendering*.

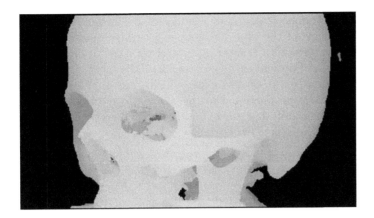

FIGURE 8.7: Depth shading is a simple shading technique that assigns a gray value to the pixel to be rendered based upon its distance from the origin of the ray. The further away a voxel lies from the imaging plane, the brighter it gets. Depth shading does not give a photorealistic impression, but it adds a visual clue and can be used if simple structures are to be rendered. This image was created using AnalyzeAVW. Image data courtesy of the Dept. of Radiology, Medical University Vienna.

Again, $\{\vec{x}\}$ is the set of voxels lying in the beam's path, and $\vec{x}_{\text{Render Plane}}$ is the end point of the ray. The voxel with the greatest distance to the image plane defines a surface; it is also the first voxel which lies above a rendering threshold encountered by the ray. Its distance gives the gray value of the pixel in the rendering plane the ray aims at. What is remarkable about Equation 8.5 when comparing it to Equations 8.4 and 8.3 is the fact that ρ, the intensity of the voxel, does not play a role here since depth shading is, in fact, a *surface rendering* technique.

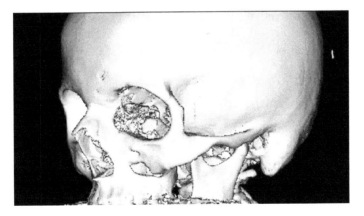

FIGURE 8.8: The same volume as in Figure 8.7, rendered by a surface shader. This image was created using AnalyzeAVW. Image data courtesy of the Dept. of Radiology, Medical University Vienna.

An important consequence is the fact that we do not need the gray value information from voxels anymore – we just need some information on the surface. A binary dataset containing a segmented volume is absolutely sufficient for surface rendering. In order to achieve a more natural view of the object when using surface rendering, we have to place our light sources in the coordinate system used, and we have to employ a *lighting model* that provides a simulation of optical surface properties. The most simple model is actually *Lambertian shading*; it is based on *Lambert's law*, which states that the intensity of reflected light from a diffuse surface is proportional to the cosine of the viewing angle. If we have a normal vector $\vec{n}$ on our ideal diffuse surface, and the view direction is given by a vector $\vec{v}$, the intensity I of reflected light is given by:

$$I = I_{\max} \frac{\vec{n} \bullet \vec{v}}{\|\vec{n}\| \|\vec{v}\|} \tag{8.6}$$

$I_{\max}$ is the maximum intensity, emitted in the direction of the normal vector $\vec{n}$ of the reflecting surface. The cosine of the angle between vectors $\vec{v}$ and $\vec{n}$ is given by the inner product of the vectors, divided by the norms of the vectors – recall Equation 5.12. With such a simple model, we can simulate the behavior of a surface. If we go back to the introduction of this chapter, we are now trying to simulate a camera rather than an x-ray machine.

Equation 8.6 is basically all we need to generate a realistic rendering of a surface. The normal to a surface voxel can be determined, for instance, by inspecting the neighboring voxels. Consider a 26-connected surrounding of a surface voxel.[3] The ray defines a subset of these 26-connected voxels – the ones in front and directly behind the surface voxel are, for instance, irrelevant. Using a finite difference similar to Equation 5.7, allows for computing two non-collinear gradients; let's call those ∇_x and ∇_y. Figure 8.9 illustrates two such gradients for seven voxels which are 26-connected to a surface voxel hit by one of the rays in the raycasting process.

If we have the position vector to a surface voxel $\vec{x}_{ijk} = (x_i, y_j, z_k)^T$ at hand and our beam approaches in the z-direction, we have to select those 26-connected non-zero voxels that give two non-collinear gradients; the difference vectors between four neighbors, which can be aligned in x- and y-directions (as in Example 8.5.6, where a surface shading is demonstrated), or which can be determined by the two gradients with the largest norm, give the central differences $\vec{\nabla}_x$ and $\vec{\nabla}_y$ in vector notation. These two gradients span a local plane with the surface voxel $\vec{x}_{ijk}$ in the center. The normal vector on this local planar segment is given by the *outer* or *cross product* of $\vec{\nabla}_x$ and $\vec{\nabla}_y$. It is computed as

$$\vec{\nabla}_x \times \vec{\nabla}_y = \begin{pmatrix} \nabla_{x_1} \\ \nabla_{x_2} \\ \nabla_{x_3} \end{pmatrix} \times \begin{pmatrix} \nabla_{y_1} \\ \nabla_{y_2} \\ \nabla_{y_3} \end{pmatrix} = \begin{pmatrix} \nabla_{x_2} \nabla_{y_3} - \nabla_{x_3} \nabla_{y_2} \\ \nabla_{x_3} \nabla_{y_1} - \nabla_{x_1} \nabla_{y_3} \\ \nabla_{x_1} \nabla_{y_2} - \nabla_{x_2} \nabla_{y_1} \end{pmatrix} \tag{8.7}$$

In order to make this normal vector a unit vector of length 1, we may furthermore compute $\vec{n}_e = \frac{\vec{n}}{\|\vec{n}\|}$. If we also derive a unit vector $\vec{r}$ in the direction of the beam, we may compute the illumination of the plane segment associated with a single surface voxel $\vec{x}_{ijk}$ according to Equation 8.6 as $I = \vec{r} \bullet \vec{n}_e$. Example 8.5.6 implements such a rendering on a segmented binary volume of 1 mm³ voxel size. The result can be found in Figure 8.26.

This technique, where a normal vector is assigned to each surface element, is called *flat shading*. In our case, the surface element is one face of a voxel; a refinement can be achieved by using a finer resolution in voxel space. If we switch to visualization of *surface models*, where the surface is represented by geometric primitives such as triangles, flat shading may produce an even more coarse surface since a single element can be relatively large – more on this subject comes in Section 8.4.1.

---

[3]If you already forgot about connectedness, you may take a quick look at Figure 5.9.

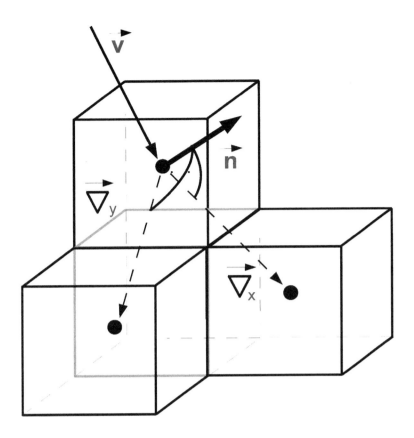

FIGURE 8.9: Computing two surface gradients for a surface voxel hit by a ray. The other non-zero voxels in the 26-connected neighborhood are used to compute two gradients ∇_x and ∇_y, which give the slope to the nearest other voxels belonging to the surface.

8.4.1 Surface extraction, file formats for surfaces, shading and textures

For most of this book, we have dealt with image elements; in the 2D case, we call them *pixels*, and in the 3D case, we are dealing with *voxels*. The representation of volume image data as datacubes consisting of voxels is, however, not very widespread outside the medical domain. 3D graphics as shown in computer games and computer-aided design (CAD) programs rely on the representation of *surfaces* rather than voxels. These surfaces are given as geometric primitives (usually triangles), defined by node points (or *vertices*) and normal vectors. The advantage of this technical surface presentation is evident – surface rendering as introduced in Section 8.4 can be performed directly since the normal vectors and the area to be illuminated are directly defined. A computation of gradients and normal vectors is therefore not necessary since this information is already available in the surface presentation. Furthermore, modern graphics adapters are optimized for fast computation of renderings from such surface models, and well-developed application programmer interfaces (API) like OpenGL exist for all kinds of rendering tasks.

While all of this sounds great, there is also a severe drawback. *Man does not consist of surfaces.* In order to get a nice surface, one has to segment the organ or anatomic structure

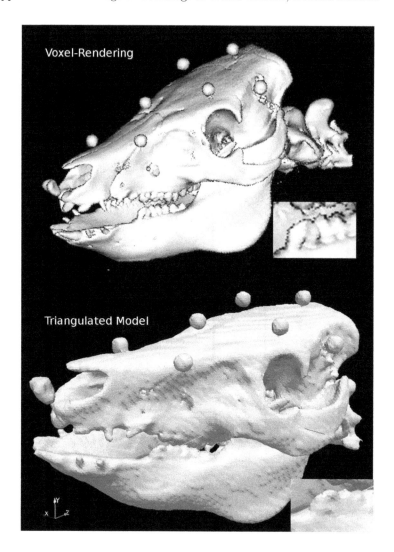

FIGURE 8.10: A comparison of voxel and triangulated surface rendering. The upper image of the well-known pig skull was generated from a voxel model of 0.5 mm^3 using AnalyzeAVW. The lower rendering shows the triangulated surface model generated using the surface-extraction module of AnalyzeAVW. The upper volume has a total size of 346.8 MB, whereas the binary file containing the 367061 triangles used for the lower rendering is only 13.1 MB large. A loss in detail in the lower image is evident – just inspect the enlarged section of the mandibular molars.

of interest – from Chapter 6 we know that this can be a tedious task. The great advantage of volume rendering techniques, which are introduced in Section 8.3.1, is actually the fact that segmentation is *not* necessary, although some sort of "soft" segmentation step is introduced in the *transfer function*. Furthermore, we lose all the information on tissue stored in the gray value of every single voxel. Another problem lies in the discretization of the surface – compared to the technical structures like screws and mechanical parts displayed in a CAD program, biological structures are of greater complexity, and the segmentation and computation of a mesh of geometric primitives usually lead to a simplification of the surface which may further obfuscate relevant anatomical detail. An example showing a rendering of our well-known porcine friend is given in Figure 8.10. Still there are some fields of application where triangulated anatomical models are extremely helpful:

Fast rendering: Real-time visualization, for instance in augmented reality or surgical simulation, is easily achieved by using appropriate hardware available at a more than reasonable price. Acceleration boards for voxel representations do exist but never gained wide acceptance in the field.

Collision detection: Connected to the problem of simulation is the problem of real-time collision detection. In a rendering environment, usually no feedback is given if two surfaces intersect. Using a voxel-representation, it may be pretty time consuming to detect whether two surfaces collide or not. Collision detection is nevertheless relevant in applications like surgical planning, or in applications where a robot or a simple manipulator is used during an intervention. Using triangulated surfaces allows the use of fast collision detection algorithms. An example can be found in Figure 8.11.

Finite element modelling: If we want to simulate the mechanical behavior of tissue, we have to use a simulation software based on the numerical computation of partial differential equations; this technique is generally called finite element modelling (FEM), and it was already mentioned in Section 9.2.2. FEM requires a 3D mesh generated from surface models or voxel volumes. The mechanical properties to be simulated are associated with the mesh elements.

Rapid prototyping: Finally, it is possible to generate 3D plastic models out of volume data by rapid prototyping or a similar technique. An example for such a model can be found in Figure 6.8. The input data for such a 3D printer is usually a triangulated mesh.

Therefore, it may be a good idea if we would find a way to transform a segmented, binary voxel volume into a set of geometric primitives forming a surface. In its most basic form, *triangulation* of a voxel surface takes place by

identifying voxels that belong to a surface – these are those voxels that have less than six neighbors.

assigning rectangles or triangles that represent the surface.

storing the resulting geometric primitives in an adequate form.

This method is generally referred to as a *cuberille* approach, and it is implemented in Example 8.5.8. The result of this example – the triangulation of a binary segmented voxel model of a human pedicle – is shown in Figure 8.32. The result is rather blocky and cannot be considered a state-of-the-art triangulation. Nevertheless it illustrates the principle of a triangulation algorithm in a simple manner.

A more sophisticated triangulation algorithm should actually take care of smoothing the sharp edges of the voxel surface. Such an algorithm is the *marching cubes* algorithm. Let us illustrate the principle of this method in 2D; if we consider a binary image of a segmented structure, there are four possible elements that form a boundary of the shape when looking at areas of 2×2 pixels. These are shown in Figure 8.12. The four elements shown below the actual binary shape are the only elements that can form an outline – if you consider all of their possible positions, you will come to the conclusion that fourteen

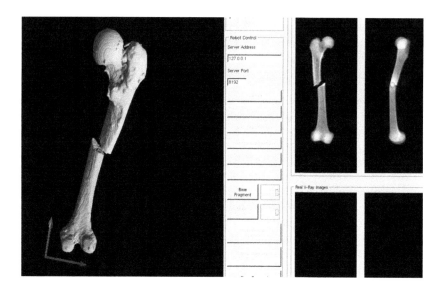

FIGURE 8.11: A screenshot of software for simulating long bone fractures. The user can apply an arbitrary fracture to a model of a bone derived from CT. The manipulation of the fragments in 3D is visualized using triangulated mesh models shown in the left part of the image. A *collision detection* algorithm, which keeps the fragments from intersecting each other, is also implemented. Meanwhile, simulated lateral and anterio-posterior DRRs are rendered as well from a smaller version of the original CT-volume (right hand side). The purpose of this training tool was to provide a simple demonstration for the context of 3D manipulation of bone fragments and the resulting x-ray images.

possible shapes are derived from these elements. If one wants to determine the outline of the shape, it is a feasible approach to check whether one of the fourteen shapes fits an arbitrary 2×2 subimage. If this is the case, one can assign a line segment representing the outline of the appropriate image element. This is called a *marching squares* algorithm. In 2D, this approach is however of little interest since we can always determine the outline of a binary 2D shape by applying a Sobel-filter as introduced in Chapter 5 or another edge-detection algorithm, which is by far more elegant.

The interesting fact is that this method can be generalized to 3D, which results in the aforementioned marching cubes algorithm. Here, the volume is divided in cubic subvolumes of arbitrary size. There are 256 different possibilities to populate the eight corners of these cubes. If we omit the possibilities which are redundant since they can be generated by rotating a generic shape, we end up with fifteen different configurations. This is very similar to the situation illustrated in Figure 8.12, where fourteen possible 2D configurations can be derived from four generic shapes. The advantage of the marching cubes algorithm lies in the fact that it can be easily scaled – choose large cubes as subvolumes, and you will get a coarse grid. Small cubes result in a fine grid. Two out of fifteen possible configurations with associated triangles are shown in Figure 8.13. An actual implementation of the marching cubes algorithm simply consists of a lookup-table that contains the fifteen basic shapes and a rather straightforward algorithm that assigns the appropriate set of triangles appropriate for the shape encountered in a given cube.

Once a surface is parameterized using graphics primitives, it can be stored by using one of the numerous file formats for surface models. As opposed to image file formats

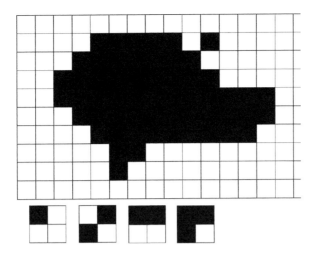

FIGURE 8.12: When looking at the possible configurations of pixels forming an outline of a binary 2D shape, we can identify four basic shapes. By rotating these basic shapes, it is possible to identify all straight line segments forming the shape. These line segments form the outline of the shape – the algorithm that does this for a 2D image is called the *marching squares* algorithm.

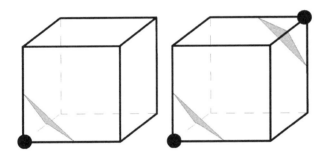

FIGURE 8.13: Two out of fifteen possible configurations for the marching cubes algorithm. The black circles denote occupied edge points in the cubic subvolumes. In 3D triangulation algorithm, the volume is divided into cubic subvolumes. Dependent on the number of cube edges populated with non-zero voxels, certain triangle sets are assigned. The result is a smooth triangulated surface.

introduced in Chapter 3, we do not have to take care of gray values here. A typical format, which is also used for storing the results of our triangulation effort in Example 8.5.8, is the *Surface Tessellation Language* (STL). It is a standard that is readable by most programs for computer-aided design, stereolithography, and surface visualization. It exists in an ASCII-encoded text type and a binary form. The general shape of an ASCII-STL file is as follows:

```
solid name
```

```
facet normal xₙ yₙ zₙ
outer loop
vertex x₁ y₁ z₁
vertex x₂ y₂ z₂
vertex x₃ y₃ z₃
endloop
endfacet
...endsolid name
```

First, a name is assigned to a surface, which is called a *solid* here. The triangles called *facets* are defined by a normal vector pointing to the outside of the object; orientation is defined by a *right-hand rule* here. When visiting all edgepoints of the facet in a counterclockwise direction (just as if you are bending the fingers of your right hand to form the *right-hand rule* known from physics), the normal vector points in the direction of the thumb. The description of each facet is given within the two keywords `facet ...` and `endfacet`. When all facets are described, the file ends with the keyword `endsolid`. The most important requirement is that two out of the three `vertex` coordinates must match for two adjacent triangles. STL is therefore a rather uneconomic format since many coordinates are to be repeated. Furthermore, we face the usual problem when storing numerical data as ASCII – the files become very big since, for instance, an `unsigned int`, which usually occupies two bytes in binary form and can take the maximal value 65536, requires up to five bytes in ASCII-format. A binary version of STL therefore exists as well. Other file formats for triangulated surfaces are, for instance, the *Initial Graphics Exchange Specification* (IGES) or the *Standard for the Exchange of Product model data* (STEP); they are, however, organized in a similar manner.

8.4.2   Shading models

Another problem with triangulated surfaces lies in the fact that triangles covering large, planar areas may appear rather dull when using a simple flat shading model as in Equation 8.6; in medical image processing, this is not as big a problem as in technical surfaces since the surface encountered in the body are usually not very regular, and a fine representation can be achieved by using volumes with a fine voxel grid. However, if one wants to improve the appearance of a model triangulated using a rather coarse grid, it may be useful to *interpolate additional normal vectors* in dependence of the normal vectors associated with a surface facet. Figure 8.14 illustrates this principle, which is also known as *Phong* shading. Example 8.5.9 implements an indirect interpolation for our simple raycaster from Example 8.5.6, and the effect can be seen in Figure 8.35. If one interpolates the *color of pixels* in the image plane between vertices instead of the normal vectors, we are speaking of *Gouraud* shading.

Finally, one may render 2D patterns, so-called *textures* on the graphic primitives to increase the 3D effect. This is of great importance for instance in computer games, surgical simulation, and other visualization applications. However, in basic medical imaging, textures do usually not play a very important role.

8.4.3   A special application – virtual endoscopy

Finally, a special rendering technique called *virtual endoscopy* is introduced. An endoscope is an optical instrument with a small wide-angle camera that can be inserted into the body. Various types of flexible and rigid endoscopes for neurosurgery, ENT-surgery and, above

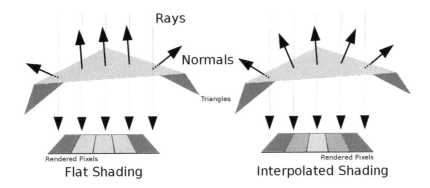

Rays

Normals

Triangles

Rendered Pixels

Rendered Pixels

Flat Shading

Interpolated Shading

FIGURE 8.14: The principle of Gouraud-shading. When rendering a large triangle that is hit by several rays aiming at neighboring pixels in the render plane, we may end up with rather large, dull areas on the rendered image. If the normal vectors for the respective rays are interpolated between the neighboring geometric primitives, we will get a smoother appearance of the rendered surface.

all, gastrointestinal interventions exist. It is also possible to take histological samples or to inject drugs using these devices. Given the ergonomics of an endoscope, it is sometimes difficult to orientate oneself during an endoscopic intervention. Therefore it is interesting, for training purposes as well as visualization, to simulate endoscopic views. Since the endoscope is, technically speaking, a wide-angle camera, this can be performed using a perspective surface rendering technique. A special problem here is the simulation of barrel distortion, an optical property of wide-angle lenses that is also known as the fisheye effect. Figure 8.15 shows such a virtual endoscopy – here, we take a look in cranial direction through the cervical spine of our pig CT dataset into the calvaria; the rendering threshold is chosen in such a manner that no soft tissue is visible. Virtual endoscopy has gained some importance in the early detection of colon cancer, where it is sometimes used to generate endoscopy-like views from CT data of the lower abdomen.

8.5   PRACTICAL LESSONS

8.5.1   A perspective example

`Perspective_8.m` illustrates the perspective projection of a cube's eight cornerpoints. The cube has 10 pixels sidelength. The origin of the cube is located at $(10, 10, 0)^T$. The distance of the viewer, located on the z-axis of the coordinate system is given by `fdist`. You are encouraged to play with different values of `fdist`. Some of the possible output can be found in Figure 8.16.

First, we have to the define the cornerpoints of the cube; there is little to be discussed in this part of the script.

```
1:>clear;
2:> cube=zeros(4,8);
3:> cube(1,1)= 10;
4:> cube(2,1)= 10;
5:> cube(4,1)= 1;
6:> cube(1,2)= 20;
```

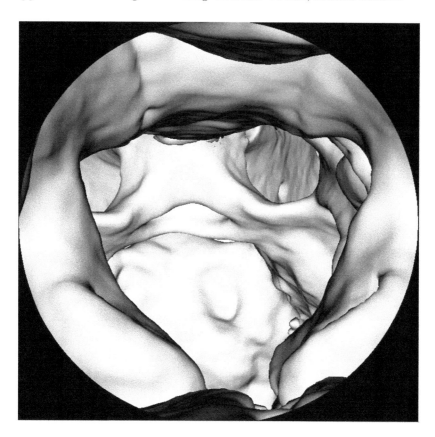

FIGURE 8.15: A virtual endoscopy of the spinal canal of the pig dataset, rendered from CT. Basically speaking, this is a surface rendering that, in addition, simulates the barrel distortion induced by the wide angle optics of a conventional endoscope. Image data courtesy of the Dept. of Radiology, Medical University Vienna.

```
 7:> cube(2,2)= 10;
 8:> cube(4,2)= 1;
 9:> cube(1,3)= 10;
10:> cube(2,3)= 20;
11:> cube(4,3)= 1;
12:> cube(1,4)= 20;
13:> cube(2,4)= 20;
14:> cube(4,4)= 1;
15:> cube(1,5)= 10;
16:> cube(2,5)= 10;
17:> cube(3,5)= 10;
18:> cube(4,5)= 1;
19:> cube(1,6)= 20;
20:> cube(2,6)= 10;
21:> cube(3,6)= 10;
22:> cube(4,6)= 1;
23:> cube(1,7)= 10;
```

```
24:> cube(2,7)= 20;
25:> cube(3,7)= 10;
26:> cube(4,7)= 1;
27:> cube(1,8)= 20;
28:> cube(2,8)= 20;
29:> cube(3,8)= 10;
30:> cube(4,8)= 1;
```

Next, we define an image `img` to hold the rendering, and the distance of the eyepoint to the viewing plane `fdist` is being defined. A projection matrix `projector` is set up as given in Equation 8.2. And we define two vectors to hold the coordinates of the 3D object points and the rendered 2D points.

```
31:> img=zeros(30,30);
32:> fdist=100;
33:> projector=eye(4);
34:> projector(3,3)=0;
35:> projector(4,3)=-1/fdist;
36:> V=projector;
37:> worldPoints=zeros(4,1);
38:> imagePoints=zeros(4,1);
```

Finally, we carry out the projection and display the result; denote the renormalization step, which takes care of the different scale of projections in dependence of the distance to the imaging plane:

```
39:> for j=1:8
40:> for k=1:4
41:> worldPoints(k,1)=cube(k,j);
42:> end
43:> imagePoints=V*worldPoints;
44:> imagePoints=round(imagePoints/(imagePoints(4,1)));
45:> ix=imagePoints(1,1);
46:> iy=imagePoints(2,1);
47:> if (ix > 0 & ix < 30 & iy > 0 & iy < 30)
48:> img(ix,iy)=64;
49:> end
50:> end
51:> colormap(gray)
52:> image(img)
```

8.5.2   Simple orthogonal raycasting

`Raytracing_8.m` introduces a very simple version of MIP-rendering using raycasting; there is no perspective involved, therefore all rays are parallel. First, we load a volume that was scaled down and saved with 8 bit depth in order to keep the volume size manageable. The procedure of loading the volume is not new – we know it already from Example 7.6.5:

```
1:> vol=zeros(98,98,111);
2:> fp = fopen('pigSmall.img','r');
3:> for z=1:110;
```

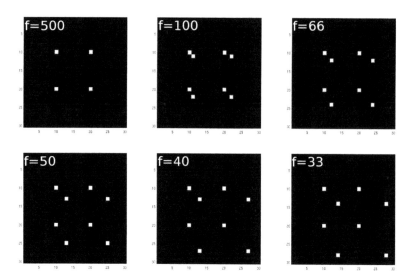

FIGURE 8.16: Sample output from `Perspective_8.m`. As the viewpoint approaches the eight corners of a cube of 10 pixels sidelength, the projection changes from a square to a sheared projection. The first image shows an orthogonal projection since the distance of the viewpoint is 50 times larger than the typical dimension of the object, therefore the projection operator approximates P_∞ given in Equation 8.1.

```
4:> z
5:> for i=1:97
6:> for j=1:97
7:> rho=fread(fp,1,'char');
8:> vol(i,j,z)=rho;
9:> end
10:> end
11:> end
```

Next, we introduce a minimum threshold `minth` for rendering; remember that such a threshold helps to keep the rendered image free from unwanted projections of low-intensity non-zero pixels that may, for instance, stem form the air surrounding the object; a matrix holding the rendered image `img` is allocated, as well as a vector `vox`. This vector holds the actual position of the ray passing through the volume:

```
12:> minth=20;
13:> img=zeros(98,98);
14:> vox=zeros(3,1);
```

Now we are ready to start the rendering process. The procedure is pretty straightforward; the ray, whose actual position is given in the `vox` vector proceeds to the volume from a starting point above the volume, following the z-axis. If it hits the image surface, it terminates. A new gray value `rho` at the actual voxel position beyond the highest gray value encountered so far is assigned the new maximum gray value `maxRho` if its value is higher than the rendering threshold `minth`. Once the ray terminates, the maximum gray value is assigned to the rendered image `img`, and the image is displayed.

```
15:> for i =1:98
16:> for j =1:98
17:> maxRho=0;
18:> for dep=1:110
19:> vox=transpose([i,j,(110-dep)]);
20:> if vox(1,1) > 0 & vox (1,1) < 98 &
vox(2,1) > 0 & vox(2,1) < 98 & vox(3,1)>0 &
vox(3,1)<111
21:> rho = vol(vox(1,1),vox(2,1),vox(3,1));
22:> if rho > maxRho & rho > minth
23:> maxRho = rho;
24:> end
25:> end
26:> end
27:> img(i,j)=maxRho;
28:> end
29:> end
30:> minint=min(min(img));
31:> img=img-minint;
32:> maxint = max(max(img));
33:> img=img/maxint*64;
34:> colormap(gray)
35:> image(img)
```

The – admittedly not very impressive – result is shown in Figure 8.17.

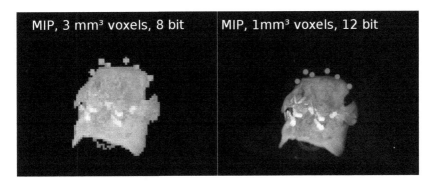

FIGURE 8.17: The output from `Raytracing_8.m` is shown on the left; it shows a frontal MIP rendered from CT data. The image quality is poor because of the small size of the volume; if one uses a more powerful rendering engine like the one of AnalyzeAVW with a volume of better resolution, one gets an image like the one shown on the right. The similarity is, nevertheless, obvious.

Besides the poor resolution, which is atributed to the memory management in MATLAB®, the view is also not very enlightening since we are looking at the snout of our patient. It would be better to rotate the volume around the y-axis so that we get a lateral view. This is, however, not a real problem since we have done this before. `RaytracingRotated_8.m` does this. It is derived from `Raytracing_8.m`; the volume is rotated, but its boundaries are maintained. The following code is inserted after reading the volume. It rotates the volume – the rotation center is the center of the volume – and writes the result to a volume `newvol` with the same boundaries as `vol`. Finally, it copies the rotated volume to `vol`, and the raycasting algorithm proceeds; the result, together with an equivalent high-quality MIP, is shown in Figure 8.18.

```
...> R=eye(4);
...> R(2,3) = 1;
...> R(3,2) = -1;
...> R(2,2)=0;
...> R(3,3)=0;
...> T=eye(4);
...> T(1,4)=48;
...> T(2,4)=48;
...> T(3,4)=54;
...> invT=inv(T); ...> newvol=zeros(98,98,111);
...> oldvox=zeros(4,1);
...> newvox=zeros(4,1);
...> for i=1:97
...> for j=1:97
...> for z=1:110
...> oldvox(1,1)=i;
...> oldvox(2,1)=j;
...> oldvox(3,1)=z;
...> oldvox(4,1)=1;
...> newvox=round(T*R*invT*oldvox);
...> if newvox(1,1) > 0 & newvox(1,1) < 98 &
newvox(2,1) > 0 & newvox(2,1) < 98
& newvox(3,1) > 0 & newvox(3,1) < 111
...> newvol(newvox(1,1),newvox(2,1),newvox(3,1))=
vol(i,j,z);
...> end
...> end
...> end
...> end
...> vol=newvol;
```

Additional Tasks

Inspect the result when changing `minth`.

Change the script so that it produces a summed voxel rendering instead of a MIP. A possible output can be found in Figure 8.19.

8.5.3 Viewpoint transforms and splat rendering

In `Splatting_8.m`, we implement splatting – the projection of voxels onto the imaging plane using the operator P from Equation 8.1 – as an alternative rendering method. If we just load the volume dataset from Example 8.5.2, the whole code looks like this:

```
1:> vol=zeros(98,98,111);
2:> fp = fopen('pigSmall.img','r');
```

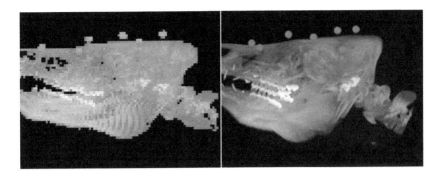

FIGURE 8.18: A MIP derived by raytracing, after rotation of the object. A high-quality version with a similar object orientation rendered with AnalyzeAVW can be seen on the right.

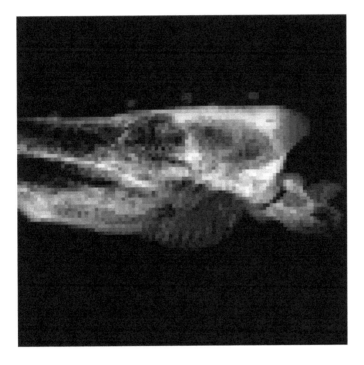

FIGURE 8.19: A summed voxel shading rendered with a modified version of Raytracing_8.m. The orientation of the volume is similar to Figure 8.18.

```
3:> for z=1:110;
4:> for i=1:97
5:> for j=1:97
6:> rho=fread(fp,1,'char');
7:> vol(i,j,z)=rho;
8:> end
9:> end
10:> end
```

A MIP rendering using splat rendering looks rather similar to Example 8.5.2. We derive a projection operator P and apply it to all voxel positions vox. If the projected gray value is higher than the one already encountered in the rendering plane img, it replaces the gray value.

```
11:> img=zeros(98,98);
12:> minth=20;
13:> P=eye(4);
14:> P(3,3)=0;
15:> vox=zeros(4,1);
16:> pos=zeros(4,1);
17:> for i=1:97
18:> for j=1:97
19:> for z=1:110
20:> vox=transpose([i,j,z,1]);
21:> pos=P*vox;
22:> rho=vol(i,j,z);
23:> if pos(1,1) > 0 & pos(1,1) < 98 & pos(2,1) > 0 & pos(2,1) < 98
24:> if rho > img(pos(1,1),pos(2,1)) & rho > minth
25:> img(pos(1,1),pos(2,1)) = rho;
26:> end
27:> end
28:> end
29:> end
30:> end
31:> minint=min(min(img));
32:> img=img-minint;
33:> maxint = max(max(img));
34:> img=img/maxint*64;
35:> colormap(gray)
36:> image(img)
```

One may ask about the benefit of this approach since the result looks pretty similar to Figure 8.17. The strength of splat rendering as a volume-driven method however lies in the fact that it does not need the whole volume data set. If we load a scaled version of the volume that was used to generate Figure 8.7 with $215 \times 215 \times 124 = 5731900$ voxels and 2 bit depth, we can directly introduce the rendering threshold of -540 HU in the volume and save the volume as a $N \times 4$ matrix; the columns of this matrix consist of the three voxel coordinates and the associated gray value. This vector that still contains most of the gray scale information, has only $N = 2579560$ columns – these are all the voxels above the rendering threshold. The volume was preprocessed and saved in a file named VoxelVector.dat. Since it is stored as ASCII-text, you can directly inspect it using a text editor. The fact that it was saved as text did, however, blow up the data volume considerably. MATLAB reads this matrix, and a more sophisticated version of Splatting_8.m called BetterSplatting_8.m uses this data, which is loaded in a quick manner. It implements a MIP-rendering routine in only 23 lines of code. First, the matrix VoxelVector.dat is loaded, a projection operator is assigned, and vectors for the 3D voxel coordinates (named vox) and the coordinates on the rendered image (called pos) are allocated:

```
1:> vect=zeros(2579560,4);
2:> vect=load('VoxelVector.dat');
```

```
3:> img=zeros(215,215);
4:> P=eye(4);
5:> P(3,3)=0;
6:> vox=zeros(4,1);
7:> pos=zeros(4,1);
```

Next, we visit each column in the matrix containing the processed volume, which was thresholded at -540 HU; the gray values were shifted in such a manner that the lowest gray value is 0; finally, the resulting rendering is displayed; a selection of possible outputs is presented in Figure 8.20:

```
8:> for i=1:2579560
9:> vox=transpose([vect(i,1),vect(i,2),vect(i,3),1]);
10:> pos=P*vox;
11:> rho=vect(i,4);
12:> if pos(1,1) > 0 & pos(1,1) < 215 &...
pos(2,1) > 0 & pos(2,1) < 215
13:> if rho > img(pos(1,1),pos(2,1))
14:> img(pos(1,1),pos(2,1)) = rho;
15:> end
16:> end
17:> end
18:> minint=min(min(img));
19:> img=img-minint;
20:> maxint = max(max(img));
21:> img=img/maxint*64;
22:> colormap(gray)
23:> image(img)
```

For the impatient, there is another voxel matrix `VoxelVectorBone.dat`. It introduces a rendering threshold of 250 HU; only 360562 or approximately 16% of the voxel data are used; applying a perspective summed voxel rendering using this dataset results in Figure 8.21, which is still pretty convincing and is rendered pretty fast compared to Example 8.5.2. Aliasing artifacts, which are basically round-off-errors, become evident here; in more sophisticated approaches these are suppressed by various blurring techniques.[4]

Additional Tasks

Introduce perspective to `BetterSplatting_8.m`. Do not forget renormalization of the resulting homogeneous vector.

Change the script `BetterSplatting_8.m` to implement viewpoint transforms. Start with translations, and compare the effect of the operation TP to PT. Next use small rotations applied to P and comment on the effect.

8.5.4   Volume rendering using color coding

Starting from Example `BetterSplatting_8.m`, we can modify the script in such a manner that we get a color-coded volume rendering, which resembles the rendering from Figure 8.5.

---

[4]An example for an efficient blurring technique can be found in W. Birkfellner, R. Seemann, M. Figl et al. Wobbled splatting–a fast perspective volume rendering method for simulation of x-ray images from CT, Phys Med Biol, 50(9):N73-84, (2005).

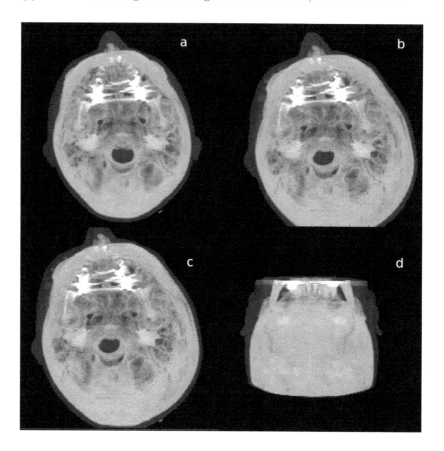

FIGURE 8.20: Possible outputs from `BetterSplatting_8.m`. **a** shows an orthogonal splat rendering; if a perspective is introduced (in this case, the viewpoint is localized at a distance of 1000 voxels from the imaging plane), the result is Figure **b**. A translation of $t = (-12.7, -12.7, 0, 1)^T$ applied to the perspective projection operator P results in Figure **c**. A rotation of 90°of the volume gives Figure **d**. Image data courtesy of the Dept. of Radiology, Medical University Vienna.

`VolumeSplatting_8.m` is the script in question. First of all, we will again clear all variables in the workspace and load our prepared CT-dataset `VoxelVector.dat`:

```
1:> clear;
2:> vect=zeros(2579560,4);
3:> vect=load('VoxelVector.dat');
```

Next, we have to assign some memory for three images containing the red, green and blue subimage named `imgr`, `imgg` and `imgb`. If you already forgot about how to compose color image, you may go back to Section 3.2.2:

```
4:> imgr=zeros(215,215);
5:> imgg=zeros(215,215);
6:> imgb=zeros(215,215);
```

Now, we will fully utilize our knowledge about spatial transforms to align the volume in such a manner that we look into the eyes of our specimen:

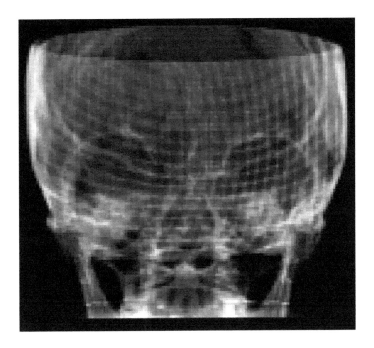

FIGURE 8.21: A summed voxel rendering from the volume `VoxelVectorBone.dat`, which was preprocessed in such a manner that it only contains the voxels with a gray value of more than 250 HU. Splat rendering can generate a DRR like this from the volume vector in a rather rapid manner. Aliasing artifacts, which are inherent to volume driven approaches and which have to be suppressed by blurring techniques, are, however, clearly visible. Image data courtesy of the Dept. of Radiology, Medical University Vienna.

```
 7:> P=eye(4);
 8:> P(3,3)=0;
 9:> Ry=eye(4);
10:> Ry(1,1)=0;
11:> Ry(1,3)=1;
12:> Ry(3,1)=-1;
13:> Ry(3,3)=0;
14:> Rz=eye(4);
15:> Rz(1,1)=-1;
16:> Rz(2,2)=-1;
```

What happens here? First, the matrix P is our rendering operator – the projection matrix known from Equation 8.1, which does the orthogonal rendering for us since we are again dealing with a splatting example. Next, we have a rotation matrix Ry, which is the result of a rotation by 270° around the y-axis, as one can verify by inserting this value into Equation 7.13. The next matrix Rz is the result of inserting a value of 180° around the z-axis (see also Equation 7.14). What follows is a translation to make sure that the center of rotation is identical with the center of the center of the volume (see also, for instance, Example 7.6.2); this is matrix T.

```
17:> T=eye(4);
18:> T(1,4)=107;
```

```
19:> T(2,4)=107;
20:> T(3,4)=82;
21:> RM=P*T*Rz*Ry*inv(T);
```

The one matrix that is finally of interest is the matrix RM; it takes care of rotation for each voxel so that we are "face-to-face" with the dataset instead of looking down on it in a cranio-caudal direction like in some of the images shown in Figure 8.20, it shifts the origin of rotation in an appropriate manner, and the rendering matrix is also in there already. For those who are interested, the full matrix now looks like this:

$$
\mathrm{RM} = \begin{pmatrix} 0 & 0 & -1 & 189 \\ 0 & -1 & 0 & 214 \\ 0 & 0 & 0 & 0 \\ 0 & 0 & 0 & 1 \end{pmatrix} \tag{8.8}
$$

Next, we assign some memory for the position of the rendered pixel, and we enter a for-loop that visits each voxel stored in vect, and we apply the matrix RM to the location of the voxel. Finally, the gray value rho associated with each voxel is stored.

```
22:> pos=zeros(4,1);
23:> for i=1:2579560
24:> pos=RM*(transpose([vect(i,1),vect(i,2),...
vect(i,3),1]));
25:> rho=vect(i,4);
```

What follows is a pretty straightforward routine, which is basically already known, for instance, from Example 8.5.2. We carry out a DRR-rendering (see also Equation 8.4). After taking care that the rendered pixels are within the range of the images imgr, imgg and imgb, we render

a voxel with a gray value between 250 and 1250 into imgr – therefore all soft tissue with a Hounsfield-density below 226 will be rendered as a red pixel. Denote that the volume contained in VoxelVector.dat was shifted in intensity from the Hounsfield scale to an unsigned 12 bit range, therefore the rendering threshold 250 corresponds to -774 HU.

a voxel with gray value between 1250 and 1750 into imgr and imgg. Voxels in this intensity range are rendered as yellow pixels.

a voxel with a gray value above 1750 (which is equivalent to a Hounsfield density of 726) into all three images. These voxels will be displayed as white pixels.

In fact, we implement a very simple version of a transfer function as shown in Figure 8.6 in this case.

```
26:> if pos(1,1) > 0 & pos(1,1) < 215 & pos(2,1) > 0 & pos(2,1) < 215
27:> if (rho > 250) & (rho < 1250)
28:> imgr(pos(1,1),pos(2,1))=imgr(pos(1,1),...
pos(2,1))+rho;
29:> end
30:> if (rho >= 1250) & (rho < 1750)
31:> imgr(pos(1,1),pos(2,1))=imgr(pos(1,1),...
pos(2,1))+rho;
```

```
32:> imgg(pos(1,1),pos(2,1))=imgg(pos(1,1),...
pos(2,1))+rho;
33:> end
34:> if (rho >= 1750)
35:> imgr(pos(1,1),pos(2,1))=imgr(pos(1,1),...
pos(2,1))+rho;
36:> imgg(pos(1,1),pos(2,1))=imgg(pos(1,1),...
pos(2,1))+rho;
37:> imgb(pos(1,1),pos(2,1))=imgb(pos(1,1),...
pos(2,1))+rho;
38:> end
39:> end
40:> end
```

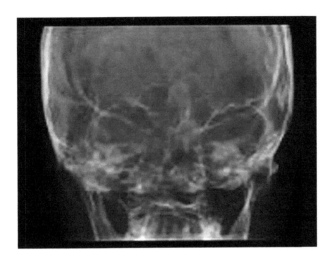

FIGURE 8.22: The output from the script `VolumeSplatting_8.m`, a color-coded volume rendering similar to Figure 8.5. The original MATLAB output is in color. Again, for the sake of keeping the printing cost within reasonable limits, we print this image in grayscale. However, the color version can be found on the accompanying CD. Image data courtesy of the Dept. of Radiology, Medical University Vienna.

After the image is rendered, we have to scale the three color channels `imgr`, `imgg` and `imgb` to an intensity range from $0 \ldots 1$, which is the common representation for color. You may also recall Example 4.5.2, where we did something similar. However, we do not have to assign a lookup table using the `colormap` routine when displaying such an RGB-image. Beyond that, we know that our volume is saved as unsigned 16 bit values. Therefore, we can also omit the usual step of subtracting the minimum grayvalue prior to scaling the intensity range.

```
41:> maxint = max(max(imgr));
42:> imgr=imgr/maxint;
43:> maxint = max(max(imgg));
44:> imgg=imgg/maxint;
45:> maxint = max(max(imgb));
46:> imgb=imgb/maxint;
```

Finally, we have to insert the single color channel images into one RGB-color image, and this image is displayed. The result (whose color version can be found on the accompanying CD), is shown in Figure 8.22.

```
47:> colorimg=zeros(215,215,3);
48:> for i=1:215
49:> for j=1:215
50:> colorimg(i,j,1)=imgr(i,j);
51:> colorimg(i,j,2)=imgg(i,j);
52:> colorimg(i,j,3)=imgb(i,j);
53:> end
54:> end
55:> image(colorimg)
```

Our example is somewhat simplistic – we do not really use subtleties such as opacity or voxel location to create our image. However, you may compare this image to a grayscale image that is generated by simple summed voxel shading without color coding.

Additional Tasks

Draw a graph of the intensity transfer function for this example similar to Figure 8.6.

8.5.5 A simple surface rendering – depth shading

Based on `Splatting_8.m`, we can also introduce the most simple of all surface rendering techniques – *depth shading*, introduced in Figure 8.7; here, a transfer function $\mathcal{T}_{DS}$ as given in Equation 8.5 is used. What looks complicated at a first glance is actually pretty simple; for all voxels with coordinates $\vec{x}$ on a ray aiming at the pixel $\vec{x}_{\text{Image Plane}}$, we determine the maximum gray value to be proportional to the voxel with the largest distance to the image plane. In other words: voxels far away from the image plane are brighter than voxels close to the image plane.

To some extent, depth shading is pretty similar to MIP. But it does not determine a gray value from the content of the volume to be rendered but from the geometrical properties of the voxels relative position to the image plane. To some extent, depth shading is a little bit similar to the distance transform, introduced in Section 5.3.2.

Let's take a look at the code; in the script `DepthShading_8.m`, the volume is read and the volume transform matrix is set up, just as we did in `Splatting_8.m`; here, we do not shift the projection operator, but we transform the origin of volume rotation prior to rendering:

```
1:> vect=zeros(360562,4);
2:> vect=load('VoxelVectorBone.dat');
3:> img=zeros(215,215);
4:> P=eye(4);
5:> P(3,3)=0;
6:> vox=zeros(4,1);
7:> pos=zeros(4,1);
8:> R=eye(4);
9:> R(1,1)=0;
10:> R(1,3)=1;
11:> R(3,1)=-1;
```

```
12:> R(3,3)=0;
13:> T=eye(4);
14:> T(1,4)=107;
15:> T(2,4)=107;
16:> T(3,4)=82;
17:> invT=inv(T);
```

The only difference to `Splatting_8.m` is implemented here. We rotate each voxel in the appropriate position, compute the projected position, and determine the gray value `rho` as the absolute value of the z-coordinate in the 3D voxel position. This is equivalent to the distance of the voxel to the image plane since our projection operator `P` is set up in such a manner that it splats all voxels to the x-y plane of the volume coordinate system. Next, we check whether another rendered voxel has a higher intensity (and therefore stems from a position at a greater distance to the rendering plane); if this is not case, the gray value is stored at the pixel position, just as we did in Examples 8.5.2 and 8.5.3 when rendering MIPs. Finally, the result is displayed like so many times before:

```
18:> for i=1:360562
19:> vox=T*R*invT*...
(transpose([vect(i,1),vect(i,2),vect(i,3),1]));
20:> pos=P*vox;
21:> rho=abs(vox(3,1));
22:> if pos(1,1) > 0 & pos(1,1) < 215 &
pos(2,1) > 0 & pos(2,1) < 215
23:> if rho > img(pos(1,1),pos(2,1))
24:> img(pos(1,1),pos(2,1)) = rho;
25:> end
26:> end
27:> end
28:> minint=min(min(img));
29:> img=img-minint;
30:> maxint = max(max(img));
31:> img=img/maxint*64;
32:> colormap(gray)
33:> image(img)
```

The result, which is very similar to Figure 8.7, can be found in Figure 8.23. Depth shading is not a very sophisticated surface rendering technique, but is useful for simple rendering tasks, and it directly leads us to surface rendering using voxel surface, which will be explored in Example 8.5.6.

Additional Tasks

Depth shading assigns a brightness to each surface voxel in dependence of its distance to the viewer. Therefore, the *lighting model* of depth shading is similar to a setup where each surface voxel glows with the same intensity. The intensity of a point light source in dependence of the viewers distance, however, follows the *inverse square law* – it decreases in a quadratic fashion. A physically correct depth shading method would therefore map the square of the distance between surface voxel and viewpoint. Can you modify `DepthShading_8.m` in such a fashion that it takes this dependence into account? The result can be found in Figure 8.24.

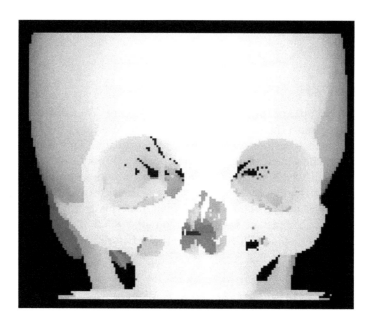

FIGURE 8.23: The output of `DepthShading_8.m`, where a depth shading is computed using a splat rendering technique. For your convenience, this illustration was rotated by 180°compared to the original image as displayed by `DepthShading_8.m`. Image data courtesy of the Dept. of Radiology, Medical University Vienna.

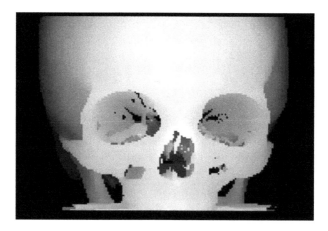

FIGURE 8.24: If one takes the lighting model of depth shading seriously, it is necessary to apply the *inverse square law* to the brightness of each surface voxel – the brightness of a surface voxel therefore depends on the square of the distance to the viewpoint. A small modification in `DepthShading_8.m` takes this into account; the result is, however, not very different from the simple implementation with a linear model, shown in Figure 8.23. Image data courtesy of the Dept. of Radiology, Medical University Vienna.

8.5.6 Rendering of voxel surfaces

In `SurfaceShading_8.m`, we expand the concept of depth shading to render more realistic surfaces. For this purpose, we go back to orthogonal raycasting and apply a simple flat shading model to a volume already segmented using a simple thresholding operation; again, we will use a volume of the skull CT. A threshold was introduced in such a manner that it only contains voxels with binary values. Only the bone remains here. This time, the non-zero voxels are stored in a file containing an $N \times 3$ matrix named `VoxelVectorThreshold.dat`. The non-zero voxel coordinates are read, rotated to the same position as in Example 8.5.5, and stored in a $215 \times 215 \times 215$ volume `vol`.

```
1:> vect=zeros(360562,3);
2:> vect=load('VoxelVectorThreshold.dat');
3:> vol=zeros(215,215,215);
4:> vox=zeros(3,1);
5:> R=eye(4);
6:> R(1,1)=0;
7:> R(1,3)=1;
8:> R(3,1)=-1;
9:> R(3,3)=0;
10:> T=eye(4);
11:> T(1,4)=107;
12:> T(2,4)=107;
13:> T(3,4)=62;
14:> invT=inv(T);
15:> for i=1:360562
16:> vox=round(T*R*invT*...
(transpose([vect(i,1),vect(i,2),vect(i,3),1])));
17:> if vox(1,1) > 0 & vox(1,1) < 216 & ...
vox(2,1) > 0 & vox(2,1) < 216 & vox(3,1) > 0 & ...
vox(3,1) < 216
18:> vol(vox(1,1),vox(2,1),vox(3,1)) = 1;
19:> end
20:> end
```

Now we have a volume, and we can apply a raycasting technique just as we did in Example 8.5.2. The difference lies in the way we assign a gray value to the new intermediate image called `hitmap`. We proceed along a beam which is parallel to the z-axis towards the imaging plane by an increment `dep`; if a non-zero voxel is encountered in `vol`, the ray is clipped, and the z-coordinate is stored in `hitmap`. If the ray does not encounter a voxel, it is terminated once it reaches the x-y-plane of the coordinate system. Figure 8.25 shows a surface plot of `hitmap`.

```
21:> hitmap=zeros(215,215);
22:> img=zeros(215,215);
23:> for i=1:215
24:> for j=1:215
25:> hit=0;
26:> dep=215;
27:> while hit == 0
28:> if vol(i,j,dep) > 0
```

```
29:> hit=1;
30:> hitmap(i,j)=dep;
31:> end
32:> dep=dep-1;
33:> if dep < 1
34:> hit=1;
35:> end
36:> end
37:> end
38:> end
```

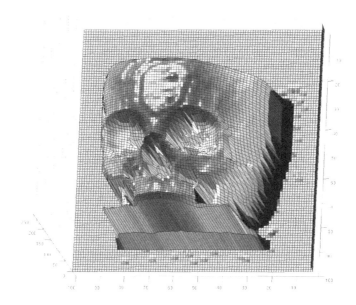

FIGURE 8.25: The surface representation of `hitmap`, generated using MATLAB's `surf` function. `hitmap` stores the z-coordinate when a beam hits a voxel surface of the volume `vol`. Based on this data, a surface normal is computed, and a lighting model can be applied. Basically speaking, the `surf` function already does this. Image data courtesy of the Dept. of Radiology, Medical University Vienna.

The next step is to apply a lighting model. For this purpose, we have to compute the normal vector on every surface voxel we already encountered. In order to do so, we have to allocate memory for a few vectors:

```
39:> normal=zeros(3,1);
40:> beam=transpose([0,0,1]);
41:> gradx=zeros(3,1);
42:> grady=zeros(3,1);
```

`normal` will become the normal vector. `beam` is the unit vector in the direction of the ray, which proceeds parallel to the z-axis towards the image plane. `gradx` and `grady` are two gradients in x- and y-direction – see also Figure 8.9 for an illustration. These are computed as finite differences between the neighboring pixels of a pixel at position $\vec{x} = (i, j)^T$ in `hitmap`.

However, these gradients are three-dimensional; they are given by the 2D coordinate of a surface voxels projection in the planar image `hitmap` *and* the z-value stored in `hitmap`. The gradient in x-direction as a finite difference (remember Chapter 5) is given as:

$$\text{gradx} = \nabla \begin{pmatrix} i \\ j \\ \text{hitmap(i,j)} \end{pmatrix} = \begin{pmatrix} i+1 \\ j \\ \text{hitmap(i+1,j)} \end{pmatrix} - \begin{pmatrix} i-1 \\ j \\ \text{hitmap(i-1,j)} \end{pmatrix} \quad (8.9)$$

`grady` is computed in a similar way. The surface normal, `normal`, is the outer or cross-product of `gradx` and `grady`. In MATLAB, this product is computed by calling the function `cross`. In order to determine the tilt of the surface relative to the beam, we compute the inner product of `normal` and `beam`. Remember Chapter 5 – in a Cartesian coordinate system, the inner product of two vectors is given as $\vec{a} \bullet \vec{b} = \|\vec{a}\| \|\vec{b}\| \cos(\alpha)$ where α is the angle enclosed by the two.

Our lighting model is simply given by an ambient light that is reflected according to the cosine of its angle of incidence – see Equation 8.6. Here, the light beam is identical to the view direction `beam` (just like a headlight). The inner product, computed in MATLAB by calling `dot`, of the normal vector `normal`, scaled to length 1, and `beam` gives us the amount of reflected light. Let's take a look at the code:

```
43:> for i =2:214
44:> for j =2:214
45:> if hitmap(i,j) > 1
46:> gradx=transpose([(i+1),j,hitmap((i+1),j)]) -
transpose([(i-1),j,hitmap((i-1),j)]);
47:> grady=transpose([i,(j+1),hitmap(i,(j+1))]) -
transpose([i,(j-1),hitmap(i,(j-1))]);
48:> normal=cross(gradx,grady);
49:> refl=dot(normal,beam)/(norm(normal));
50:> img(i,j) = 64*refl;
51:> end
52:> end
53:> end
54:> colormap(gray)
55:> image(img)
```

Here, we do just as told. The cross-product of the x- and y-gradients gives us the normal to the surface segment defined by the non-zero voxel encountered by the ray aiming at the image plane and its direct neighbors. The inner product of `beam` and `normal` gives a value between 1 and zero. Multiplying the maximum intensity by the cosine gives us an image intensity between 0 and 64. This can be directly displayed. We don't want to render the image plane itself, therefore only positions in `hitmap` larger than one are taken into account. Figure 8.26 shows the result of `SurfaceShading_8.m`.

Additional Tasks

Plot `hitmap` instead of `img`. Does the output look familiar?

Can you change the appearance of the image by varying the light? It is actually just one line of code; a possible result is shown in Figure 8.27.

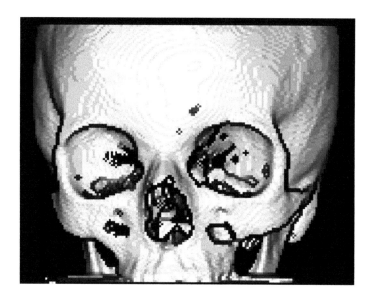

FIGURE 8.26: The result of `SurfaceShading_8.m`. By using a simple lighting model, which is actually the cosine of an incident ray of light parallel to the ray cast through the volume and the surface normal, we get a surface rendering from a segmented binary voxel volume. Image data courtesy of the Dept. of Radiology, Medical University Vienna.

Once you have mastered the first task here, it is pretty straightforward to combine `DepthShading_8.m` and `SurfaceShading_8.m` to produce a perspective surface rendering. Can you think of a simple method to reduce the aliasing artifacts visible in Figure 8.27? Alternatively, one can also implement perspective raycasting. In such a case, all rays proceed from the eyepoint to a pixel on the render plane.

8.5.7 A rendering example using 3DSlicer

Of course, we can also explore the possibilities of the 3D visualization also by means of 3DSlicer. For this purpose, one can for instance simply download a sample dataset by pressing the button "Download Sample Data" in the startup screen; in Fig. 8.28, we see the dialog which allows for downloading sample datasets. In the given case, a CT dataset of the abdominal region (called "CTAbdomen" in the module *Sample Data*) was loaded. On this dataset, one can try various visualization options. However, it makes sense to use a CT since the good contrast of bone compared to soft tissue allows for a decent visualization.

Next, one should switch to the module "Volume Rendering", which can be selected in the uppermost menu on the main screen. Next, the rendering has to be made visible using the "eye icon" in the left menu, and by selecting a preset, for instance "CT-AAA" in the pull-down menu "Display". Fig. 8.29 shows the looks of this setup in Slicer 4.2.2-1.

By rolling the mouse wheel and by moving the mouse with the left mouse button pressed, one can manipulate the view of the rendering. Choosing different volume rendering presets will also result in different views - Fig. 8.30 gives an example.

By switching to the display preset "CT-Bones" and by making the sincle slices "visible" (via the "eye icon" in the submenus of the single CT-slices), one can also show the spatial orientation of the reformatted images in the rendering (see also Fig. 8.31).

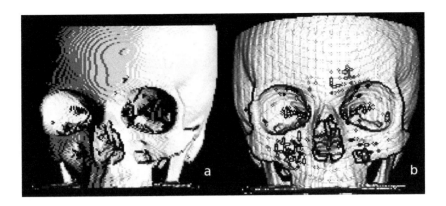

FIGURE 8.27: Some possible results from the additional tasks; in **a**. a different visualization of the volume data set is achieved by changing the direction of the incoming light. In **b**, a perspective surface shading is generated from depth shading derived in Example 8.5.5. The artifacts already visible in Figure 8.21 become even more prominent since no countermeasures against aliasing are taken. Image data courtesy of the Dept. of Radiology, Medical University Vienna.

8.5.8 Extracting a surface using the cuberille algorithm

In `Triangulation_8.m`, we find a very simple implementation of a surface triangulation technique referred to as the cuberille algorithm. It simply assigns a rectangle (or, in our case, two triangles forming a rectangle) to every voxel surface in a segmented binary volume that does not have a neighbor. The volume data of a segmented pedicle are stored as coordinate triplets in a simple text file named `PedicleSegmented.dat` in the `LessonData` folder. It consists of 16922 coordinates for non-zero voxels. The file is written in plain text, and you can inspect it using a simple text editor. Since indices in MATLAB start with 1 instead of 0, we have to add one to each coordinate; this results in a vector `pos`, which is stored in a $59 \times 57 \times 27$ volume named `vol`:

```
1:> vect=zeros(16922,3);
2:> vect=load('PedicleSegmented.dat');
3:> pos = zeros(3,1);
4:> vol=zeros(60,58,27);
5:> for i=1:16922
6:> pos(1,1)=round(vect(i,1))+1;
7:> pos(2,1)=round(vect(i,2))+1;
8:> pos(3,1)=round(vect(i,3))+1;
9:> vol(pos(1,1),pos(2,1),pos(3,1))=1;
10:> end
```

Next, we remove all stray voxels (this is the voxels that don't have any neighbors) for the sake of simplicity. We are also not interested in the voxels that have six nearest neighbors since these cannot be part of a surface; the result of this operation is stored in a new volume named `cleanvol`:

```
11:> cleanvol=zeros(60,58,27);
12:> for i=2:59
13:> for j=2:57
```

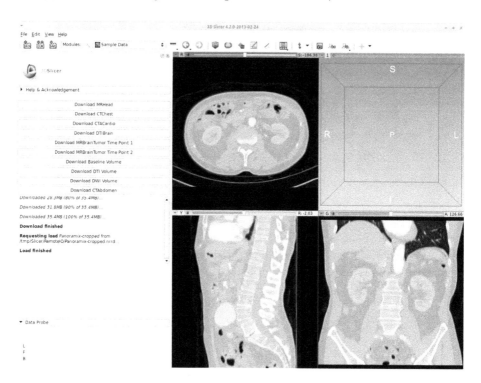

FIGURE 8.28: When clicking the module "Sample Data" in 3DSlicer, one can download a number of datasets for demonstration purposes. For rendering, it makes sense to try a CT dataset first since the high contrast of bone allows for simple segmentation and visualization. In this case, the dataset "CTAbdomen" was loaded. After finishing the download, the main screen of 3DSlicer should resemble this illustration.

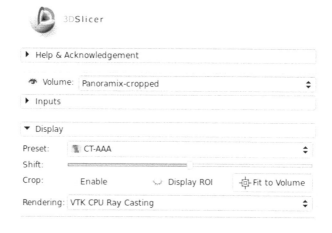

FIGURE 8.29: The settings for displaying a volume rendering in 3DSlicer Ver. 4.2.2. The result can be found in Fig. 8.30.

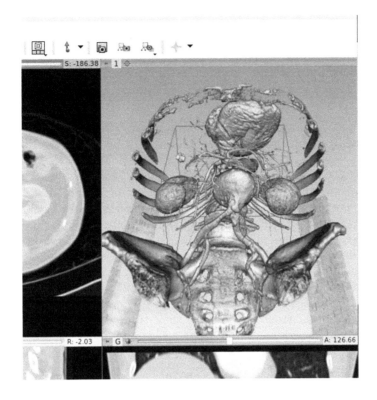

FIGURE 8.30: A rendering generated using 3DSlicer with the "CT-AAA" preset.

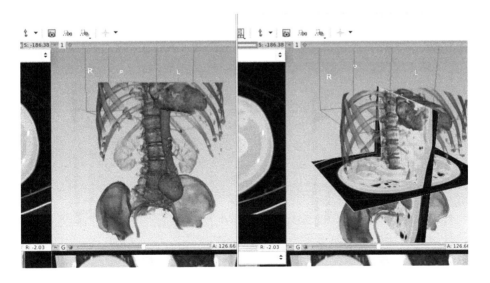

FIGURE 8.31: A rendering from 3DSlicer with the "CT-Bones" preset, with and without the slices from the orthogonal views visible.

```
14:> for k=2:26
15:> if vol(i,j,k) > 0
```

```
16:> noOfNeighbors=vol(i+1,j,k)+vol(i-1,j,k)+
vol(i,j+1,k)+vol(i,j-1,k)+vol(i,j,k+1)+vol(i,j,k-1);
17:> if (noOfNeighbors > 0) & (noOfNeighbors <= 5)
18:> cleanvol(i,j,k) = 1;
19:> end
20:> end
21:> end
22:> end
23:> end
```

Now, we can assign triangles to every surface without a neighbor; since visualization of triangulated models is a rather widespread problem, a large number of viewers is available, and therefore we do not show the result of our efforts, but rather than that we save the list of triangles in an ASCII-encoded STL-file named `PedicleSurface.stl`. In order to identify the neighbors, we also define three unit vectors `evecx`, `evecy`, and `evecz`. By consecutively subtracting and adding these unit vectors to a non-zero voxel position `voxvec`, we can scan all six nearest neighbors of this voxel. If the result `resvec` of this simple computation – the subtraction and addition of the unit vectors – is zero, we find a surface, and this face of the voxel is stored as two triangles in the STL-file. The total number of triangles is stored in a counter variable named `trianglecount`. We only show the first of six such computations – the remaining five are similar:

```
24:> fp=fopen('PedicleSurface.stl','w');
25:> fprintf(fp,'solid PedicleSurface\n');
26:> evecx=transpose([1,0,0]);
27:> evecy=transpose([0,1,0]);
28:> evecz=transpose([0,0,1]);
29:> voxvec=zeros(3,1);
30:> resvec=zeros(3,1);
31:> trianglecount = 0;
32:> for i=2:59
33:> for j=2:56
34:> for k=2:26
35:> if cleanvol(i,j,k) > 0
36:> voxvec(1,1)=i;
37:> voxvec(2,1)=j;
38:> voxvec(3,1)=k;
39:> resvec=voxvec-evecx;
40:> if cleanvol(resvec(1,1),resvec(2,1),
resvec(3,1)) == 0
41:> fprintf(fp,'facet normal 0.0 0.0 0.0\n');
42:> fprintf(fp,'outer loop\n');
43:> vertexstring=sprintf('vertex %f %f %f\n',
double(i),double(j),double(k));
44:> fprintf(fp,vertexstring);
45:> vertexstring=sprintf('vertex %f %f %f\n',
double(i),double(j+1),double(k));
46:> fprintf(fp,vertexstring);
47:> vertexstring=sprintf('vertex %f %f %f\n',
double(i),double(j),double(k+1));
48:> fprintf(fp,vertexstring);
```

```
49:> fprintf(fp,'endloop\n');
50:> fprintf(fp,'endfacet\n');
51:> fprintf(fp,'facet normal 0.0 0.0 0.0\n');
52:> fprintf(fp,'outer loop\n');
53:> vertexstring=sprintf('vertex %f %f %f\n',
double(i),double(j+1),double(k));
54:> fprintf(fp,vertexstring);
55:> vertexstring=sprintf('vertex %f %f %f\n',
double(i),double(j+1),double(k+1));
56:> fprintf(fp,vertexstring);
57:> vertexstring=sprintf('vertex %f %f %f\n',
double(i),double(j),double(k+1));
58:> fprintf(fp,vertexstring);
59:> fprintf(fp,'endloop\n');
60:> fprintf(fp,'endfacet\n');
61:> trianglecount=trianglecount+2;
62:> end
...
...:> end
...:> end
...:> end
...:> end
...:> trianglecount
...:> fprintf(fp,'endsolid PedicleSurface\n');
...:> fclose(fp);
```

Next, we should take a look at the result of our efforts; for this purpose, we need a viewer for surface models. A very powerful freeware software for this purpose is *ParaView*, a joint effort of Kitware[5] Inc. and several national laboratories in the United States. Paraview can simply be downloaded and started; other viewer applications such as *Blender* are also available in the public domain. Once we've loaded the PedicleSurface.stl into Paraview and all parameters are computed, we can inspect our model from all sides; a possible result can be found in Figure 8.32.

Additional Tasks

In the LessonData folder, you may find a binary STL-file named PedicleSmooth.stl. This file was generated using a Marching Cubes method with variable cube size. Inspect it using your STL-viewer and compare the looks to PedicleSurface.stl. A possible output can be found in Figure 8.33.

8.5.9   A demonstration of shading effects

If you have done your homework in Example 8.5.6 properly, you might already have noticed that the hitmap image is nothing but a depth shading. Since the position of the first surface voxel is encoded in this 2D-image, we can derive the 3D gradients spawning the normal vector and generate a realistic surface rendering from this information. However, we have

---

[5]Kitware is also the home of the heroes that brought us such splendid things as VTK, ITK, and IGSTK. Their homepage is www.kitware.com.

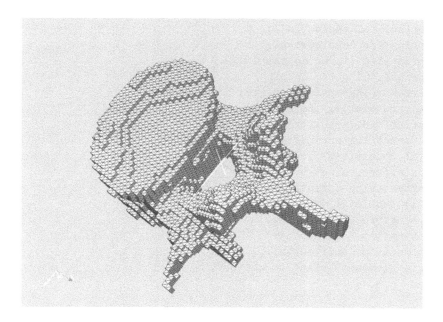

FIGURE 8.32: The result of our humble cuberille triangulation algorithm implemented in `Triangulation_8.m`, saved in `PedicleSurface.stl`; the screenshot was taken from *ParaView*. The blocky appearance is an inevitable result of the cuberille algorithm that simply assigns two triangles to every visible voxel surface. Image data courtesy of the Dept. of Radiology, Medical University Vienna.

used flat shading. The illumination of every voxel is simulated from its 2D counterpart in `hitmap`. Given the fact that our volume is rather coarse, the result as shown in Figure 8.26 is blocky and does not look very attractive. For this reason, we may apply a more sophisticated shading model similar to *Gouraud-* or *Phong-shading*. As we have learned from Section 8.4, we have to interpolate either the grid of normal vectors or the color of the shading to get a smooth appearance. We will implement such a technique (which is not exactly equivalent to the aforementioned shading algorithms, but illustrates the way these work) by manipulating `hitmap`. Therefore we have to run `BetterShadingI_8.m`, which is derived from `SurfaceShading_8.m`; this script saves `hitmap` as a .PGM file as we already did in Example 3.7.2 and terminates without rendering; the first part of the script is copied from `SurfaceShading_8.m` until `hitmap` is generated; the `hitmap` image is stored in a PGM file named `IntermediateHitmap.pgm`, which can be opened using GIMP or another standard image processing program like Photoshop:

```
...:> pgmfp = fopen('IntermediateHitmap.pgm','w');
...:> str=sprintf('P2\n');
...:> fprintf(pgmfp,str);
...:> str=sprintf('215 215\n');
...:> fprintf(pgmfp,str);
...:> maximumValue=max(max(hitmap))
...:> str=sprintf('%d\n',maximumValue);
...:> fprintf(pgmfp,str);
...:> for i=1:215
```

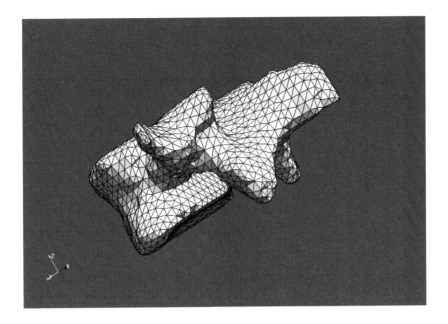

FIGURE 8.33: The result of rendering `PedicleSmooth.stl`, a surface model of the same pedicle as in Figure 8.32, generated by a more sophisticated algorithm based on the Marching Cubes algorithm implemented in AnalyzeAVW. Image data courtesy of the Dept. of Radiology, Medical University Vienna.

```
...:> for j=1:215
...:> str=sprintf('%d ',hitmap(i,j));
...:> fprintf(pgmfp,str);
...:> end
...:> end
...:> fclose(pgmfp);
```

We can now do everything we need to get a better rendering in GIMP. The single steps to be carried out are as follows:

Rotate the image by 180° in order to provide an image that is not displayed heads-up.

Interpolate the image to a larger image size. In order to generate the renderings given in Figure 8.35, the image was cropped and scaled to 900×729 pixels using cubic interpolation.

The interpolation already provides some type of low-pass filtering; we can emphasize this by adding an additional blurring using a 5×5 Gaussian blur kernel. By doing so, we distribute the gray values in a smooth manner; the gradients computed from this smoothed image are smoothed as well, and this provides the shading effect.

The resulting image is stored again, this time as a binary PGM. Such a PGM has starts with P5, as you may recall from Chapter 3. The header is 54 bytes long. If you run into trouble saving the smoothed `IntermediateHitmap.pgm` file, you may as well use the pre-generated image files `hmap.pgm` and `hmapblurred.pgm` files provided in the `LessonData/8_Visualization` folder in the following `BetterShadingII_8.m` script. `hmap.pgm` and `hmapblurred.pgm` are shown in Figure 8.34. You can, of course, also use the scripts from Examples 7.6.2 and 5.4.1 to achieve the same effect.

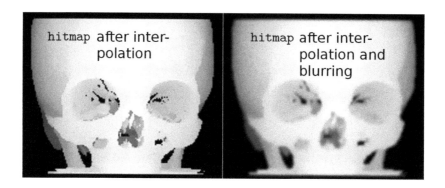

FIGURE 8.34: `hmap.pgm` and `hmapblurred.pgm`; these images are generated from the `hitmap` image from `BetterShadingI_8.m` by carrying out the interpolation and blurring steps from Example 8.5.9. A surface rendering of these images results in Figure 8.35. Image data courtesy of the Dept. of Radiology, Medical University Vienna.

The modified `hitmap` images are now rendered in a second script named `BetterShadingII_8.m`; loading the binary PGM files `hmap.pgm` and `hmapblurred.pgm` is carried out similar to Example 3.7.2. The PGM header is 54 bytes long and is skipped:

```
...:> fp=fopen('hmap.pgm','r');
...:> hitmap=zeros(900,729);
...:> fseek(fp,54,'bof');
...:> hitmap(:)=fread(fp,(900*729),'uint8');
...:> hitmap=transpose(hitmap);
...:> fclose(fp);
```

The remainder of the script applies a surface rendering routine on the 900×729 image; it is directly copied from Example 8.5.6. The result can be found in Figure 8.35. A significant improvement in image quality could be expected if we use a finer voxel resolution than the $1 \times 1 \times 1\text{mm}^3$ dimension used in the `VoxelVectorThreshold.dat` volume. However, the shading technique used here is some sort of trick; we use the depth shading to compute the 3D gradients as we did before in Example 8.5.6. By interpolation, we increase the number of rays aiming at the rendering plane, and the gradients to be computed are interpolated by the blurring step.

Additional Tasks

Why does this example resemble a Phong-shading? At least we are interpolating gray values in the rendered image, which is the principle of Gouraud shading!

What happens if one applies an intensity scaling operation to `IntermediateHitmap.pgm`?

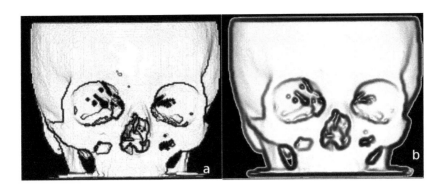

FIGURE 8.35: Additional interpolation of shading effects such as Gouraud- and Phong shading improve the appearance of a rendered model further. This rendering was generated using the same data as in Figure 8.26. However, the appearance is smoother and less blocky thanks to a manipulation of the `hitmap` image. The manipulations we applied to the intermediate depth shading `IntermediateHitmap.pgm` somewhat resemble Phong-shading. Image data courtesy of the Dept. of Radiology, Medical University Vienna.

8.6 SUMMARY AND FURTHER REFERENCES

Rendering is an important tool for conveying information; in clinical practice, it is mainly appreciated by non-radiologists, who are usually not trained to a great extent to retrieve diagnostic information from slices. Still, the most important visualization techniques from a diagnostic point of view remain windowing and reformatting rather than rendering. Volume rendering, which in many cases does not require an explicit segmentation step, deserves special consideration for such visualization tasks. Surface rendering from voxel surfaces or triangulated meshes does require segmentation and may furthermore suffer from geometrical inaccuracy. Still, it is an important tool for fast visualization and the production of tangible models using rapid prototyping. In practice, one usually does not have to develop a rendering or triangulation algorithm from scratch since these are available as well-tested and widespread application programmers interfaces.

Literature

J. D. Foley, A. van Dam, S. K. Feiner, J. F. Hughes: Computer Graphics: Principles and Practice in C, Addison-Wesley (1995)

J. K. Udupa, G. T. Herman: 3D Imaging in Medicine, Second Edition, CRC Press, (2000)

B. Preim, D. Bartz: Visualization in Medicine, Morgan-Kaufmann, (2007)

M. Hadwiger, J. M. Kniss, C. Rezk-Salama, D. Weiskopf: Real-time Volume Graphics, A. K. Peters, (2006)

R. S. Wright, B. Lipchak, N. Haemel: OpenGL SuperBible: Comprehensive Tutorial and Reference, Addison-Wesley (2007)

W. Schroeder, K. Martin, B. Lorensen: Visualization Toolkit: An Object-Oriented Approach to 3D Graphics, Kitware, (2006)

CHAPTER 9

Registration

Wolfgang Birkfellner

CONTENTS

9.1	Fusing information	297
9.2	Registration paradigms	299
	9.2.1 Intra- and intermodal registration	299
	9.2.2 Rigid and non-rigid registration	301
9.3	Merit functions	302
9.4	Optimization strategies	313
9.5	Some general comments	315
9.6	Camera calibration	316
9.7	Registration to physical space	319
	9.7.1 Rigid registration using fiducial markers and surfaces	319
	9.7.2 2D/3D registration	321
9.8	Evaluation of registration results	322
9.9	Practical lessons	323
	9.9.1 Registration of 2D images using cross-correlation	323
	9.9.2 Computing joint histograms	325
	9.9.3 Plotting the mutual information merit function	327
	9.9.4 Chamfer matching	328
	9.9.5 Optimization	329
	9.9.6 The direct linear transform	335
	9.9.7 Marker based registration	337
9.10	Summary and further references	338

9.1 FUSING INFORMATION

In Chapter 7, we dealt with all types of spatial transforms applicable to images. Besides visualization and interpolation purposes, these operations provide the core formalism for *image registration* or *image fusion*. From the very beginning of this book, it was emphasized that medical imaging modalities do *not* provide images of the patient's anatomy and physiology. They do record certain physical properties of tissue. What sounds very philosophic is indeed a very general property of perception. We do only see what we can see – this forms our reality and our image of the world. But modern medical imaging devices enhance the limits of our perception. Less than forty years ago, the introduction of CT replaced invasive methods like exploratory laparotomy in case of unclear lower abdominal pain; MR gives stunning images of soft tissue where CT fails to achieve good image contrast. US allows for quick imaging not using ionizing radiation, and specialized probes allow even for using US inside the body. PET and SPECT visualize pathologies before these show up as anatomical changes by mapping metabolism and physiology. Still this plethora of information is worthless if it cannot be connected. This is mainly the task of well-trained experts in radiology, but the fact that most modern modalities produce 3D volume image data does not simplify the task of fusing information from different imaging sources. This is the domain of registration algorithms, where a common frame of reference for multiple data sources is established.

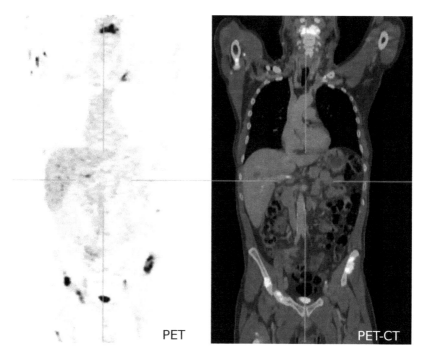

FIGURE 9.1: An image sample from a combined PET/CT system. Registration of the PET and the CT volume is automatically achieved by taking both volume datasets in a scanner that is capable of recording both tracer concentration and x-ray attenuation. Image data courtesy of the Dept. of Nuclear Medicine, Medical University Vienna.

The main problem lies in the fact that the reference coordinate system of a volume dataset does not reference the patient – it references the scanner. Changing patient position between two imaging sessions is, however, necessary in many cases. The position of a patient in an MR scanner during a head scan is governed by the shape of the receiver coil and the gradients, whereas patient pose in a CT or PET scanner is governed by the patient's principal axes. Combined modalities like PET/CT solve this problem; the poor anatomic image information from PET, especially in body regions other than the brain, renders exact fusion of PET and CT or MR difficult, and the information from the CT scan can even be used to improve volume reconstruction in the PET scan. Figure 9.1 gives a sample of the capabilities of a modern PET/CT system, and PET/MR systems are subject to clinical investigation. However, it is not that simple to combine modalities. A CT/MR scanner would be a very clumsy and difficult device, given the fact that the avoidance of ferromagnetic materials in the CT and the appropriate shielding of electromagnetic fields from the CT scanner is a rather delicate task. It would also be uneconomic to use such a system; a CT can handle more patients within a given period of time compared to an MR-tomograph.

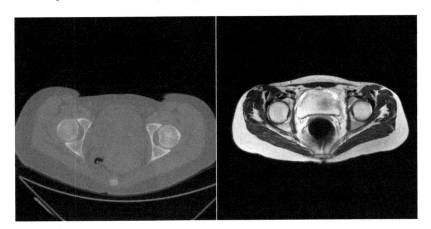

FIGURE 9.2: Two slices of the same patient at the same location, the hip joint. The left image shows the CT image, the right image is taken from the MR scan. Differences in the field-of-view and patient orientation are evident. Registration algorithms compensate for these discrepancies by finding a common frame of reference for both volume datasets. Image data courtesy of the Dept. of Radiology, Medical University Vienna.

Fusion of images – that is, finding a common frame of reference for both images – is therefore a vital task for all kinds of diagnostic imaging. Besides fusing images for tasks such as comparison of image series, we can co-register the coordinate system of an external device such as a robot or a LINAC. It is also possible to merge abstract information, such as eloquent areas in the brain from a generalized atlas, to patient specific image information. In this chapter, we will introduce the most important methods and paradigms of registration. In general, all *registration algorithms* optimize parameters of *rigid motion* and internal dof (for deformable registration) until a measure that compares images is found to be optimal. The choice of this measure, which we will simply call *merit function*, depends on the specific registration task.

9.2 REGISTRATION PARADIGMS

In general, registration algorithms determine a volume transformation from identifying common features in two coordinate systems. These features can be intrinsic (that is features that are inherent to the image data) and extrinsic. Extrinsic features are usually markers attached to the patient; these markers, usually called *fiducial markers*, are identified in both frames of reference, but cause considerable additional clinical effort and are usually not available for retrospective studies. Registration algorithms can also be categorized by the type of image data or frames of reference they operate on. Let's take a closer look at this classification.

9.2.1 Intra- and intermodal registration

In *intramodal* registration, we are registering images that stem from the same modality; an example is CT-to-CT registration of volumes acquired at different times. Such a procedure is extremely helpful when doing time series evaluation, for instance when tracking the effect of chemo- or radiotherapy on tumor growth. Here, a number of CT images is taken at different points in time. The one quantity of interest is tumor size, which can be identified easily provided a sufficient uptake of contrast agent. But with varying orientation of the patient, segmentation of the tumor and, above all, assessment of the direction of tumor growth or shrinkage becomes extremely cumbersome. By registration of the volumes, this task is greatly simplified since all slices can be viewed with the same orientation.

When fusing image data from different modalities, we are dealing with *intermodal* registration. A classical example is MR/CT fusion; an example of MR/CT fusion using an similarity measure named *normalized mutual information* (NMI) in AnalyzeAVW can be found in Figure 9.3. It is evident that different merit functions are necessary for this type of application. In *intramodal* registration, it may be sufficient to define a measure that compares the voxel gray values ρ at identical positions in the base and match volume. In intermodal registration, such an approach is bound to fail since the physical principle for the imaging modalities is different; therefore, there is no reason why a bright voxel in one volume should correspond to a bright voxel in the other volume. Our already well-known pig is actually the result of a series of experiments for multi-modal image registration. In total, the cadaver was scanned using T_1, T_2 and proton density sequences in MR as well as multislice CT and CBCT; after registration of those volumes, a single slice was selected and the images were blended. The result of this operation was stored as an MPG-movie. It can be found in the accompanying CD in the folder `MultimediaMaterial` under the name `7_MultimodalRegistration.mpg`.

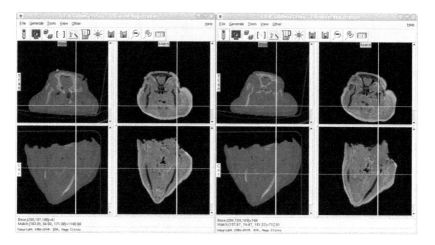

FIGURE 9.3: Two screenshots from the registration tool of AnalyzeAVW. On the left side, we see two slices of the MR and the CT scan, unregistered. Gross orientation is similar, but discrepancies are clearly visible. Besides soft tissue deformation, it is also evident that rigid structures such as the calvaria of the well-known pig scan do not coincide. After initiating the registration algorithm (in this case, an implementation of normalized mutual information), the two images match. The resulting volume transformation matrix V can be seen in Figure 9.4. Image data courtesy of the Dept. of Radiology, Medical University Vienna.

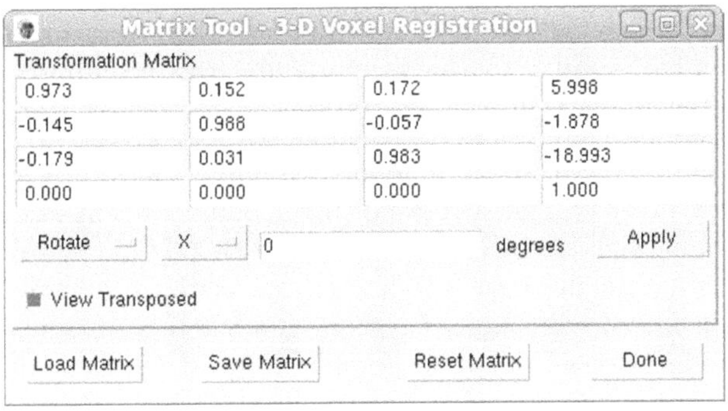

FIGURE 9.4: The volume transformation as produced by the AnalyzeAVW registration tool (see Figure 9.3).

We will learn about specific merit functions in Section 9.3. Example 9.9.1 implements a very simple merit function computation for a rotated intramodal image; the merit function here is Pearson's cross correlation coefficient, which we already know from Equation 7.16. Figure 9.21 shows the merit function for this very simple 2D-registration approach in one rotational dof.

9.2.2 Rigid and non-rigid registration

Rigid registration refers to algorithms that are confined to finding an affine transformation in three or six dof; affine transformations were extensively handled in Chapter 7. However, tissue may change its shape, and the relative position of inner organs may vary. Even the simple registration example shown in Figure 9.3 reveals this. In the registered transversal and coronal slices, we see that bony structures coincide very well. The soft tissue does not – this is simply due to the fact that the poor little piglet was decapitated before we scanned it. The head was sealed in a body bag, but in the case of the CT scan, it was lying in a plastic tub, whereas in the case of the MR, it was tucked into a head coil. The soft tissue was therefore deformed, and while the NMI-based registration algorithm of AnalyzeAVW does its job well (since it perfectly aligns the rigid anatomical structures), it cannot compensate for those deformations.

In *non-rigid registration*, the affine transformation is only a first step in alignment of volumes. The fine-tuning is handled by adding additional, internal dof, which handle the deformation as well. A non-rigid registration algorithm is therefore not a completely different approach to the registration problem; it relies on the same merit functions and optimization schemes, and it can be intra- or intermodal. What is added is actually a model that governs the deformation behavior. In other words, we need additional assumptions on how image elements are allowed to migrate. The formalism to describe this displacement is a deformation field. Each image element is displaced by a vector that indicates the direction and amount of displacement.

The distinctive feature for deformable registration methods is the way of modelling this displacement. In general, the mesh defining the displacement field is given, and local differences in the base and the match image are evaluated using a merit function; the local difference in the image define the amount of displacement for a single image element. The algorithms for modelling the displacement field can be put into the following categories:

Featurelet-based approaches: The most trivial approach is to sub-divide the image to smaller units, which are registered as rigid sub-units. The resulting gaps in the image are to be interpolated, similar to the volume-regularization approach mentioned in Section 7.2. This technique is also called *piecewise rigid registration.*

B-Spline-based approaches: In short, a spline is a numerical model for a smooth function given by a few pivot points. A mesh of pivot points is defined on the image, and the merit function chosen produces a force on the B-spline. The original meaning of the word *spline* is a thin piece of wood, used for instance in building the body of boats. Such a thin board will bulge if a force is applied to it, and its shape will be determined by the location of the pivot points – that is, the shape of the board under pressure depends on the location of its pivot points. It will be definitely different if its ends are clamped to a fixed position, or if they are allowed to move freely. The same thing happens to the B-spline. It can model deformation in a smooth manner, but huge local deformation will have a considerable effect on remote areas of the image.

Linear elastic models: For small deformations, it is permissible to treat the surface under deformation as an elastic solid. Local differences again apply a force on the elastic solid until an equilibrium is reached. The linearity assumption is only valid for small deformations, as one might know from real life. The advantage of this linear model, however, lies in the fact that non-local effects such as in the case of B-splines should not occur, but on the other hand, huge deformations cannot be compensated for.

Viscous fluid models: A generalization to the linear elastic model is the viscous fluid model, where strong local deformations are allowed; one can imagine a viscous fluid model as honey at different temperatures – it may be rather malleable or very liquid. Such a model allows for strong local deformations at the cost of registration failure if a large deformation occurs because of a flawed choice of internal parameters.

Finite-element models: In finite-element modelling (FEM), a complex mesh of the whole image is constructed, with well defined mechanical properties on interfaces of materials with different properties; in such a model, bone can be modelled as rigid, whereas other anatomical structures are handled as viscous fluids or as linear elastic models. The power of such an approach is evident since it models the structure of an organism. The drawback is the fact that a full segmentation of the volume of interest is necessary, and that constructing the mesh and solving the partial differential equations of a FE-model can be extremely labor- and time-intensive.

9.3 MERIT FUNCTIONS

In general, merit functions in registration provide a *measure on the similarity of images*; therefore, these functions are also referred to as similarity measures or cost functions. In general, these have the following properties:

They yield an optimum value if two images are aligned in an optimal manner; it is therefore evident that a merit function for intramodal registration may have completely different properties than an merit function for a special intermodal registration problem.

The capture (or convergence) range of the merit function should be as wide as possible. In other words, the merit function has to be capable of distinguishing images that are only slightly different from those that are completely different, and a well-defined gradient should exist for a range of motion as large as possible.

Merit functions for image fusion can be defined as intensity-based, or as gradient-based. The latter rely on differentiated images such as shown in Figure 7.21.

In general, merit functions assume a common frame of reference, and one of the two images "moves" by means of a volume transform; the merit function compares the gray values in the images *at the same position* in this common frame of reference. Figure 9.5 illustrates this concept.

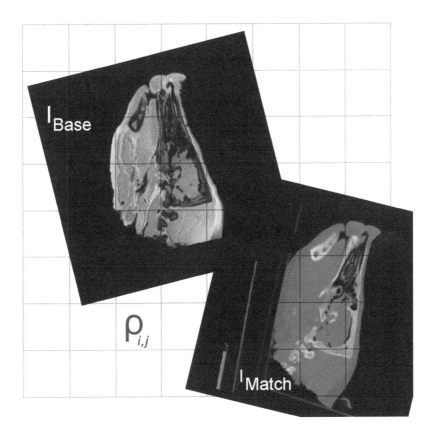

FIGURE 9.5: Merit functions compare gray values ρ_{ij} in a common frame of reference. The images I_{Match} and I_{Base} move in this common frame of reference, but the gray value is taken at the same location in the common coordinate system.

A number of intensity-based merit functions were defined, and most of them are basically statistical measures for giving a measure of mutual dependence between random variables. In these cases, the intensity values ρ are considered the random variables, which are inspected at the location of image elements which are assumed to be the same. This directly leads to a very straightforward and simple measure, the *sum of squared differences*:

$$\mathcal{M}_{\text{SSD}} = \frac{1}{N} * \sum_{}^{N} \left(\rho_{\text{Base}}(x,y,z) - \rho_{\text{Match}}(x,y,z) \right)^2 \tag{9.1}$$

where N is the total number of pixels. The inner mechanics of this measure are evident; if two gray values ρ differ, the squared difference will be non-zero, and the larger the difference for all image elements, the larger the sum of all squared differences will be. It is evident that this measure will work best for completely identical images with the same histogram content, which only differ by a spatial transform. A more versatile merit function can be defined by using Equation 7.16; in this case, the correlation coefficient of paired gray values $\rho_{\text{Base}}(x, y, z)$ and $\rho_{\text{Match}}(x, y, z)$ is computed. Pearson's cross-correlation assumes a *linear* relationship between the paired variables, it does not assume these to be identical. This is a clear progress over $\mathcal{M}_{\text{SSD}}$ given in Equation 9.1. Still it is confined by definition to intramodal registration problems. And, to add some more real life problems, one can usually not assume that the gray values ρ in two intramodal images follow a linear relationship. Nevertheless, a merit function $\mathcal{M}_{\text{CC}}$ can be pretty useful sometimes, and a sample implementation is given in Example 9.9.1.

Another possibility to compare intramodal images is to take a look at the difference image I_{diff} of two images, and to assess the disorder in the result. Such a measure is *pattern intensity*, given here only for the 2D case:

$$
\begin{aligned}
\mathcal{M}_{\text{PI}} &= \sum_{x,y}^{N} \sum_{d^2 \leq r^2} \frac{\sigma^2}{\sigma^2 + \left(I_{\text{diff}}(x, y) - I_{\text{diff}}(u, v)\right)^2} \\
d &= (x - u)^2 + (y - v)^2 \\
\sigma &= \text{Internal scaling factor}
\end{aligned}
\tag{9.2}
$$

d is the diameter of the local surrounding of each pixel; if this surrounding is rather homogeneous, a good match is assumed. This measure, which has gained some popularity in 2D/3D registration (see Section 9.7.2), assesses the local difference in image gray values of the difference image I_{diff} within a radius r, thus giving a robust estimate on how chaotic the difference image looks like. It is very robust, but also requires an excellent match of image histogram content; furthermore, it features a narrow convergence range and therefore can only be used if one is already pretty close to the final registration result. The internal scaling factor σ is mainly used to control the gradient provided by $\mathcal{M}_{\text{PI}}$.

So far, all merit functions were only suitable for intramodal registration (and many more exist). A merit function that has gained wide popularity due to the fact that it can be applied to both inter- and intramodal registration problems is *mutual information*.[1] This measure from information theory gives a measure for the statistical dependence of two random variables which is derived from a *probability density function* (PDF) rather than the actual gray values ρ given in two images. This sounds rather theoretic, but in practice, this paradigm is extremely powerful. The PDF – we will see later on how it can be obtained – does not care whether a voxel is tinted bright, dark or purple; it just measures how many voxels carry a similar value. Therefore, a PDF function can be derived for each image, and the mutual information measure is defined by comparing these functions in dependence of a registration transformation. In general information theory, mutual information (MI) is defined as:

$$
MI = E\left(P\left(I_{\text{Base}}, I_{\text{Match}}\right)\right) \ln \frac{P\left(I_{\text{Base}}, I_{\text{Match}}\right)}{P\left(I_{\text{Base}}\right) P\left(I_{\text{Match}}\right)}
\tag{9.3}
$$

where $E\left(P\left(I_{\text{Base}}, I_{\text{Match}}\right)\right)$ is the expectation value of the *joint PDF* – noted as $P\left(I_{\text{Base}}, I_{\text{Match}}\right)$ in Equation 9.3 – of the two images I_{Base} and I_{Match}, and $P\left(I_{\text{Base}}\right)$ and

---

[1] As a sidenote, it should be mentioned that statistical measure was also introduced by C. Shannon, of whom we already have heard in Chapter 5.

$P(I_{\text{Match}})$ are the PDF for the gray values in the single images. So far, this definition is not very useful as long as we do not know what the expectation value of a PDF is, and how the single and joint PDFs are derived. So what exactly is a PDF? A PDF is a function that gives the *probability to encounter a random variable x in sampling space*. For a random variable that follows the normal distribution, the PDF is given as the Gaussian. For an image, a nice approximation of a PDF is the *histogram*, which we already know from Section 4.3.

The *joint histogram* is a 2D function that maps from a 2D-domain, namely the gray values of the images I_{Base} and I_{Match}, to a statistic that measures the occurrence of a similar gray value *at the same pixel (or voxel)*. Note that the gray values need not be the same; the basic idea of mutual information lies in the fact that areas with similar content will have a *similar distribution* of gray values. If we define a measure that becomes optimal if the joint histogram is as well-organized as possible, we can assume an optimum match of the images I_{Match} and I_{Base}. Ex. 9.9.2 computes the joint histogram for an image and itself (where the disorder in the joint histogram is minimal), and the same image after slight rotation and translation. Figure 9.6 shows the result.

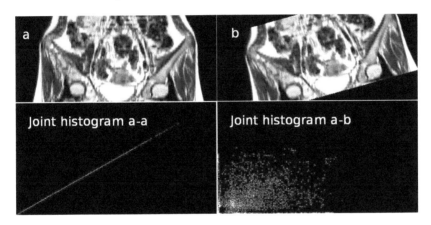

FIGURE 9.6: The output from the `JointHistogram_9.m` script in Example 9.9.2. In the upper row, we see two MR images, which can be found in the `LessonData` folder and are named `OrthoMR` (**a**) and `OrthoMRTransf` (**b**). They are the same images, but they differ by a small rotation and translation. The lower images show the output of the `JointHistogram_9.m` script in Example 9.9.2 – first, the joint histogram of image **a** and itself is computed (lower left). We see a low level of disorder in the histogram since all gray values are well correlated and aligned nicely on the line of identity in the joint histogram. The joint histogram of images **a** and **b** look worse; the common occurrence of similar gray values is scarce, and the cells with high counts in the histogram are more scattered (lower right). Disorder – measured by Shannon's entropy – is higher here. The surface plots of these joint histograms can be found in Figure 9.8. Image data courtesy of the Dept. of Radiology, Medical University Vienna.

In order illustrate the idea of a joint histogram, we can introduce it also with a simple example from statistics; let us consider a group of people. Among those, four are girls and five are boys. Furthermore, three of them are milk drinkers, and the other six prefer beer. The histogram for this distribution is to be found in Figure 9.7.

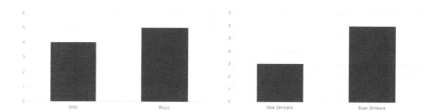

FIGURE 9.7: A statistical example for illustrating the joint histogram. Out of a group of nine people, four are female. Furthermore, three group members prefer non-alcoholic beverages. A joint histogram of this statistical collective is given in Table 9.1.

	Girls	Boys	Total
Milk drinkers	2	1	3
Beer drinkers	2	4	6
Total	4	5	9

TABLE 9.1: The 2 x 2 table for our simple example of girls and boys, drinking beer or milk. The central part of this table is a joint histogram of the two properties, similar to the Figures 9.6, 9.8 and 9.9. Later in this chapter, we will illustrate the concept of "disorder" (or *entropy*) using this example.

Now let us take a look at the joint histogram of this group. Such a joint distribution is the well-known 2×2 table, shown in Table 9.1. Later in this chapter, we will return to this table and illustrate the concept of entropy using this example.

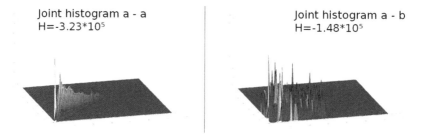

FIGURE 9.8: Surface plots of the joint histograms given in Figure 9.6. The first histogram – which is the joint histogram of the MR image **a** from Figure 9.6 with itself – shows that the histograms are *not* scatterplots. Rather than that, different bins show different heights. The second surface plot shows the joint histogram of the MR image and its rotated counterpart (image **b** from Figure 9.6). Apparently, more bins are non-zero, but the overall height is much lower – note that the z-axes have a different scale. The bin height ranges from 0 to 350 in the left plot, whereas the bin height in the right plot does not exceed 4. Shannon's entropy as given in Equation 9.4 was also computed for both histograms. It is considerably lower for the well-ordered left histogram, as expected.

Back to images. Figure 9.6 shows an ideal case for a joint histogram. In an intramodal image with similar gray values, the optimal joint histogram becomes a straight line; if we would compute the correlation coefficient according to Equation 7.16, we would get a value of 1 since the joint histogram can be considered a scatterplot in this case – it is not exactly scatterplot since a scatterplot does not weight common values of ρ within a given bin higher. If all values align nicely along a line, Pearson's correlation coefficient yields an optimum value. Therefore, we could ask ourselves why $\mathcal{M}_{CC}$ should be any worse than a MI-based merit function $\mathcal{M}_{MI}$. The answer is easily given when taking a look at Figure 9.9. Here, an MR and a CT slice from a co-registered dataset were rotated against each other; if the rotation angle is $0°$, the match is optimal. The associated joint histogram, however, does not align to a straight line. This is not surprising since the functional relationship between MRI- and CT- gray values is neither linear, and it is not even monotonous. The mutual information measure can nevertheless assess the disorder in the joint histogram, just as the correlation coefficient does in the case of a linear relationship in a scatterplot.

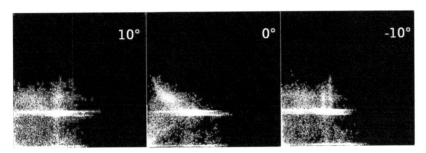

FIGURE 9.9: The joint histogram of two registered slices from the `LessonData` folder, `CT.jpg` and `T1.jpg`. The images were rotated against each other with an angle of -10°, 0°, and 10°; while the joint histogram for the optimum case (rotation angle 0°, middle image) does not look like the lower left image in Figure 9.6, since the images are taken from different modalities, it is optimal in terms of disorder, as one can see when computing the mutual information as a merit function. A series of joint histograms for this multimodal case can be found in Example 9.9.2 when running `MultimodalJointHistogram_9.m`.

In Figure 9.9, we see that there is a subtle change in the appearance of the joint histogram; since we only apply a rotation, we always have a rather large overlapping area. If we perform a translation, the number of densely populated areas does obviously change to a greater extent, with large sparsely populated areas. A script that performs such a translation for the CT- and MR-datasets named `MultimodalJointHistogramTranslation_9.m` can be found in the `LessonData`-folder. The joint histograms for overlap and translations in y-direction of -100 and 100 pixels can be found in Figure 9.10.

We see that a well-ordered histogram is characterized by the fact that most points in the joint histograms are accumulated in a few areas. This is independent of the range of gray values – a scaling operations would just stretch the joint histogram, or it would move the densely populated areas to other positions in the joint histogram. A measure for this disorder in a PDF P, which we will call *entropy*[2] from now on, is *Shannon's entropy*:

$$H = -\sum_i P_i \ln(P_i) \tag{9.4}$$

Without expanding in mathematical detail, it is evident why Equation 9.4 is a good measure for entropy (or disorder, as we called it previously). A joint histogram with densely

---

[2]The term entropy stems from thermodynamics, where it is used as a measure to quantify irreversible processes. In other words, the higher the entropy, the higher the disorder in a thermodynamic system.

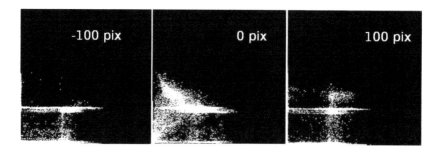

FIGURE 9.10: Another example for the joint histogram of two registered slices from the `LessonData` folder, `CT.jpg` and `T1.jpg`. This time, one of the slices was translated by -100 pixels, and by 100 pixels. Since the overlap of the images is less than in the case of image rotation (see Figure 9.9), the disorder in the joint histogram is increased, resulting in visibly less densely populated areas in the joint histogram. Again, a series of joint histograms for this multimodal case can be found in Example 9.9.2 when running `MultimodalJointHistogramTranslation_9.m`.

	Girls	Boys	Total
Milk drinkers	0	3	3
Beer drinkers	4	2	6
Total	4	5	9

TABLE 9.2: An alternative 2 x 2 table for beer- or milk-drinking girls and boys. While the total numbers stay the same, this distribution shows lesser disorder since we can make quite likely conclusions about the other property from a given property.

populated bright areas (that is, bins with a high count of occurrences) show a lesser degree of chaos than a sparsely populated joint histogram with a "dark" appearance. A high count – that is a bright spot in the joint histogram – increases H, but the logarithm – a function that grows at a very slow rate for higher values, as we have seen in Example 4.5.3 – as a second factor defining the elements of H suppresses this growth very effectively. Furthermore, the sum of counts in two joint histograms of high and low entropy should be the same. As a consequence, the histogram with low entropy has only a few non-zero elements, and the high value of P_i is damped by the term $\ln(P_i)$. The chaotic histogram, on the other hand, has many summands with a low value P_i and this value is not damped by the logarithmic term.

Our simple example given in Figure 9.7 and Table 9.1 might help to understand this concept. For the sample of beer- and milk-drinking boys and girls, we can also compute Shannon's entropy:

$$H = -(2\ln(2) + \ln(1) + 2\ln(2) + 4\ln(4)) = -8.317 \tag{9.5}$$

A possible joint distribution with lesser entropy would be the following – all girls drink beer and some boys drink milk or beer. The total numbers have not changed – we still have the same number of males and females, and the number of milk or beer drinkers also stays the same. Therefore, we have the following joint histogram: Computing Shannon's entropy gives the following result when neglecting non-populated cells in the joint histogram since

$ln(0) = -\infty$:

$$H = -(3\ln(3) + 4\ln() + 2\ln(2)) = -10.227 \qquad (9.6)$$

The Entropy in this case is obviously lower than the one given in Equation 9.5, which was derived from the distribution in Table 9.2 despite the fact that the total numbers are the same. The reason for this lies in the fact that – if one knows one property of a random person from our sample – one can make more likely conclusions about the other property. If we encounter a girl from our group, we do know that she prefers beer. This is order in a statistical sense. The same holds true for our joint histograms of images – in a well registered image, we can conclude the gray value in the match image from the gray value in the base image, no matter what their actual value is.

Equation 9.4 also lies at the very foundation of ($\mathcal{M}_{\mathrm{MI}}$), the *mutual information* merit function; while Equation 9.4 by itself is already a fine merit function, the related formulation of a mutual-information merit function based on Equation 9.3 has become popular. We define a merit function that utilizes mutual information as follows:

$$\mathcal{M}_{\mathrm{MI}} = H\left(I_{\mathrm{Base}}\right) + H\left(I_{\mathrm{Match}}\right) - H\left(I_{\mathrm{Base}}, I_{\mathrm{Match}}\right) \qquad (9.7)$$

Without expanding on joint entropy, Shannon entropy, Kullback-Leibler distances[3] and more information about theoretical measures, we may simply believe that Equation 9.7 is a measure for the common information in two images, which is optimal if the two images are aligned.

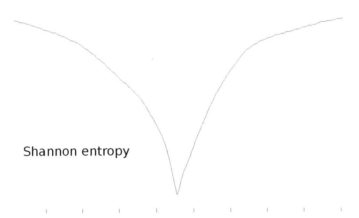

Shannon entropy

FIGURE 9.11: The Shannon entropy for the joint histogram as computed in `Multimodal-JointHistogram_9.m` in Example 9.9.2. The abscissa shows the angle of relative rotation of the `T1.jpg` and `CT.jpg` from the `LessonData` folder, which ranges from -90° to 90°. Again, an optimum is encountered when the two images match at a relative rotation of 0°. The corresponding joint histogram is shown in the middle of Figure 9.9.

The true power of $\mathcal{M}_{\mathrm{MI}}$ lies in the fact that it does not care about gray values; it retrieves all information from the PDF, which is basically given by the histogram. Therefore, it is a truly multimodal merit function. In Example 9.9.3 we plot the cross-section for the 3D merit function $\mathcal{M}_{\mathrm{MI}}$ when rotating and translating the `T1.jpg` and `CT.jpg` slices. The shape of the merit function can be found in Figure 9.12. Many more refinements of merit functions

---

[3]The Kullback-Leibler distance, defined as $\sum P_A \ln \frac{P_A}{P_B}$ gives a measure for the similarity of two arbitrary PDFs P_A and P_B.

for multimodal image registration exist, for instance it is possible to derive the PDF using the so called *Parzen-window method*. The basic idea – minimization of entropy in a joint PDF of the images – however, always stays the same. For the sake of completeness, we should also add the definition of a variation of $\mathcal{M}_{\mathrm{MI}}$ called *normalized mutual information*:

$$\mathcal{M}_{\mathrm{NMI}} = \frac{H\left(I_{\mathrm{Base}}\right) + H\left(I_{\mathrm{Match}}\right)}{H\left(I_{\mathrm{Base}}, I_{\mathrm{Match}}\right).} \tag{9.8}$$

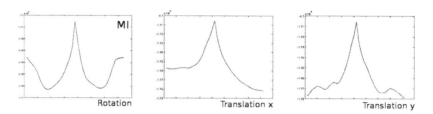

FIGURE 9.12: The output from the script `PlotMutualInformation2D_9.m` in Example 9.9.3. The shape of $\mathcal{M}_{\mathrm{MI}}$ is plotted when changing all three dof of rigid motion in 2D separately for the two sample images `T1.jpg` and `CT.jpg`. Despite the fact that this representation is ideal and that a clear maximum of $\mathcal{M}_{\mathrm{MI}}$ can be seen, local optima are visible and may cause a failure of the registration procedure.

Multimodal matching always necessitates that the gray value ρ in corresponding image elements is replaced by a more general measure; the joint entropy in PDFs derived from images is one possibility. Another possibility is the use of gradient information in an image; if we recall the edge-detection mechanisms as presented in Chapter 5 and Example 7.6.6, we see that the edge image itself retains only very little information on gray levels; one can even segment the filtered edge-image, so that only a map of ridge lines remains. Figure 9.14 illustrates this operation on our already well-known pig slices `CT.jpg` (the base image) and `T1.jpg` (the match image) from Figure 9.23.

As we can see from Figure 9.14, the differences in image intensities usually do not interfere with the delineation of edges (with some exceptions, like the additional edges in MR that stem from the better soft-tissue contrast). If we can design a merit function based on these gradient images, we may have another merit function for multimodal image fusion at hand. Such a measure is *chamfer matching*; it uses a binary image for I_{Match} that was made using a Sobel filter and intensity thresholding such as shown in Figure 9.14, and a distance transform (see Section 5.3.2) of I_{Base} that was processed in the same manner. Figure 9.15 shows the distance transform of `T1.jpg` after differentiation and intensity thresholding.

The chamfer matching merit function $\mathcal{M}_{\mathrm{CM}}$ is simply defined as:

$$\mathcal{M}_{\mathrm{CM}} = \sum_{x,y} D\left(I_{\mathrm{Base}}(x,y)\right) \tag{9.9}$$

$$x, y \quad \ldots \quad \text{Pixels in } I_{\mathrm{Match}} \text{ with } \rho > 0$$

$$D\left(I_{\mathrm{Base}}\right) \quad \ldots \quad \text{Distance transform of } I_{\mathrm{Base}}$$

Equation 9.9 can be understood as follows; $D\left(I_{\mathrm{Base}}\right)$ – the distance transform from Section 5.3.2 – defines *grooves* in the binary gradient image I_{Base}, and if I_{Match} "drops" into those grooves, $\mathcal{M}_{\mathrm{CM}}$ becomes optimal. A plot of $\mathcal{M}_{\mathrm{CM}}$ is computed in Example 9.9.4. This merit

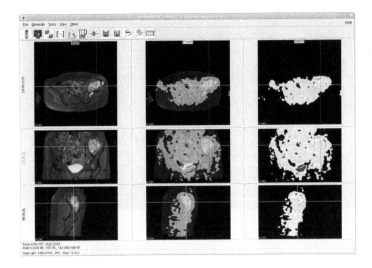

FIGURE 9.13: A more complex clinical example of multimodal image registration. Here, a PET and an MR scan of a sarcoma in the pelvis was registered. Since PET provides very little anatomic information, a direct registration of MR and PET data in the abdominal area often fails. However, it is possible to register the MR data with the CT data that came with the PET-scan from a PET-CT scanner using normalized mutual information; in this case, the implementation of AnalyzeAVW was used. The registration matrix obtained is applied to the PET data since these are provided in the same frame of reference as the CT data. Image data courtesy of the Dept. of Radiology and the Dept. of Nuclear Medicine, Medical University Vienna.

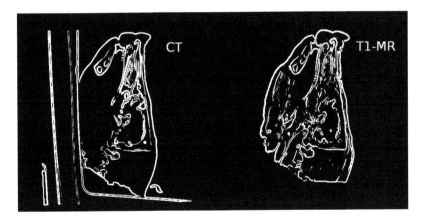

FIGURE 9.14: `CT.jpg` and `T1.jpg` after Sobel-filtering, optimization of image depth and thresholding. After this process, the differences in gray values in the two images disappear, and only gradient information remains. Applying a gradient-based measure to such an image allows for multi-modal image registration without computing joint histograms or using an intensity based measure.

function has a severe drawback – it only works well if we are already close to the solution

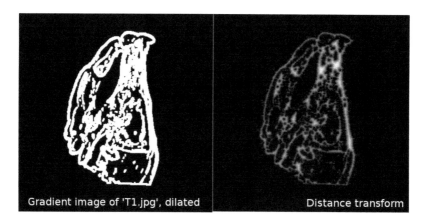

FIGURE 9.15: `T1.jpg` after Sobel-filtering, intensity thresholding, and dilation (left). This image can be found in the `LessonData` folder as `T1_EdgeImageDilated.jpg`. The right image shows its distance transform (`DT_ChamferMatch.jpg` in `LessonData`). The image is an intermediate result of Example 9.9.4. In the chamfer-matching algorithm, the sum of the entries in the distance transform of I_{Base} at the location of non-zero pixels in I_{Match} is computed while I_{Match} moves over the base image.

of the registration problem. Another example of such a merit function is Equation 9.3. In Section 9.4, we will discuss this problem to a further extent.

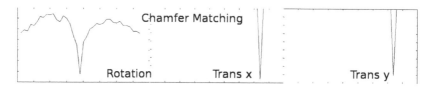

FIGURE 9.16: The results of Example 9.9.4; this is a plot of the chamfer matching merit function in 3 dof through the solution of the registration problem. The plots can be directly compared to Figure 9.12, derived in Example 9.9.3. As we can see, numerous local minima exist and for translation, there is no wide gradient. Therefore it is necessary to start the optimization algorithm close to the expected solution, since otherwise, finding the minimum is unlikely.

Finally, we can also compare images by employing an orthonormal series expansion, of which we heard in Chapter 5. Remember that every coefficient in such an expansion is unique; if we compare corresponding coefficients of the same order, we can compare images. If we compare the norms of the components in a Fourier transform, we are able to decouple translation and rotation since translation is only a complex phase in the Fourier-domain. The norm of a complex number does not know about complex phases, and therefore such a merit function would be translation-invariant. However, merit functions based on series expansions tend to be computationally expensive, and by nature, they are confined to binary or strictly intramodal image data. But if we would like to solve the registration problem when facing a merit function as shown in Figure 9.9, it might be a viable way to solve the rotation problem first and finding an optimum translation afterwards.

Here ends our presentation of merit functions; many more exist, and some of them provide valuable additional tools in our arsenal for specialized tasks. However, we have learned about the basic types of the most important methods for comparing images. What we have not yet dealt with is the question of finding an optimum in the merit function, rather than presenting functions that exhibit a known optimal value.

9.4 OPTIMIZATION STRATEGIES

The plots from Figs. 9.6, 9.9, 9.10, 9.11, 9.12 and 9.16 all presented a somewhat misleading idea of the general shape of a merit function. Here, only one dof was varied, whereas the others were kept constant at the correct value. Furthermore, we only deal with rather harmless images showing the same region of our object, and all images were in 2D. If we switch to 3D, we end up with merit functions that are dependent on six parameters (for instance three quaternions – the fourth one is defined by the requirement that the quaternions are normalized – and three dof in translation). The graphical representation of a function $\mathcal{M}(\Delta x, \Delta y, \Delta z, q_1, q_2, q_3) = r$, where r is a real-valued scalar is nevertheless a considerable task. It is even more difficult to find an optimum in a six-dimensional valley. This is the task of an *optimization algorithm*.

The optimization problem can be imagined as a salad bowl and a marble. If we have a nice, smooth salad bowl and a nice, smooth marble, the marble can be released at any point and it will find its way to the minimum under the influence of gravity. Nature always does so, and an Irish physicist, W. R. Hamilton, even made that a general principle, the principle of least action. Another creation of Sir William Rowan Hamilton we have already encountered – he has also opened our eyes to the world of quaternions.

In our less than perfect world, we may however encounter problems in optimization. Our salad bowl may be a masterpiece of design, shaped like a steep cone with a very small opening (like a champagne glass), whereas we have to use a football in order to solve this problem because of a sudden shortage of marbles. The principle of least action is still valid, but we will not see the football roll to the deepest point of the salad bowl. Other salad bowls may have a very rough and sticky surface, and our marbles may be small and our marble could be badly damaged because of being a veteran of fierce marbling contests in the past. The salad bowl is the merit function, and the marble is the optimization algorithm, grossly speaking. I will not further expand on the problems of n-dimensional salad bowls.

Optimization algorithms can be categorized as *local* and *global algorithms*. The problem with all optimization algorithms is that they can fail. Usually, the algorithm starts at a given position and tries to follow the gradient of the merit function until it reaches an optimum. Note that we do not care whether we face a maximum or a minimum, since every merit function showing a maximum can be turned over by multiplying it with -1. Since the merit function is only given on discrete pivot points, we have no chance of knowing whether this optimum is the absolute optimum (the optimal value the merit function reaches over its domain), or if there is another hidden optimum. The mathematical counterpart of the saladbowl/marble allegory is the simplex algorithm, also called Nelder-Mead method. Here, the marble is replaced by a simplex, which can be considered an n-dimensional triangle. If our simplex is one-dimensional and is supposed to find the minimum of a simple one-dimensional function $f(x) = y$, it is a segment of a straight line; this simplex crawls down the function $f(x)$, and its stepwidth is governed by the gradient of $f(x)$. Once the simplex encounters a minimum, it reduces its stepwidth until it collapses to a point. Figure 9.17 illustrates this algorithm in a humble fashion.

The simplex-algorithm is one of many optimization methods; other algorithms like

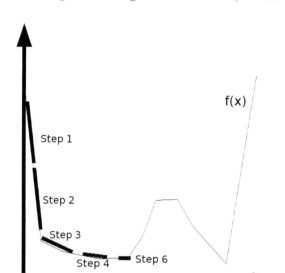

FIGURE 9.17: A simple illustration of the Nelder-Mead or simplex algorithm, a local optimization algorithm; a simplex in one dimension is a section of straight line that follows the gradient of a function; as the simplex approaches a minimum, $\frac{d}{dx}f(x) \simeq 0$ is true, and the simplex makes smaller steps until it collapses to a point since the gradient to the right is ascending again and the algorithm terminates. It cannot find the global minimum to the right, but it is stuck in the local minimum.

Powell's method, Levenberg-Marquardt, conjugate gradient and so on are well-documented in numerous textbooks. All these algorithms are *local optimizers* – they are good at finding the obvious nearest minimum, and some of them require the computation of derivative functions, whereas others do not. The simplex is of special interest for us since it is incorporated in MATLAB® as `fminsearch`, and Example 9.9.5 demonstrates it.

Global optimizers try to tackle the problem of finding – as the name implies – global optima. The simplest type of a global optimization method is a full search in the parameter space with decreasing stepwidth. Imagine you have a set of N starting parameters $\vec{p}$, and a gross area you want to explore. The area is claimed by defining a starting interval Δp_i; next, one computes all values of the merit function $\mathcal{M}(\vec{p}')$ for all possible combinations of parameters $\vec{p}' \in \{(p_1 - \Delta p_1, p_2, p_3, \dots p_N), \dots (p_1, \dots, p_N + \Delta p_N)\}$. The result is an array of merit function values, and one can easily find the minimum in this array. In a subsequent step, the starting parameter set $\vec{p}$ is replaced by the parameters that yield the smallest value, and one continues with a smaller set of interval $\Delta p'$ and so on. Given the proper choice of starting values and proper intervals, this method may converge at huge computational cost. If we choose the simplest implementation of such a parameter space search, which is an interval that only looks once to the left and to the right of each starting parameter, we end up with 3^N evaluations of the N-dimensional merit function $\mathcal{M}$. More sophisticated methods try to solve the problem in a stochastic manner – the best known algorithm of this type is *simulated annealing*, where an N-dimensional random walker charts the manifold defined by $\mathcal{M}$ and decreases its momentum as it gathers more samples of $\mathcal{M}$. Another class of algorithms are referred to as genetic algorithms, where seeds are placed randomly in parameter space. Figuratively speaking, the seeds in the fertile plains of $\mathcal{M}$ multiply, whereas the ones on the barren plateaus slowly vanish. Still, global optimization algorithms are usually slow, and it is not guaranteed that they converge to a global minimum. One thing that all optimizers have in common is the fact that they are highly dependent on internal parameters such as termination criteria and stepwidths.

9.5 SOME GENERAL COMMENTS

Registration, despite the considerable complexity of a full-featured implementation of a high-performance registration tool, is the more pleasant part of medical image processing compared to segmentation. After all, $\mathcal{M}_{\mathrm{MI}}$ is a measure that works as a good basic approach for many registration problems. Therefore it would be reasonable to use mutual information, combined with global optimizers and maybe a deformation model for coping with non-rigid deformations, for all registration problems.

In real life, this does not work. While mutual information is an excellent measure, it also sacrifices information by omitting the actual gray values from the images after forming the PDF; if the joint histogram is sparsely populated, for instance due to lacking information in one of the images, the measure is likely to fail. An example is MR/PET registration, one of the first applications for this measure in neuroscience. Fusing MR and PET images of the brain works well since a high and specific uptake of tracer yields lot of information. If one tries to accomplish the same with PET images of the body, the difficulties are considerable. This has led to the development of PET/CT, and PET/MR is a further development under research for the time being.

If a combined scan is not feasible, it may be a good idea to resort to registration techniques using external markers (see also Section 9.7.1). Another problem related to sparse histogram population, which results in an inconclusive optimum for the Shannon entropy, is often encountered in 2D/3D registration (see Section 9.7.2), where six dof of motion in 3D are retrieved from planar images. Therefore one is well advised to consider alternatives, especially when dealing with intramodal registration problems, to improve the robustness of the registration algorithm by utilizing more stringent merit functions.

Another challenge lies in the evaluation of registration algorithms; we will encounter the well-accepted measures of *target registration error* (TRE) and *fiducial registration error* (FRE) in Section 9.8. However, it is also interesting to explore the reliability of an implementation, which is not only dependent on the merit function used, but also on the clinical application area, the imaging modalities used, and the configuration of the optimization algorithm used; a validation of a registration algorithm can, for most practical purposes, only be carried out by repeated runs of the algorithm with randomly changing starting positions, which may be confined to different maximal values. And it should take place on as many datasets as available.

Another problem that is ignored pretty often lies in the fact that we are optimizing for parameters which are given in different units. Rotations are given in *radians* or *degrees*, and translations are given in voxels, pixels, or millimeters. The optimization algorithm scales itself to the function slope, but it is not necessarily aware that a change in $1°$ in rotation may have a way more dramatic effect on the image compared to a translation of 1 pixel.

So what can be done to achieve good registration results? Here is a small checklist:

Initialization: As we can see in Example 9.9.5, it is advisable to start the registration close to expected solution; one may, for instance, position the volumes or images manually. Or it is possible to move the volumes to the same center of gravity – a *principal axes transform* may also help to obtain an initial guess for the relative rotation of the images.

Appropriate choice of the merit function: The nature of the registration problem governs the choice of the merit function. In general, one may consider other statistical measures than mutual information if a intramodal registration problem is given. Gradient based methods tend to have a smaller capture range than intensity–based methods.

Appropriate choice of optimization methods: Global optimizers tend to require lots of computational time while a correct result is not guaranteed. One may try a good implementation of a local algorithm first. Sometimes, a multiscale approach is proposed. Here, the volumes are scaled down and the registration problem is handled on this coarse stage first before proceeding to finer resolution. This approach is, however, not always successful – it may as well lead to local optima and considerable runtime.

Avoid additional degrees-of-freedom: It is of course possible to match images of different scale using an additional scaling transformation, and of course one could always try to carry out a deformable registration in order to avoid errors from changing soft tissue. Don't do this – additional dof increase the risk of winding up in local optima.

Restriction to relevant image content: This is an often underestimated aspect. It is very helpful to constrain the area in I_{Base} used for merit function validation. This does not only refer to the spatial domain, but also to intensities. A lower bound in intensity can, for instance, improve robustness by suppressing noise and structures that stem from the imaging modality such as the table in CT. And it can be helpful to exclude parts of the body which moved relative to each other; an example is the registration of abdominal scans such as shown in Figure 9.2, where it is advisable to exclude the femora since these are mobile relative to the pelvis.

9.6   CAMERA CALIBRATION

Another important technique, especially for image-guided therapy (Section 7.5) and visualization (Chapter 8) is the determination of projection parameters of a 3D body to a 2D imaging plane. The shape of the projection image will, of course, be determined by the actual pose of the 3D body, which can be described by an affine rigid body transformation in homogeneous coordinates, and by the position of the projection source and the projection screen relative to the 3D-body. In Chapter 8, we have learned how to produce such projected images from 3D datasets. In *camera calibration*, the inverse problem is being treated – how can we determine both the 3D-position of an object and the properties of the camera – that is, any projection system including x-ray machines and head-mounted displays – from the projected image? In the most simple (and common) of all cases, we just want to know about the reference coordinate system and the distance of the focal spot (or the eyepoint) of our camera; this can be determined by projecting single points with a known 3D-position onto a projection screen (which can be an x-ray image detector or a display as well). Figure 9.18 illustrates this problem.

In order to tackle the camera calibration problem, we have to remember another matrix, which is the projector P. In mathematics, each matrix that fulfills the requirement $P = P^2$ is called a projection. Let's go to Figure 9.18 – the effect of $P\vec{u}_i$ is the 2D image of the markers. If we project this image again, nothing will change. A projection matrix that maps 3D positions $\vec{u}_i$ to 2D positions $\vec{w}_i$ to the x-y plane of a Cartesian coordinate system where

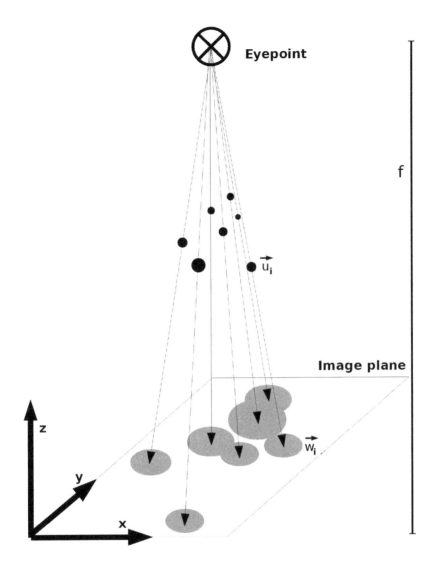

FIGURE 9.18: An illustration of the camera calibration problem. In this example, the imaging plane is located in the x-y plane of a Cartesian coordinate system. The normal distance of the eyepoint – the source of projection – is located at a distance **f** from the imaging plane. The known coordinates of the fiducial markers $\vec{u}_i$ are projected onto the plane, and their coordinates are given as $\vec{w}_i$. The task is to determine **f** and an affine transformation that locates the eyepoint in the coordinate system.

the eyepoint is located at the the z-axis at a distance **f** is given as:

$$P = \begin{pmatrix} 1 & 0 & 0 & 0 \\ 0 & 1 & 0 & 0 \\ 0 & 0 & 0 & 0 \\ 0 & 0 & -\frac{1}{\mathbf{f}} & 1 \end{pmatrix} \tag{9.10}$$

One can easily verify that P is a projector indeed. The projector operates on a point $\vec{u}_i$

by multiplication. If we want to apply the volume transformation V on that point prior to projection, we have to compute $PV\vec{u}_i = \vec{w}_i$. You may remember that, in order to change the position of the eyepoint by another volume transformation V', we have to compute $V'PV\vec{u}_i = \vec{w}'$. Since we deal with a projection in homogeneous coordinates here, we have to add a rescaling step to $\vec{w}'$ to get coordinates $\vec{w}$ – remember that the fourth element of vector giving homogeneous coordinates has to be 1, which is not the case when applying an operator like P.

In the camera calibration problem, we know a set of N planar projected coordinates $\vec{w}_i \in \{\vec{w}_0 \ldots \vec{w}_N\}$ and the associated 3D coordinates $\vec{u}_i \in \{\vec{u}_0 \ldots \vec{u}_N\}$. We have to find out about V and **f**. A simple algorithm to achieve this is called the *Direct Linear Transform* (DLT). It is easily formulated using homogeneous coordinates; a 3D coordinate $\vec{u}$ is transformed by a 4×4 matrix $PV = D$, where P is given in Equation 9.10 and V is our well-known affine transformation matrix from Section 7.3.2, as:

$$D\vec{u} = \vec{v} \tag{9.11}$$

It is, however, necessary to renormalize the resulting vector $\vec{v}$ by computing $\vec{w} = \frac{\vec{v}}{v_4}$. We omit the z-variable since it is of no importance for the projected screen coordinates; therefore we have a resulting pair of screen coordinates:

$$\vec{w}' = \begin{pmatrix} w_1 \\ w_2 \\ 0 \\ 1 \end{pmatrix}. \tag{9.12}$$

All we have to find out is the twelve components of matrix D; by expanding the matrix product and using Equation 9.12 we can rewrite Equation 9.11 as:

$$D_{11}u_1 + D_{12}u_2 + D_{13}u_3 + D_{14} = w_1 * v_4 \tag{9.13}$$
$$D_{21}u_1 + D_{22}u_2 + D_{23}u_3 + D_{24} = w_2 * v_4 \tag{9.14}$$
$$D_{41}u_1 + D_{42}u_2 + D_{43}u_3 + D_{44} = v_4 \tag{9.15}$$

We can insert Equation 9.15 in Eqs. 9.13 and 9.14, which gives us two equations with twelve unknowns $D_{11}, D_{12}, D_{13}, D_{14}, D_{21}, D_{22}, D_{23}, D_{24}, D_{41}, D_{42}, D_{43}$, and D_{44}. These can be rewritten as a 12×2 matrix:

$$\begin{pmatrix} u_1 & u_2 & u_3 & 1 & 0 & 0 & 0 & 0 & -w_1u_1 & -w_1u_2 & -w_1u_3 & -w_1 \\ 0 & 0 & 0 & 0 & u_1 & u_2 & u_3 & 1 & -w_2u_1 & -w_2u_2 & -w_2u_3 & -w_2 \end{pmatrix} \begin{pmatrix} D_{11} \\ D_{12} \\ D_{13} \\ D_{14} \\ D_{21} \\ D_{22} \\ D_{23} \\ D_{24} \\ D_{41} \\ D_{42} \\ D_{43} \\ D_{44} \end{pmatrix} = \vec{0} \tag{9.16}$$

where $\vec{0}$ is a vector containing zeros only. If we have at least six points $\vec{u}_i$, we can augment the matrix from Equation 9.16 by adding more rows; let us call this matrix S and the vector containing the components of matrix D is called $\vec{d}$. Equation 9.16 becomes a homogeneous system of equations $S\vec{d} = 0$, which can be solved using, for instance, a *linear least squares* method. Example 9.9.6 demonstrates this. A number of more sophisticated variations of this algorithm exist; these can also compensate for distortions in the projection images such as the radial distortion in wide angle optics, or for the higher order distortion encountered in analog image intensifiers used in C-arms. But, at least for the calibration of modern amorphous silicon x-ray imaging detectors, the DLT is usually fine.

9.7   REGISTRATION TO PHYSICAL SPACE

So far, we have talked about image-fusion; we have learned that we can merge images of the same origin and from different modalities, and that we can enhance the affine transformation in six dof by adding internal dof of deformation, which is governed by various models. But in a number of applications (remember Section 7.5), it is necessary to map a coordinate system defined in physical space to an image coordinate system. Application examples include the registration of a patient, whose coordinate system is defined by a rigidly attached tracker probe, to an MR or CT-volume. Another example includes the registration of a robot's internal frame-of-reference to a patient, who is either fixated by molds or other devices, or who is tracked as well. In the following sections, a few techniques for registration to physical space will be introduced.

9.7.1   Rigid registration using fiducial markers and surfaces

Until now, we have dealt with intensity based registration; if intensity based algorithms fail, one may resort to explicit landmarks, which can either be prominent anatomical features, or explicitly attached so-called *fiducial markers*. This is an extremely important technique, not only in image processing, but also in image-guided therapy, where a match between patient and image data is to be achieved. Figure 9.19 shows the so-called Vogele-Bale-Hohner mouthpiece, a non-invasive device for registration using fiducial markers. The mouthpiece is attached to the patient by means of a personalized mold of the maxillary denture. A vacuum pump evacuates the mold, therefore the mouthpiece is held in position in a very exact manner. The strength of this setup is certainly fusion of anatomical image data and SPECT or PET datasets, where an intensity-based algorithm often fails due to a lack of common information in the images.

In the best of all cases, the coordinates of the markers match each other. If the transformation matrix is composed as a rotation followed by a translation ($V = TR$) one can immediately determine three dof of translation by computing the centroid of the marker pairs according to Equation 6.1 in both frames of reference. The difference of the two centroids gives the translation vector. After translation of the marker positions so that the centroids of the point pairs $\{\vec{p}_1, \vec{p}_2, \ldots, \vec{p}_N\}$ and $\{\vec{p'}_1, \vec{p'}_2, \ldots, \vec{p'}_N\}$ match, a rotation matrix R that merges the positions best can be determined if the markers are not *collinear* – in other words, the points must not lie on a line. And we do need at least three of them. Let P_{Base} be the set of coordinates in the base reference frame, and P'_{Match} be the matching set of points in the coordinate system to be registered after they were translated to the centroid. This can, however, also be done inside the algorithm. In this setup, the center of rotation is the centroid of the base point set.

One of the most widely used algorithms for matching ordered point sets was given by Horn.[4] It matches two ordered point sets P_{Base} and P_{Match} by minimizing

$$\mathcal{M} = \frac{1}{2} \sum_{i=1}^{N} \|\vec{p}_{\text{Base}_i} - V\vec{p}_{\text{match}_i}\|^2 \tag{9.17}$$

where V is the well-known affine volume transformation matrix. After computing the centroids $\vec{\bar{p}}_{\text{Base}}$ and $\vec{\bar{p}}_{\text{Match}}$, one can define a 4×4 covariance matrix C

---

[4]B. K. P. Horn: Closed-form solution of absolute orientation using unit quaternions, J. Opt. Soc. Am. A 4(4), 629ff. (1987). Here we give the formulation used in P. J. Besl, N. D. McKay, A method for Registration of 3-D Shapes, IEEE Trans PAMI 15(2), 239ff. (1992).

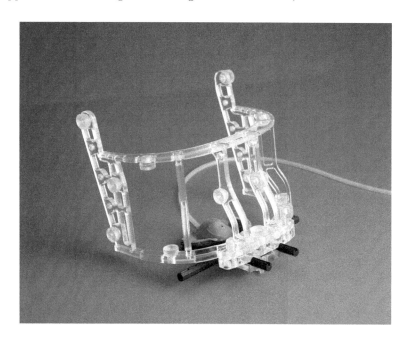

FIGURE 9.19: The Vogele-Bale-Hohner mouthpiece, a device for non-invasive registration using fiducial markers. The mouthpiece is personalized by means of a dental mold. A vacuum pump ensures optimum fit of the mouthpiece during imaging. Image courtesy of Reto Bale, MD, University Clinic for Radiology, University of Innsbruck, Austria.

of the point sets as

$$C = \frac{1}{N} \sum_{i=1}^{N} \left(\vec{p}_{\mathrm{Match}_i} - \vec{\bar{p}}_{\mathrm{Match}} \right) \left(\vec{p}_{\mathrm{Base}_i} - \vec{\bar{p}}_{\mathrm{Base}} \right)^{T} \tag{9.18}$$

Next, an anti-symmetric matrix $A = C - C^T$ is formed from C; the vector Δ is given by $\Delta = (A_{23}, A_{31}, A_{12})^T$. Using this vector, one can define a 4×4 matrix Q:

$$Q = \left(\begin{array}{cc} \mathrm{tr}\, C & \Delta^T \\ \Delta & C + C^T - \mathrm{tr}\, C \mathbf{I}_3 \end{array} \right) \tag{9.19}$$

$\mathrm{tr}\, C$ is the *trace* of matrix C, the *sum of all diagonal elements*. $\mathbf{I}_3$ is the 3×3 identity matrix. If we compute the eigenvectors and eigenvalues of Q and select the eigenvector that belongs to the biggest eigenvalue, we have four quaternions. A rotation matrix R can be derived by using Equation 7.19. These are the parameters of the optimum rotation that match the point sets. The translation is derived, as already mentioned before, by computing:

$$\vec{t} = \frac{1}{N} \sum_{i=1}^{N} \vec{p}_{\mathrm{Match}_i} - R\vec{p}_{\mathrm{Base}_i} \tag{9.20}$$

Example 9.9.7 implements such a computation.

A logical next step would be to enhance the method to non-ordered point sets. This is for instance important if one wants to match surfaces, which are digitized and given as node points. Matching two such meshes is a widespread problem, for instance in image-guided therapy. If one segments a body surface from a CT- or MR-scan, it is possible to generate a mesh of the resulting surface (as presented in Chapter 8), consisting of node points. Another modality such as a surface scanner, which produces a 3D surface by scanning an object using optical technologies for instance, can produce another mesh of the patient surface in the operating room. Surface data can also be collected, for instance, by tracked ultrasound probes, where a 3D point is assigned to a 2D point in the US-image by tracking the scanhead using some sort of position measurement device (see Section 7.5). By matching the surface as scanned and the segmented surface, it is possible to achieve a match of the patients position in the treatment suite to the volume image; in such a case, the node points of the meshes are matched by using a point-to-point registration technique, but the point sets are not ordered.

An enhancement of the method as presented in Eqs. 9.18–9.20 is the so-called *iterative closest point* (ICP) algorithm, which was presented in the already mentioned paper by P. Besl and N. McKay. In the ICP-algorithm, the distance d between a single point $\vec{p}$ and a surface S is defined as $d(\vec{p}, S) = \min_{\vec{x} \in S} \|\vec{x} - \vec{p}\|$. Computing such a minimum distance is not new to us – we have done this before in Example 6.8.7. The result of this search for closest points is an *ordered* set of corresponding points from S which are closest to the points $\vec{p}$ in our matching surface, which is given as a set of points $\vec{p}$. What follows is a point-to-point registration as shown before. The next step is to repeat the procedure, with a new set of closest points as the results. This procedure can be repeated until a termination criterion is met – usually this is the minimal distance between closest points.

The ICP-algorithm, which had numerous predecessors and refinements, also lies at the base of *surface-based* registration algorithms. If one tries to match two intramodal datasets, a feasible way is to segment surfaces in both volumes is to segment these surfaces, create a mesh, and apply an ICP-type of algorithm. This is generally referred to as surface registration; it is, however, usually inferior to intensity-based algorithms such as mutual information measure based methods. First, it requires segmentation, which can be tedious; second, the ICP algorithm is sensitive to outliers. A single errant node point, generated by a segmentation artifact for instance, can screw up the whole procedure.

9.7.2   2D/3D registration

Registration of the patient to image data is not confined to point- or surface-based methods; it can also be achieved by comparing image data taken during or prior to an intervention with pre-interventional data. An example of such an algorithm is the registration of a patient to a CT-dataset using x-ray data. If one knows the imaging geometry of an x-ray device, for instance by employing a camera-calibration technique (see Section 9.6), If the exact position of the x-ray tube focus is known relative to the patient (for instance by using a tracker, or from the internal encoders of an imaging device), one can derive six dof of rigid motion by varying the six parameters for the registration transformation. The fact that x-ray is a central projection with a perspective (which is governed by parameter f in Equation 9.10) is of the utmost importance in this context since a motion to and from the x-ray tube focus changes the scale of the projection. In a 2D/3D registration algorithm, DRRs are produced iteratively, and a merit function is used to compare the DRR to the actual x-ray image. Once an optimum match is achieved, the registration parameters are stored and give the optimum transform. This type of registration algorithm is usually more complex and sometimes tedious compared to 3D/3D registration since the optimization problem is not well defined. Multimodal and non-rigid 2D/3D registration are also open challenges.

Figure 9.20 shows a reference x-ray, a DRR before registration and the overlay of the two. In the folder `MultimediaMaterial`, you will also find a MPG-movie named `7_2D_3DRegistration.mpg` which shows a 2D/3D registration algorithm at work.[5] The movie shows the series of DRRs and the merit function; after convergence, an overlay of the DRR and the reference x-ray is displayed.

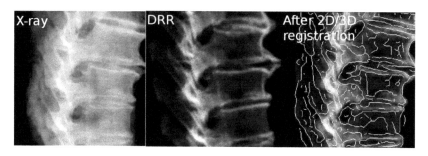

FIGURE 9.20: Three images of a spine reference-dataset for 2D/3D image registration. We see the reference x-ray on the left, the DRR generated from the initial guess, and the registration result. An edge image of the x-ray is overlaid over the final DRR after 2D/3D registration.

9.8 EVALUATION OF REGISTRATION RESULTS

As usual in medical image processing, many algorithms can be defined, but they tend to be worthless if a substantial benefit for clinical applications cannot be shown. Therefore, evaluation is a crucial problem here. The most important measure for registration is, of course, the accuracy of the registration method. Such a measure was introduced initially for image-guided therapy, but it also fits general registration problems perfectly well. It is the *target registration error* (TRE).[6] In image fusion, points (that must not be the fiducial markers in the case of marker based registration) randomly chosen from the base volume are transformed to the match volume (or vice versa), and the average or maximal Euclidean distance of the two positions in the base and match coordinate system is computed. It is however important to sample more than one point, and to distribute them evenly over the whole volume.

In image-guided therapy, the issue is a little bit more complex. Here, a fiducial marker has to be localized in patient space by means of a tracker or a similar device, which has an intrinsic error. This initial localization error is called *fiducial localization error* (FLE). The FLE does of course affect the precision of a marker-based registration method. After computing the registration transform from the marker positions, the euclidean distance between the markers in the target volume and their transformed positions is given by the *fiducial registration error* (FRE), which is sometimes reported by a IGT-software suite as a measure for the quality of the registration. This measure is, however, misleading. If the original distribution of markers is positioned in a more or less collinear manner, the quality

---

[5]A detailed description of the dataset used in this illustration can be found in E. B. van de Kraats, G. P. Penney, D. Tomazevic, T. van Walsum, and W. J. Niessen: Standardized evaluation methodology for 2-D-3-D registration, IEEE Trans Med Imaging, 24(9):1177-89, (2005).

[6]The classic treatise on these things is, for instance C. R. Maurer Jr, J. M. Fitzpatrick, M. Y. Wang, R. L. GallowayJr, R. J. Maciunas, and G. S. Allen: Registration of Head Volume Images Using Implantable Fiducial Markers, TMI 16(4), pp. 447-462, (1997).

of the registration may, for instance, be pathetic despite an excellent FRE. It is therefore also necessary to determine a TRE in addition to the FRE; since the localization of a target is usually carried out by a tracker, the tracker accuracy may affect TRE as well.

Besides accuracy, it is also necessary to report the range of convergence for a measure; this can be done by a random sampling of starting points within a certain initial TRE, and a comparison of resulting TREs. A report on failed registrations (where the algorithm does not converge or produces a result worse than the initial TRE) and on algorithm runtimes is also mandatory. Finally, a validation should be carried out on phantom datasets which allow for determination of a ground truth such as our pig-dataset we tormented to such a large extent in this chapter. It is actually from such a dataset since it carries multimodal fiducial markers.

9.9 PRACTICAL LESSONS

9.9.1 Registration of 2D images using cross-correlation

CC2DRegistration_9.m is a script derived from Example 7.6.1. In this example, we rotate a single 2D image by an angle $\phi \in \{-90° \ldots 90°\}$ and compute Pearson's cross-correlation coefficient given in Equation 7.16 as a merit function. The values for the merit function in dependence of the rotation angle are stored in a vector ccvals. The single MR-slice of our already well-known pig head (see also Figure 7.12) is loaded and a matrix rotimg is allocated for the rotated image. Furthermore, the vector ccvals is declared:

```
1:> img=imread('PorkyPig.jpg');
2:> rotimg=zeros(300,300);
3:> ccvals=zeros(181,1);
```

Next, we enter a loop where the rotation angle ϕ is varied from -90° to 90° in 1° steps. The rotation matrix is defined. We perform a nearest neighbor interpolation by transforming the new coordinates newpix in rotimg back to the original image img. Furthermore, we also rotate the image around its center, therefore the center of the image is transformed to the origin of the coordinate system by a vector shift; after rotation, the coordinates are shifted back. The result is a rotated image such as shown in Figure 7.14 from Example 7.6.2.

```
4:> for angle=-90:90
5:> rotmat=zeros(2,2);
6:> rotmat(1,1)=cos(angle*pi/180);
7:> rotmat(1,2)=-sin(angle*pi/180);
8:> rotmat(2,1)=sin(angle*pi/180);
9:> rotmat(2,2)=cos(angle*pi/180);
10:> invrotmat=transpose(rotmat);
11:> oldpix=zeros(2,1);
12:> newpix=zeros(2,1);
13:> shift=transpose([150,150]);
14:> for i=1:300
15:> for j=1:300
16:> newpix(1,1)=i;
17:> newpix(2,1)=j;
18:> oldpix=round((invrotmat*(newpix-shift))+shift);
19:> if (oldpix(1,1) > 0) & (oldpix(1,1) < 300) &
(oldpix(2,1) > 0) & (oldpix(2,1) < 300)
```

```
20:> rotimg(i,j)=img(oldpix(1,1),oldpix(2,1));
21:> end
22:> end
23:> end
```

Next, we compute the correlation coefficient; since we are only interested in the optimum of this simple merit function, we do not care about normalization factors and so on. Furthermore, the merit function becomes maximal for an optimum match; it is therefore inverted by displaying its negative value. Finally, the contents of the merit function vector ccvals are displayed. We store the result of the merit function evaluation in an array ccvals. Since we change the angle of rotation from -90 to 90°, we have to add 91 to the variable angle for proper indexing. A plot of ccvals can be found in Figure 9.21.

```
24:> meanImg=mean(mean(img));
25:> meanRotImg=mean(mean(rotimg));
26:> ccdenom=0.0;
27:> ccnomImg=0.0;
28:> ccnomRotImg=0;
29:> for i=1:300
30:> for j=1:300
31:> ccdenom=ccdenom+double(((img(i,j)-meanImg)*
(rotimg(i,j)-meanRotImg)));
32:> ccnomImg=ccnomImg+double(((img(i,j)-meanImg)^2));
33:> ccnomRotImg=ccnomRotImg+double(((rotimg(i,j)-
meanRotImg)^2));
34:> end
35:> end
36:> ccvals((angle+91),1)=-ccdenom/
(sqrt(ccnomImg)*sqrt(ccnomRotImg));
37:> end
38:> plot(ccvals)
```

In a full-fledged implementation of a registration algorithm, a minimum for all three dof would be computed by an optimization algorithm, thus producing the parameters for a registration matrix V.

Additional Tasks

Implement a translation rather than a rotation, and inspect the result.

Implement intramodal merit functions other than cross correlation from Section 9.3.

A modified script, More2DRegistration_9.m compares two registered slices of the porcine phantom taken with different types of CT; the first one is a slice from the already well-known multislice CT dataset, the other one was taken using a CBCT machine attached to a linear accelerator. While this is an intramodal image registration problem, the imaging characteristics of the two machines are different concerning dose, dynamic range of the detector, and tube voltage. Inspect the results for the intramodal merit functions in this script. Two examples for $\mathcal{M}_{SSD}$ and $\mathcal{M}_{CC}$ are given in Figure 9.22.

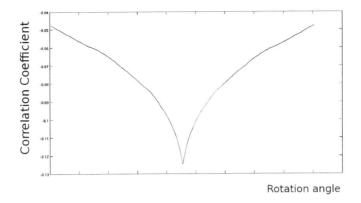

FIGURE 9.21: The output of Example 9.9.1. When rotating the image from Figure 7.12 from -90° to 90° and computing the correlation coefficient as given in Equation 7.16, we get an optimum correlation if the two images match; this is, of course, the case for a rotation of 0°. A registration algorithm computes the spatial transform to match two images by optimizing all dof until a minimum in the merit function is found.

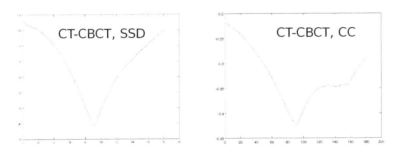

FIGURE 9.22: Two sample outputs from modified versions of `More2DRegistration_9.m`, where two registered slices of a CBCT and a CT were rotated against each other, and the result was evaluated using Equation 9.1, the sum of squared differences, and $\mathcal{M}_{CC}$ – the merit function based on Pearson's cross correlation coefficient. While $\mathcal{M}_{SSD}$ performs fine (left side), $\mathcal{M}_{CC}$ exhibits an local minimum at approximately 140° that may even lead to a failure in a registration process.

9.9.2 Computing joint histograms

In `JointHistogram_9.m`, we compute the joint histogram for an MR image of a female pelvis. The images can be found in the `LessonData` folder as `OrthoMR` and `OrthoMRTransf`. They are stored as DICOM-images since the greater depth helps to make the result of joint histogram computation more evident. First, we load the two images `img` and `rimg`, and we allocate a matrix that holds the joint histogram `jhist`:

```
1:> fp=fopen('OrthoMR','r');
2:> fseek(fp,2164,'bof');
3:> img=zeros(380,160);
4:> img(:)=fread(fp,(380*160),'short');
```

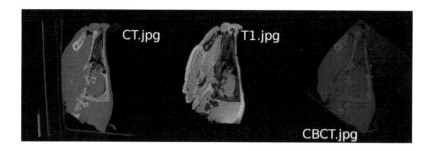

FIGURE 9.23: Three sample slices from co-registered volumes; `T1.jpg` is taken from an MR-volume, whereas `CT.jpg` and `CBCT.jpg` are from CT-volumes. The images are used in Examples 9.9.1, 9.9.2 and 9.9.3.

```
 5:> fclose(fp);
 6:> fp=fopen('OrthoMRTransf','r');
 7:> fseek(fp,960,'bof');
 8:> rimg=zeros(380,160);
 9:> rimg(:)=fread(fp,(380*160),'short');
10:> fclose(fp);
11:> jhist=zeros(900,900);
```

Next, we compute the joint histogram of `img` with itself; each pixel location $(i, j)^T$ is visited, and a scatterplot of the gray values `rho1` and `rho2` is produced. Since our indices in `jhist` start with one rather than zero, we increment `rho1` and `rho2` by one for easier indexing. The joint histogram `jhist` gives the statistics of occurrence in this scatterplot. In order to improve the visibility of the gray values in the joint histogram, we compute the logarithm of `jhist`, just as we did in Example 4.5.3. After inspecting the result, we are prompted to proceed:

```
12:> for i=1:380
13:> for j=1:160
14:> rho1=img(i,j)+1;
15:> rho2=img(i,j)+1;
16:> jhist(rho1,rho2)=jhist(rho1,rho2)+1;
17:> end
18:> end
19:> jhist=log(jhist);
20:> maxint=double(max(max(jhist)));
21:> jhist=jhist/maxint*255;
22:> colormap(gray)
23:> image(jhist)
24:> foo=input('Press RETURN to advance to the
joint histogram of the different images...\n');
```

Now, the same procedure is carried out using `img` and `rimg`. The result can be found in Figure 9.6.

```
25:> jhist=zeros(900,900);
26:> for i=1:380
27:> for j=1:160
```

```
28:> rho1=img(i,j)+1;
29:> rho2=rimg(i,j)+1;
30:> jhist(rho1,rho2)=jhist(rho1,rho2)+1;
31:> end
32:> end
33:> jhist=log(jhist);
34:> maxint=double(max(max(jhist)));
35:> jhist=jhist/maxint*255;
36:> colormap(gray)
37:> image(jhist)
```

Additional Tasks

MultimodalJointHistogram_9.m is a combination of JointHistogram_9.m and More2DRegistration_9.m. It displays the joint histogram for CT.jpg and T1.jpg when rotating the images against each other with an angle of $\phi \in \{-90^o \ldots 90^o\}$ with steps of 10°. Run the script and inspect the result (see also Figure 9.9). In addition, compute joint entropy according to Equation 9.4 for in the script and plot it. The output should look similar to Figure 9.11.

MultimodalJointHistogramTranslation_9.m is essentially the same script as MultimodalJointHistogram_9.m, but it does not perform a rotation but a translation in y-direction by an amount $\Delta y \in \{-100 \ldots 100\}$ pixels by a stepwidth of 10 pixels. The overlapping area of the two images is smaller in this case, and the differences in the joint histogram are more evident. Figure 9.10 shows some of the results.

9.9.3 Plotting the mutual information merit function

PlotMutualInformation2D_9.m, is directly derived from More2DRegistration_9.m and MultimodalJointHistogramTranslation_9.m. It computes the cross-section of the merit function $\mathcal{M}_{\mathrm{MI}}$ through the known optimal registration in all three dof of rigid motion in 2D; for the sake of brevity, we only take a look at the part where the $\mathcal{M}_{\mathrm{MI}}$ is computed; the remainder is basically identical to the scripts from Example 9.9.2. First, a vector mi is defined, which holds the values for the merit function; then, the histograms and joint histograms are derived:

```
...:> mi=zeros(37,1);
...
...:> jhist=zeros(256,256);
...:> histImg=zeros(256,1);
...:> histRotimg=zeros(256,1);
...:> for i=1:388
...:> for j=1:388
...:> rho1=img(i,j)+1;
...:> rho2=rotimg(i,j)+1;
...:> jhist(rho1,rho2)=jhist(rho1,rho2)+1;
...:> histImg(rho1)=histImg(rho1)+1;
...:> histRotimg(rho2)=histRotimg(rho2)+1;
...:> end
...:> end
```

The histograms are derived for each step in translation; basically speaking, this is not necessary since the histogram of the base image does not change. It is done here nevertheless to keep the code compact. Next, we compute Shannon's entropy for the histograms of img and rotimg, which are in fact the PDFs $P(I_{\text{Base}})$ and $P(I_{\text{Match}})$ from Equation 9.7. $\mathcal{M}_{\text{MI}}$ is computed and stored in the vector mi. We elegantly circumvent the problem that $\ln(0) = -\infty$ by computing H (which is named shannon... in the script) only for non-zero values:

```
...:> shannonBase=0;
...:> shannonMatch=0;
...:> shannonJoint=0;
...:> for i=1:256
...:> for j=1:256
...:> if jhist(i,j) > 0
...:> shannonJoint=shannonJoint+jhist(i,j)*
log(jhist(i,j));
...:> end
...:> end
...:> if histImg(i) > 0
...:> shannonBase=shannonBase+histImg(i)*
log(histImg(i));
...:> end
...:> if histRotimg(i) > 0
...:> shannonMatch=shannonMatch+histRotimg(i)*
log(histRotimg(i));
...:> end
...:> end
...:> shannonBase=-shannonBase;
...:> shannonMatch=-shannonMatch;
...:> shannonJoint=-shannonJoint;
...:> mi((a+19),1)=shannonBase+shannonMatch-
shannonJoint;
```

Figure 9.12 shows the output for the three movements, which all cross the optimum position in the middle.

Additional Tasks

Implement Equation 9.8 and compare the outcome.

9.9.4 Chamfer matching

For matching the thresholded gradient images of CT.jpg and T1.jpg, we need a distance transform of I_{Base}, which is computed by the script DTChamfermatch_9.m. This script is directly derived from DistanceMap_4.m from Example 5.4.11 and will therefore not be discussed here. Since the inefficient implementation of the distance transform in DistanceMap_4.m causes a long runtime, we have also stored the result as DT_ChamferMatch.jpg in the LessonData folder. The base image derived from T1.jpg and its distance transform can be found in Figure 9.15. The actual chamfer matching merit function is computed in `PlotChamferMatch2D_9.m`, which is derived from `PlotMutualInformation2D_9.m`. Again, we only comment on the changes in the script compared to its predecessor; first, we read the distance transform image `DT_ChamferMatch.jpg`, which is our base image. The image that undergoes the transformation is called `otherimg` – this is the thresholded gradient image `CT_EdgeImage.jpg`. An array for the resulting chamfer matching merit function $\mathcal{M}_{\mathrm{CM}}$ named `cf` is also allocated:

```
...:> img=double(imread('DT_ChamferMatch.jpg'));
...:> otherimg=double(imread('CT_EdgeImage.jpg'));
...:> rotimg=zeros(388,388);
...:> cf=zeros(37,1);
```

Next, the image undergoes a rotation by an angle $\phi \in \{-180^{o} \ldots 180^{o}\}$ by steps of 10°. The resulting image is `rotimg`. The merit function $\mathcal{M}_{\mathrm{CM}}$ is computed and stored in `cf`:

```
...:> sumInt=0;
...:> for i=1:388
...:> for j=1:388
...:> if rotimg(i,j)>0
...:> sumInt = sumInt+img(i,j);
...:> end
...:> end
...:> end
...:> cf((a+19),1)=-sumInt;
```

In short words, the value of the distance transform is summed up at the location of a non-zero pixel in `rotimg`, which is our I_{Match}. The same procedure is repeated for translation in x- and y-direction. The resulting values for $\mathcal{M}_{\mathrm{CM}}$ are found in Figure 9.16. It is evident that $\mathcal{M}_{\mathrm{CM}}$ will only provide useful registration results if the optimization procedure starts close to the solution since significant local minima and lacking gradients at a larger distance from the correct result will make optimization a very difficult task.

Additional Tasks

Develop a more efficient version of `DTChamfermatch_9.m` by replacing the euclidean metric by a so-called *Manhattan metric*; here, only the shortest distances in x- and y- direction are sought and plotted. Usually, a distance transform derived using the Manhattan-metric is sufficient for chamfer matching.

Improve the convergence radius of $\mathcal{M}_{\mathrm{CM}}$ by dilating `T1_EdgeImage-Dilated.jpg` to a larger extent prior to computing `DT_ChamferMatch.jpg` using `DTChamfermatch_7.m`. You may use the dilation filter of GIMP or the script from Example 6.8.6. Why should this help?

9.9.5 Optimization

First, we want to explore the properties and pitfalls of numerical optimization. For this purpose, we define two very simple one-dimensional functions that can be found in Figure 9.24. One is a sine, overlaid with a spike-type function producing a number of local minima and one global minimum. We will try to find out whether the MATLAB-implementation of the simplex algorithm is able to find the global minimum in dependence of its starting point. The other function is a simple spike, showing one global minimum but virtually no gradient – and we will observe what happens in such a case.

In the `SimpleOptimization_9.m`[7] example, we apply a simplex algorithm to two functions, defined in separate scripts `strangeSine.m` and `spike.m`.

As said before, we have abdicated from many of MATLAB's advanced functions for the sake of simplicity; we have not used vector notation whenever possible (at the cost of performance), we have not used the graphical user interface (GUI) functionality of MATLAB, and we have not used functions. The latter becomes necessary now since the MATLAB-function `fminsearch` utilizes function pointers. A MATLAB-function is defined in a separate script that is named like the function. A function that takes three input variables x, y and z and returns a vector with two components is defined by the following syntax:

```
function [resOne, resTwo] = myFunction(x,y,z)
...
resOne = ...
resTwo = ...
end
```

where one may do whatever he wants with x, y, and z. The first of the two functions to be optimized in this example is defined in the script `strangeSine.m` and is defined as follows:

```
1:> function [sSine]=strangeSine(x)
2:> sSi=sin(x)+3;
3:> if x > 10.8 && x < 11.2
4:> sSi=sSi-1;
5:> end
6:> sSine=sSi;
7:> end
```

This is a sine with a somewhat strange global minimum at $x = \frac{7}{2}\pi \simeq 10.99557$. The other function is defined in `spike.m`. It is a narrow inverse rect-function:

```
1:> function [spi]=spike(x)
2:> sp=1;
3:> if x > 4.95 && x < 5.05
4:> sp=0;
5:> end
6:> spi=sp;
7:> end
```

This function is zero for all values of the independent variable $x \in \{4.95\ldots5.05\}$, and one otherwise.

The script `SimpleOptimization_9.m` minimizes the two functions in dependence of a starting value `xs` using the function `fminsearch`. First, the function is plotted in a vector `minvect` over a range of approximately 7.2π or $1300°$. The result is found in Figure 9.24, together with a plot of `spike.m`. Next, the minimum for the function is sought using `fminsearch`. The function `strangeSine.m` is referenced using the @-operator; this is actually a pointer to the function `strangeSine.m`, so that the `fminsearch`-routine can call it

---

[7]This example requires the Optimization toolbox of MATLAB. It does not work very well with Octave, as we will see.

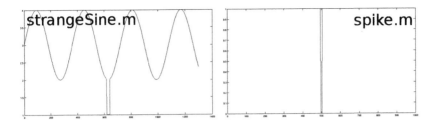

FIGURE 9.24: The functions defined in the scripts strangeSine.m and spike.m. Both show somewhat unpleasant properties; the first one features a series of local minima, the other has a gradient of zero for most of its domain.

independently. A starting point xs is provided in ascending order from 1 to 20 radians. If the starting point is close to the location of the global minimum x = 10.99557, it gives the correct solution. Otherwise, it converges to a local minimum. The found minima are plotted as a function of xs in Figure 9.25. The option '.' causes plot to show single bullets instead of a connected line.

```
 1:> mfunct=zeros(1300,1);
 2:> for xs = 1:1300
 3:> mfunct(xs) = strangeSine(xs*pi/180.0);
 4:> end
 5:> plot(mfunct)
 6:> foo = input('Press RETURN to see the minima found
 by the simplex...');
 7:> minxvect=zeros(20,1);
 8:> for xr = 1:20
 9:> minxvect(xr)=fminsearch(@strangeSine,xr)
10:> end
11:> plot(minxvect,'.')
12:> foo = input('Press RETURN to see the next
function...');
```

An interesting effect shows up when running the script using Octave instead of MAT-LAB; at least in my current version, it appears as if the implementation of the Nelder-Mead algorithm is inferior to the one in MATLAB. Octave only finds one correct minimum, very close to the solution, and fails otherwise. The output from SimpleOptimization_9.m in Octave can be found in Figure 9.26. I therefore apologize to Octave users, who may encounter severe problems with this example.

The same procedure is repeated for spike.m.

```
13:> mfunct=zeros(1000,1);
14:> for xs = 1:1000
15:> mfunct(xs) = spike(xs/100.0);
16:> end
17:> plot(mfunct)
18:> foo = input('Press RETURN to see the minima found by the simplex...');
19:> minxvect=zeros(1000,1);
20:> for xs = 1:1000
```

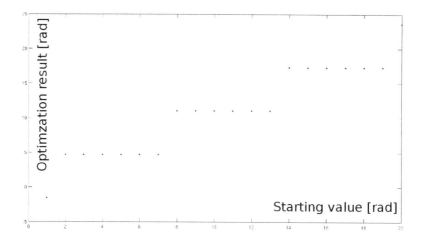

FIGURE 9.25: The optimization result of `strangeSine.m` in dependence of the starting value `xr`. Only for a limited range, the correct value (which is approximately 11) is found, otherwise the optimizer is struck in local minima.

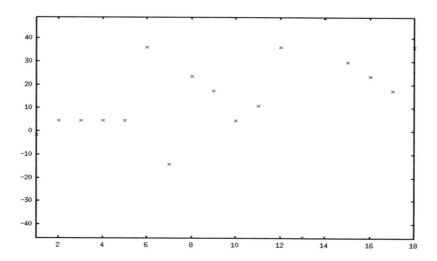

FIGURE 9.26: The result of optimizing `strangeSine.m` using the implementation of the simplex algorithm of Octave. It should look exactly like Figure 9.25. However, the internal settings of the optimizer cause a very poor convergence behavior.

```
21:> minxvect(xs)=fminsearch(@strangeSine,(xs/100));
22:> end
23:> plot(minxvect)
```

Again, the correct minimum (which is any value between 4.95 and 5.05) is only found if the starting value is close enough to the true solution of the optimization problem (see Figure 9.27).

So far, these are very simple functions; we can apply the same procedure to functions

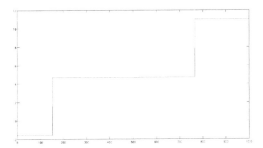

FIGURE 9.27: The result for the optimization of the inverse rect-function `spike.m`; the starting values `xs` range from 0 to 10 in steps of 0.01. Only if the starting value is close enough to the solution, the correct minimum (approximately 5) is found.

of more than one variable. This can be done for instance by modifying `PlotMutualInformation2D_9.m` from Example 9.9.3. Let us take a look at the function to be optimized; we still stick to planar 2D slices (if you have not already guessed about their nature, you may take a short look at Figure 9.23).

The merit function to be optimized takes three arguments provided in a vector `start`. This is the angle of rotation around the image center, and the translation in 2D. The script defining the merit function is `MI2D.m`. Note how the transform is carried out; first, the pixel position is shifted to the image center. Next, it is rotated, and shifted back to a corner of the image. Finally, the translation is applied. The order of transformations is TR. `MI2D.m` is not carried out by you in MATLAB – rather than that, it is called from a second script named `Optimize2D_9.m`, which will be introduced soon:

```
1:> function [mf] = MI2D(start)
2:> baseimg=imread('CT.jpg');
3:> matchimg=imread('T1.jpg');
4:> rotimg=zeros(388,388);
5:> rotmat=zeros(2,2);
6:> rotmat(1,1)=cos(start(1,1)*pi/180);
7:> rotmat(1,2)=-sin(start(1,1)*pi/180);
8:> rotmat(2,1)=sin(start(1,1)*pi/180);
9:> rotmat(2,2)=cos(start(1,1)*pi/180);
10:> invrotmat=transpose(rotmat);
11:> oldpix=zeros(2,1);
12:> newpix=zeros(2,1);
13:> shift=transpose([194,194]);
14:> tshift=transpose([(start(2,1)),(start(3,1))]);
15:> for i=1:388
16:> for j=1:388
17:> newpix(1,1)=i;
18:> newpix(2,1)=j;
19:> oldpix=round(((invrotmat*(newpix-shift))+shift)+
tshift);
20:> if (oldpix(1,1) > 0) && (oldpix(1,1) < 388) &&
(oldpix(2,1) > 0) && (oldpix(2,1) < 388)
```

```
21:> rotimg(i,j)=matchimg(oldpix(1,1),oldpix(2,1));
22:> end
23:> end
24:> end
```

The mutual information merit function is implemented in the same manner as in Example 9.9.3. An important difference lies in the fact that `fminsearch` searches for a minimum, whereas the mutual information as defined in Equation 9.7 becomes a maximum; we simply invert the merit function by multiplying it with -1.

```
25:> jhist=zeros(256,256);
26:> histImg=zeros(256,1);
27:> histRotimg=zeros(256,1);
28:> for i=1:388
29:> for j=1:388
30:> rho1=baseimg(i,j)+1;
31:> rho2=rotimg(i,j)+1;
32:> jhist(rho1,rho2)=jhist(rho1,rho2)+1;
33:> histImg(rho1)=histImg(rho1)+1;
34:> histRotimg(rho2)=histRotimg(rho2)+1;
35:> end
36:> end
37:> shannonBase=0;
38:> shannonMatch=0;
39:> shannonJoint=0;
40:> for i=1:256
41:> for j=1:256
42:> if jhist(i,j) > 0
43:> shannonJoint=shannonJoint+jhist(i,j)*
log(jhist(i,j));
44:> end
45:> end
46:> if histImg(i) > 0
47:> shannonBase=shannonBase+histImg(i)*
log(histImg(i));
48:> end
49:> if histRotimg(i) > 0
50:> shannonMatch=shannonMatch+histRotimg(i)*
log(histRotimg(i));
52:> end
53:> end
54:> shannonBase=-shannonBase;
55:> shannonMatch=-shannonMatch;
56:> shannonJoint=-shannonJoint;
57:> mf=-(shannonBase+shannonMatch-shannonJoint);
58:> end
```

The script that optimizes `MI2D.m` is comparatively simple; it is named `Optimize2D_9.m`. Again, it uses the simplex-algorithm of MATLAB. The resulting rotation matrix is displayed:

```
1:> startangle=10;
```

```
 2:> startTransX=50;
 3:> startTransY=50;
 4:> startParams=zeros(3,1);
 5:> startParams(1,1)=startangle;
 6:> startParams(2,1)=startTransX;
 7:> startParams(3,1)=startTransY;
 8:> resultParams=zeros(3,1);
 9:> resultParams=fminsearch(@MI2D,startParams)
10:> Rmat=zeros(2,2);
11:> Rmat(1,1)=cos(resultParams(1,1)*pi/180);
12:> Rmat(1,2)=-sin(resultParams(1,1)*pi/180);
13:> Rmat(2,1)=sin(resultParams(1,1)*pi/180);
14:> Rmat(2,2)=cos(resultParams(1,1)*pi/180);
15:> Rmat
```

Since the two images CT.jpg and T1.jpg are already co-registered, the correct solution is something close to $(0,0,0)^T$ for all three parameters.

Additional Tasks

Experiment with various start parameters startangle, startTransX, and startTransY.

Implement $\mathcal{M}_{CM}$ and $\mathcal{M}_{CC}$ into a variation of MI2D.m.

9.9.6 The direct linear transform

In DirectLinearTransform_9.m[8], we implement a direct linear transform as given in Equation 9.16. We do not discuss the whole script here; we will simply apply the projection operator P from Equation 9.10 with a distance $\mathbf{f}$ of fdist to a set of seven given points; these are stored as homogeneous coordinates in a matrix named sevenPoints. The projected coordinates are stored in sevenPlanarPoints. We do not apply any further transform to the points, therefore the projection operator is the only matrix we apply:

```
...:> fdist=100;
...:> projector=eye(4);
...:> projector(3,3)=0;
...:> projector(4,3)=-1/fdist;
...:> V=projector;
...:> worldPoints=zeros(4,1);
...:> imagePoints=zeros(4,1);
...:> for j=1:7
...:> for k=1:4
...:> worldPoints(k,1)=sevenPoints(k,j);
...:> end
...:> imagePoints=V*worldPoints;
...:> imagePoints=imagePoints/(imagePoints(4,1));
...:> for k=1:4
...:> sevenPlanarPoints(k,j)=imagePoints(k,1);
```

---

[8]This example requires the Optimization Toolbox of MATLAB – it does, however, work with Octave if the appropriate functions are provided in your distribution.

```
...:> end
...:> end
```

Next, we construct a matrix according to Equation 9.16; the for-loop looks a little bit complicated, but it just fills the matrix for the homogeneous equation system, which is solved by calling the MATLAB routine lsqlin; the result of this operation is fed into a 4×4 matrix calMatr, which should look like our initial transform which we used to get sevenPlanarPoints:

```
...:> smatrix=zeros(14,11);
...:> k=1;
...:> screenVector=zeros(14,1);
...:> for i=1:14
...:> if mod(i,2)  = 0
...:> smatrix(i,1)=sevenPoints(1,k);
...:> smatrix(i,2)=sevenPoints(2,k);
...:> smatrix(i,3)=sevenPoints(3,k);
...:> smatrix(i,4)=1;
...:> smatrix(i,9) =-sevenPoints(1,k)*
sevenPlanarPoints(1,k);
...:> smatrix(i,10)=-sevenPoints(2,k)*
sevenPlanarPoints(1,k);
...:> smatrix(i,11)=-sevenPoints(3,k)*
sevenPlanarPoints(1,k);
...:> screenVector(i,1)=sevenPlanarPoints(1,k);
...:> else
...:> smatrix(i,5)=sevenPoints(1,k);
...:> smatrix(i,6)=sevenPoints(2,k);
...:> smatrix(i,7)=sevenPoints(3,k);
...:> smatrix(i,8)=1;
...:> smatrix(i,9) =-sevenPoints(1,k)*
sevenPlanarPoints(2,k);
...:> smatrix(i,10)=-sevenPoints(2,k)*
sevenPlanarPoints(2,k);
...:> smatrix(i,11)=-sevenPoints(3,k)*
sevenPlanarPoints(2,k);
...:> screenVector(i,1)=sevenPlanarPoints(2,k);
...:> k=k+1;
...:> end
...:> end
...:> solution=lsqlin(smatrix,screenVector);
...:> calMatr=zeros(4,4);
...:> calMatr(1,1)=solution(1,1);
...
```

Additional Tasks

Apply an arbitrary spatial transform to sevenPoints and inspect the result.

9.9.7   Marker based registration

`MarkerRegistration_9.m` implements Eqs. 9.18–9.20. It allows you to define three points $\vec{p}_{\text{Base}_i}$ and three rotation angles `px`, `py`, `pz`, and a translation vector `trans`. The volume transform matrix V is computed, and the transformed points `Pm1`, `Pm2` and `Pm3` are computed. The whole script is a little bit lengthy, but most of it contains only trivial matrix computations; therefore we do not give it completely. Let's start with the first few lines that allow you to give some input:

```
1:> Pb1=transpose([10,0,0,1]);
2:> Pb2=transpose([10,10,0,1]);
3:> Pb3=transpose([30,30,30,1]);
4:> px=-10;
5:> py=40;
6:> pz=-30;
7:> trans=transpose([-10,20,33]);
```

Next, the point-to-point registration algorithm as given in Section 9.7.1 is implemented. We finally compute the eigenvectors of matrix Q from Equation 9.19; `V` contains the eigenvectors in columns, and `D` is a matrix with the matching eigenvalues. The index of the maximum eigenvalue is sought by computing a vector that only contains the eigenvalues. This is achieved using the `max` operator which returns a vector of the maximum element in each column. The quaternions are assigned as the elements of the eigenvector that belongs to the maximum eigenvalue. If the first scalar quaternion q_0 is negative, the whole quaternion vector is multiplied with -1 just as said in Section 7.3.4:

```
...:> ...
...:> [E,D]=eig(Q)
...:> maxvect=max(D);
...:> maxi=1;
...:> for i=1:4
...:> if maxvect(i)> maxvect(maxi)
...:> maxi=i;
...:> end
...:> end
...:> quaternions=zeros(4,1);
...:> quaternions(1,1)=E(1,maxi);
...:> quaternions(2,1)=E(2,maxi);
...:> quaternions(3,1)=E(3,maxi);
...:> quaternions(4,1)=E(4,maxi);
...:> if quaternions(1,1) < 0
...:> quaternions=-quaternions;
...:> end
```

Finally, we compute the registration matrix by using Equation 7.19 and the translation by using Equation 9.20.

Additional Tasks

Remember Equation 7.18? Can you verify this equation, which says that the quadruplet of quaternions gives the angle of rotation and the eigenvector of a rotation matrix on a simple example for V and a eigenvector-decomposition of the resulting rotation matrix?

Eqs. 9.18–9.20 give an analytical solution to the problem of minimizing Equation 9.17; one can also try to solve it numerically using `fminsearch`. Try it!

Compute the FRE for this example, and try to determine a TRE by adding points that are transformed initially, but which are not used to determine the registration matrix V.

9.10   SUMMARY AND FURTHER REFERENCES

Registration is a wide field with numerous applications; as opposed to segmentation, we have an arsenal of proved algorithms at hand that can handle most clinical problems if applied properly. We have learned about inter- and intramodal image fusion techniques, the determination of affine registration parameters from projective images, and about marker- and surface based registration. The methods presented here only provide an overview, and for performance reasons, we have only used 2D datasets. All methods do, however, directly translate to 3D. One aspect that cannot be underestimated is the proper implementation of optimization algorithms; the optimization algorithm is as important as the merit function, and its functionality can only be determined in extensive validation series on a multitude of images.

Literature

J. V. Hajnal, D. L. G. Hill, D. J. Hawkes: Medical Image Registration, CRC Press, (2001)

J. Modersitzky: Numerical Methods for Image Registration, Oxford University Press, (2004)

T. S. Yoo: Insight into Images: Principles and Practice for Segmentation, Registration, and Image Analysis, A. K. Peters, (2004)

W. H. Press, S. A. Teukolsky, W. T. Vetterling, B. P. Flannery: Numerical Recipes: The Art of Scientific Computing, Cambridge University Press (2007)

CHAPTER 10

CT Reconstruction

Michael Figl

CONTENTS

10.1	Introduction	339
10.2	Radon transform	340
	10.2.1 Attenuation	340
	10.2.2 Definition of the Radon transform in the plane	340
	10.2.3 Basic properties and examples	342
	10.2.4 MATLAB® implementation	343
10.3	Algebraic reconstruction	345
	10.3.1 A system of linear equations	345
	10.3.2 Computing the system matrix with MATLAB	346
	10.3.3 How to solve the system of equations	348
10.4	Some remarks on Fourier transform and filtering	351
10.5	Filtered backprojection	354
	10.5.1 Projection slice theorem	354
	10.5.2 Filtered backprojection algorithm	356
10.6	Practical lessons	359
	10.6.1 Simple backprojection	360
	10.6.2 Noise	362
	10.6.3 Ring artifacts	363
	10.6.4 Streak artifacts	365
	10.6.5 Backprojection revisited – cone beam CT reconstruction	365
10.7	Summary and further references	368

10.1 INTRODUCTION

In this chapter we give a rather basic introduction to CT reconstruction. The first section describes the projection process of a parallel beam CT in terms of a mathematical function, the *Radon Transform*. We then reconstruct the density distribution out of the projections first by an iterative solution of a big system of equations (algebraic reconstruction) and by filtered backprojection.

In contrast to the rest of the book some of the algorithms in this chapter are computationally expensive. Furthermore we need a procedure to rotate images in an accurate way (using, say bilinear interpolation). The code samples here use the `imrotate` function of

MATLAB's image processing toolbox.[1] A slower image rotation function called `mirotate` is provided with the lesson data on the CD accompanying the book. Sample image files in several resolutions based on the Shepp and Logan phantom are also contained on the CD. They can be used as a replacement for the toolbox function `phantom(n)` generating a Shepp and Logan phantom of size $n \times n$. To use the code examples in this chapter without the image processing toolbox, you have to replace `imrotate` by `mirotate` and `phantom(n)` by the appropriate image names.

10.2 RADON TRANSFORM

Classical x-ray imaging devices send x-ray beams through a body and display the mean density *along the entire path of the ray*. Density variations of soft tissues are rather small and are therefore difficult to see in conventional x-ray imaging. A closer look at the Beer – Lambert law, Equation 1.3, will give us an idea of what image information we really obtain by the attenuation along the entire ray. A more mathematical description of the imaging process is then given by the Radon transform.

10.2.1 Attenuation

As we know from the first chapter attenuation of an x-ray when passing a volume element with attenuation coefficient μ and length ds is described by the Beer–Lambert law:

$$I = I_0 e^{-\mu \cdot ds}, \qquad (10.1)$$

where I_0 and I are the intensities before and after the x-ray passed the volume element, respectively. If the material changes along the path of the ray, we have to iterate Equation 10.1 for different attenuation coefficients μ_i:

$$
\begin{aligned}
I &= I_0 e^{-\mu_1 \cdot ds} e^{-\mu_2 \cdot ds} \dots e^{-\mu_n \cdot ds} \\
&= I_0 e^{-\sum_i \mu_i \cdot ds} \approx I_0 e^{-\int \mu(s)\, ds}.
\end{aligned}
\qquad (10.2)
$$

The integration is done along the ray. Out of the knowledge of the x-ray intensity before and after the x-ray passed the body we can therefore compute the integral (which becomes a sum in a discrete situation) of the attenuations

$$\int \mu(s)\, ds \approx \sum \mu_i \cdot ds = \log \frac{I_0}{I}. \qquad (10.3)$$

CT-reconstruction means to derive the density (or attenuation) distribution μ out of the measured I_0/I.

10.2.2 Definition of the Radon transform in the plane

To get a simple mathematical model for a CT we confine our description to a first generation CT-scanner (see also Figs. 1.7 and 1.8) that produces parallel projections through the object at different angles. The projections are restricted to a plane, like in Figure 10.1.

A slice through the human body can be interpreted as a two-dimensional distribution of attenuation coefficients $\mu(x, y)$. In the rest of the chapter we will denote such a function by

---

[1]The image processing toolbox also provides a much more sophisticated Radon transform function `radon`, even `fanbeam` for second generation CTs, and the respective inverse transformations.

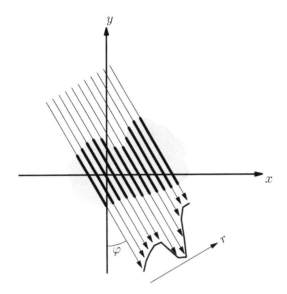

FIGURE 10.1: First generation CT scanners transmit x-rays using the same angle and different r, then change the angle. The lengths of the arrows in the figure correspond to the attenuation. The graph on the lower right therefore shows the attenuation as a function of r.

$f(x, y)$, because we will interpret it sometimes as a function, then as a density distribution, and most often as a gray scale image. The x-rays sent through the slice have different angles and different distances from the origin. For line parametrization the Hesse normal form, introduced in Section 5.3.1, is used, as can be seen in Figure 10.2.

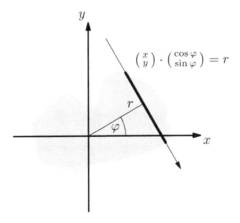

FIGURE 10.2: An x-ray beam goes through a gray body (a rather monotonic image). The normal vector of the line has an angle of φ to the x-axis and the orthogonal distance to the origin is r. The equation of the line is $x \cos \varphi + y \sin \varphi = r$.

The x-ray beam there is attenuated by every element of $f(x, y)$ along the line with the equation

$$\begin{pmatrix} x \\ y \end{pmatrix} \cdot \begin{pmatrix} \cos \varphi \\ \sin \varphi \end{pmatrix} = x \cos \varphi + y \sin \varphi = r \tag{10.4}$$

If we think of this line as the rotation of the y-axis parallel line $\begin{pmatrix} r \\ t \end{pmatrix}$, $t \in \mathbb{R}$ turned through φ degrees using a rotation matrix (see Section 7.3.1), $\begin{pmatrix} \cos\varphi & -\sin\varphi \\ \sin\varphi & \cos\varphi \end{pmatrix}$, we have a parametrization of the line by multiplying matrix and vector:

$$\begin{pmatrix} x(t) \\ y(t) \end{pmatrix} = \begin{pmatrix} \cos\varphi & -\sin\varphi \\ \sin\varphi & \cos\varphi \end{pmatrix} \begin{pmatrix} r \\ t \end{pmatrix} = \begin{pmatrix} r\cos\varphi - t\sin\varphi \\ r\sin\varphi + t\cos\varphi \end{pmatrix}, \quad t \in \mathbb{R} \tag{10.5}$$

According to Equation 10.3 the attenuation observed at the detector is given by the line integral

$$\int\limits_{\begin{pmatrix} x \\ y \end{pmatrix}\cdot\begin{pmatrix} \cos\varphi \\ \sin\varphi \end{pmatrix}=r} f(x,y)\,ds = \int\limits_{-\infty}^{\infty} f(r\cos\varphi - t\sin\varphi, r\sin\varphi + t\cos\varphi)\,dt, \tag{10.6}$$

using the parametrization from Equation 10.5. Equation 10.6 can be seen as a transformation from functions $f(x,y)$ defined in the plane $\mathbb{R}^2$ to other functions $R_f(\varphi,r)$ defined on $[0,2\pi] \times \mathbb{R}$:

$$f(x,y) \mapsto R_f(\varphi,r)$$

$$R_f(\varphi,r) := \int\limits_{\begin{pmatrix} x \\ y \end{pmatrix}\cdot\begin{pmatrix} \cos\varphi \\ \sin\varphi \end{pmatrix}=r} f(x,y)\,ds \tag{10.7}$$

This transformation is called the *Radon transform* after Austrian mathematician Johann Radon (1887–1956) who solved the problem of reconstructing the density distribution f out of the line integrals R_f in 1917.

A CT measures the attenuation along many lines of different angles and radii and reconstructs the density distribution from them. The overall attenuation in the direction of a ray is the Radon transform, Equation 10.7, but we will often think of the simple sum in Equation 10.3.

10.2.3 Basic properties and examples

Because of the linearity of integration (i.e., $\int f + \lambda g = \int f + \lambda \int g$), the Radon transform is linear as well:

$$R_{f+\lambda g} = R_f + \lambda R_g \quad \text{for } f \text{ and } g \text{ functions, and } \lambda \in \mathbb{R}. \tag{10.8}$$

Every image can be seen as a sum of images of single points in their respective gray values, we therefore take a look at the most elementary example, the Radon transformation of a point (x_0, y_0). As this would be zero everywhere, we should rather think of a small disc. Clearly the integral along lines that do not go through the point is zero and for the others it is more or less the same value, the attenuation caused by the point/disc. Now we have to find those parameters (φ, r) that define a line through (x_0, y_0). With the angle φ as the independent variable, the radial distance r is given by the line equation

$$r = x_0 \cos\varphi + y_0 \sin\varphi. \tag{10.9}$$

Therefore the Radon transform of a point/small disc is zero everywhere apart from the curve in Equation 10.9, a trigonometric curve that can be seen in Figure 10.3. The shape of this curve also motivates the name *sinogram* for the Radon transform of an image. The sinogram was already introduced in Section 1.6.

Another simple example is the transformation of a line segment. The line integral with parameters (φ_0, r_0), in the direction of the line segment, results in the sum of all points, that is the attenuations of the line segment. However all the other lines intersect just in a single point resulting in vanishing line integrals. Consequently the Radon transform is a highlighted point representing the line (φ_0, r_0) in a black image, see Figure 10.3. From this example we can also see the close relation of the Radon transform to the Hough transform for lines from Sections 5.3.1 and 5.4.10.

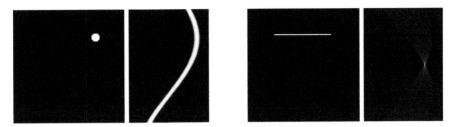

FIGURE 10.3: The image of a disc and its Radon transform with appropriate intensity windowing. The second pair of images are a line and its Radon transform. The abscissa of the Radon transform is $r = 1, \ldots, 128$, and the ordinate is $\varphi = 0, \ldots, 179$.

10.2.4 MATLAB® implementation

To implement the Radon transform using MATLAB we remember the first generation CT scanner as shown in Figure 10.1 that takes several different r steps at a fixed angle φ, and then rotates by the step $\Delta\varphi$ to the next angle.

Now we want to apply this to a discretized image given by a square MATLAB matrix. We interpret the matrix as a density distribution $f(x, y)$ with a constant density and therefore attenuation in every discretization square (i.e., matrix component, the gray value of the pixel), given by the matrix element there. Instead of $f(x, y)$ we denote the unknown gray values (density values, attenuation coefficients) simply by x_i, $i \in 1, \ldots n^2$, where n is the side length of the square image.

The Radon transform for the angle $\varphi = 0$ and the first step in r direction would be the integral along the first column, as defined in Equation 10.7, which becomes the sum of the elements in the first column, see the dashed arrow in the first column in Figure 10.4.

To simplify notation we will use the matrix R instead of the Radon transform R_f itself in the MATLAB code. As MATLAB starts matrix indices with 1 we define $R(k,1) = R_f((k-1) \cdot \Delta\varphi, (l-1) \cdot \Delta r)$, where $\Delta\varphi$ and Δr are the angle and radial step sizes. $R(1,1)$ is therefore R_f at the first angle step and the first step in r direction:

$$R(1,1) \approx x_1 + x_6 + \ldots + x_{21} \tag{10.10}$$

$R(1,2) = R_f(0, \Delta r)$, $R(1,3) = R_f(0, 2\Delta r)$, $R(1,4) = R_f(0, 3\Delta r)$ would be the sums of the elements in the second, third and fourth column, respectively.

A more general line than the one passing the first column is drawn in Figure 10.5. We can see from the figure that the beam is influenced just by a small number of squares. Of course the influence of a given square would depend on the length of the beam in the square, but for the sake of simplicity we neglect this fact. An effect similar to a ray with angle $\Delta\varphi$ could be achieved by rotating the object and having the x-ray tube and detector fixed.[2]

---

[2]This is in fact often used in Micro–CTs.

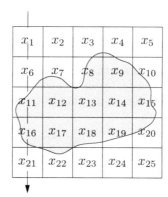

FIGURE 10.4: The area where the gray body lies is discretized, i.e., divided in 25 squares. We assume a constant density in each of the squares. The ray passing through the first column is solely attenuated by the elements $x_1, x_6, \ldots, x_{21}$. Therefore $R_f(0,0) = x_1 + x_6 + x_{11} + x_{16} + x_{21}$.

Changing the angle to $\Delta\varphi$ could be performed by rotating the image by $-\Delta\varphi$. Summing up the columns of the rotated image obtains $R_f(\Delta\varphi, 0)$, $R_f(\Delta\varphi, \Delta r)$, and so on, as can be seen in Figure 10.5.

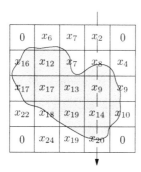 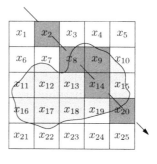

FIGURE 10.5: In the left image we see our test body rotated 45° clockwise. The matrix behind is rotated simultaneously and values outside the rotated image are set to zero. If we look at the squares in the fourth column we can see that they correspond to squares near a line with $\varphi = 45$ in the original image, as can be seen in the right image.

In the MATLAB implementation matrix rotation is done using `imrotate`. To prevent the image from changing size, we crop it to the original size. Values outside the rotated image are set to zero by default in MATLAB. The MATLAB function `sum` is then applied to the rotated image, which returns a vector containing the sums of the columns, respectively $R_f(\Delta\varphi, 0)$, $R_f(\Delta\varphi, \Delta r)$ etc.

```
1:> function R=radotra(pic,steps)
2:> R=zeros(steps,length(pic));
3:> for k=1:steps
4:>      R(k,:)= sum(imrotate(pic,...
5:>          -(k-1)*180/steps,'bilinear','crop'));
6:> end;
```

The function has two arguments: the first is the image which is assumed to be square; the second is the number of angle steps. The options in `imrotate` are the interpolation method and image cropping after rotation, as mentioned above. Output is a matrix R of size `steps*length(pic)`. Interpolation method choices are among others `'nearest'` and `'bilinear'`. Bilinear interpolation produces nicer images, whereas nearest neighbor interpolation guarantees the Radon transform to be a linear combination of the gray values x_i, $i \in 1, \ldots n^2$. In our implementation there are at most n summands for every value of the Radon transform, as they are always sums of columns of height n.

The Radon transforms of the line segment and the disc in Figure 10.3 were computed using this implementation with `'bilinear'` as interpolation method and images of the size 128×128. In Figure 10.6 the Shepp and Logan head phantom and its Radon transform (again using bilinear interpolation) can be found. The Shepp and Logan phantom can be generated using the MATLAB command `phantom(n)` with `n` indicating the side length of the square image. The phantom consists just of ellipses because the Radon transform of an ellipse can be computed analytically, see, e.g., the book by Kak and Slaney.

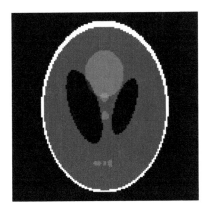 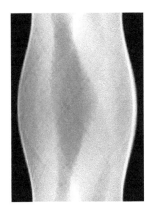

FIGURE 10.6: The Shepp and Logan head phantom and its (appropriately intensity windowed) Radon transform. The abscissa of the Radon transform is r, the ordinate is φ.

Furthermore we should keep in mind that from an algorithmic point of view there are differences between the rotation of the object and the rotation of the beam that can also lead to different results. Nevertheless the difference decreases with the granularity of the discretization.

10.3 ALGEBRAIC RECONSTRUCTION

In this section we will see how the reconstruction of the original density distribution from the Radon transform can be interpreted as the solution of a large system of linear equations, and how this system can be solved. For the EMI scanner (the first CT scanner ever built) a similar reconstruction method was used by its inventor Sir Godfrey Hounsfield. In the construction of the linear system we will use the same method we used for the implementation of the Radon transform above.

10.3.1 A system of linear equations

Let us assume a discretization of the image, resulting, like in the MATLAB implementation of the Radon transform, in a big matrix of squares as can be seen in Figure 10.4. The reconstruction task is the computation of the x_i, $i \in 1, \ldots n^2$ out of the attenuations they cause to given x-rays, i.e., out of the Radon transform.

As we have seen above nearest neighbor interpolation guarantees our MATLAB implementation of the Radon transform to be a linear combination of the gray values x_i, $i \in 1, \ldots n^2$, like in Equation 10.10 for R(1,1),R(1,2),R(1,3),...

By using 180 angle steps and n parallel beams we get $180 \times n$ linear equations in the unknowns x_i, $i \in 1, \ldots n^2$ if we construct all the rays through the image in this way. If we put the whole image as well as the Radon transform in vectors, we can reformulate this using an $(180 \times n) \times (n \times n)$ matrix S such that

$$\underbrace{\begin{pmatrix} 1 & 0 & 0 & \ldots & 1 & 0 & 0 & \ldots \\ 0 & 1 & 0 & \ldots & 0 & 1 & 0 & \ldots \\ 0 & 0 & 1 & \ldots & 0 & 0 & 1 & \ldots \\ \multicolumn{8}{c}{\cdots\cdots\cdots\cdots\cdots\cdots\cdots\cdots} \end{pmatrix}}_{S} \begin{pmatrix} x_1 \\ x_2 \\ x_3 \\ \ldots \\ x_{n^2} \end{pmatrix} = \begin{pmatrix} \texttt{R(1,1)} \\ \texttt{R(1,2)} \\ \ldots \\ \texttt{R(1,n)} \\ \texttt{R(2,1)} \\ \ldots \\ \texttt{R(180,n)} \end{pmatrix} . \tag{10.11}$$

The matrix S is called the *System Matrix* of the CT, after Russian physicist Evgeni Sistemov (1922–2003) who first introduced this notation. The system matrix completely describes the image formation process of the scanner. Please note that the matrix starts with the sums of columns, as in Equation 10.10. By the definition of matrix multiplication it is clear that the elements in a line are the coefficients of the x_i in the linear equation for R(i,j). A similar definition would have been possible even if we accounted for the way the beam crosses a square. Additional weighting factors w_{ij} would have been multiplied to the components of the matrix S. As the number of equations should be at least the number of unknowns, more angle steps have to be used for image sizes bigger than 180×180.

10.3.2 Computing the system matrix with MATLAB

The system matrix could be constructed by finding nearest neighboring squares to a line crossing the image. This could be done by basic line drawing algorithms, which can be found in introductory textbooks on computer graphics and also in Example 5.4.10. However we will do this in the same way as we implemented the Radon transform above, by rotating the image instead of the line.

For the lines of the system matrix we have to find the pixels of the image matrix that contribute to the R(1,1),R(1,2),...,R(1,n) then R(2,1),R(2,2),...,R(2,n) and R(3,1),... values of the discretized Radon transform. From Equation 10.10 we know them for the first angle, which is $\varphi = 0$. The first line of S is 1 0 0...0 1 0 0...0 1... because R(1,1)$= x_1 + x_6 + x_{11} \ldots$ the second line is 0 1 0...0,... because R(1,2)$= x_2 + x_7 + x_{12} \ldots$, the third line 0 0 1 0...0,... because R(1,3)$= x_3 + x_8 + x_{13} \ldots$, but for angles other than zero we have to use the `imrotate` function once again.

We start with an $n \times n$ test matrix T filled with the values $1, \ldots, n^2$. T is then rotated by $-\varphi$ using `imrotate` with nearest neighbor interpolation (option 'nearest'). The values in the matrix returned by `imrotate` are just the pixel numbers from the nearest squares of the rotated original matrix T or zero if the point would be outside of the original image as shown in Figure 10.7.

In the columns of the rotated matrix we find field numbers that are near to lines with angle φ through the original matrix. The situation is illustrated for a line in Figure 10.5, using x_i instead of numbers i. Summed up, the procedure to derive the system matrix consists of the following steps:

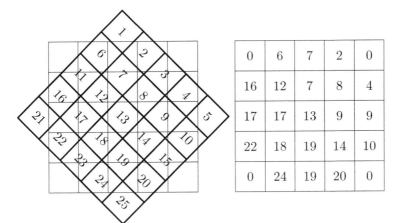

0	6	7	2	0
16	12	7	8	4
17	17	13	9	9
22	18	19	14	10
0	24	19	20	0

FIGURE 10.7: A matrix filled with the numbers $1, \ldots n^2$, rotated $45°$clockwise. In the background a pattern for the rotated matrix can be seen; the right matrix shows the pattern filled with the nearest numbers of the rotated matrix.

1. Generate a test matrix T filled with $1, \ldots n^2$.

2. Rotate it by the angle $-\varphi$ using `imrotate`.

3. The non-zero numbers in column r are the pixels of the original matrix near to a line with angle φ and distance r. The corresponding element in the appropriate line of the system matrix S has to be increased by one.

The MATLAB implementation can be found in the function `systemMatrix.m`:

```
 1:> function S=systemMatrix(side)
 2:> T = reshape(1:side^2, side,side)';
 3:> S = zeros(180*side,side^2);
 4:> for phi=0:179
 5:>   Tr=imrotate(T,-phi,'nearest','crop');
 6:>    for r=1:side      % computes R(phi,r)
 7:>     for line=1:side
 8:>      if(Tr(line,r)~=0)  S(phi*side+r,Tr(line,r))=...
 9:>         S(phi*side+r,Tr(line,r)) + 1;
10:>     end
11:>    end
12:>   end
13:> end
```

A major disadvantage of this naive approach is the memory demand for the system matrix in MATLAB. As we have seen above the matrix (for 180 angle steps) has the size $(180 \times n) \times (n \times n)$. Taking $n = 128$ (a rather small image) and a matrix of doubles (8 byte each) the matrix has about 2.8 gigabyte. From the MATLAB implementation we see that there are at most n summands (out of n^2 candidates) for every value, as they are always sums of columns of height n. Therefore only $\frac{n}{n^2} \times 100\%$ of S can be non zero. As most of the image is virtually empty (i.e., set to a gray value of 0), like areas outside the rotated image or air surrounding the object, even less values in the system matrix will be non zero. For example with $n = 64$ only about 1.3% of the values are not zero (whereas $\frac{64}{64^2} \times 100 \approx 1.56$).

In Figure 10.8 the typical structure of the matrix is shown. The image in Figure 10.8 was actually produced using $n = 16$ and only 12 different angles. About 5% of the image is not zero.

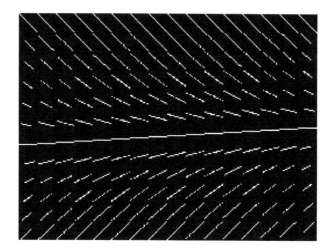

FIGURE 10.8: An example for the shape of a $(16 \times 12) \times 16^2$ system matrix produced with the MATLAB code above. Black corresponds to zero, white is 1 or 2. The dominance of the black background shows that we are dealing with a sparse matrix.

10.3.3 How to solve the system of equations

The algebraic reconstruction task consists of computing the system matrix and then solving Equation 10.11, $Sx = r$. The system matrix can be computed by knowing the geometry of the CT, like above. The variable x is a vector consisting of the image, line by line. The right hand side of the equation is the Radon transform r (denoted as a vector: $r = (\text{R(1,1)} \ \text{R(1,2)} \ \ldots)^t$). In real life r is given by measurements of the x-ray detectors in the CT, in the book we have to confine ourselves to a calculated r, for instance by our MATLAB implementation of the Radon transform applied to a phantom image.

The system matrix as defined above has $180 \times n$ lines and n^2 columns. For an image size of 32×32 we will have many more equations than unknowns, and there will most likely be no proper solution to all these equations and therefore to the system $Sx = r$. A natural generalization of a solution would be a vector x such that $\|Sx - r\|$ is minimized. Geometrically spoken we have the *image* of the matrix S, which is the set of all the Sx. This is a vector space which we will call $V = \text{im } S$ (a subspace of the codomain of S). The task is to find an element $y \in V$, that is next to a point r, where r is not necessarily in V. From Figure 10.9 we see that y is the orthogonal projection of r onto V, and therefore $r - y$ is orthogonal to V. Pythagoras' theorem shows that y is unique, see Figure 10.9. As $y \in V = \text{im } S$ we can find an x such that $y = Ax$, but x is not necessarily unique. As if S has a non–trivial kernel, i.e., if there is a vector $b \neq 0$, such that $Sb = 0$, we would have $\|S(x + b) - r\| = \|Sx - r\| = \|y - r\|$, the minimal distance, and $x + b$ would be another solution to the minimization problem. Summing up:

Linear Least Squares 1 *Given a system of equations $Sx = r$, there exists a solution x to the minimization problem*

$$\|Sx - r\| \to min.$$

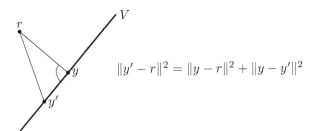

FIGURE 10.9: Given a subspace V and a vector r, then there exists a unique $y \in V$ with minimal distance to r. The vector y is the orthogonal projection of r onto the vector space V. By Pythagoras' theorem any other $y' \in V$ has a larger distance to r.

Every other solution x' can be written as

$$x' = x + w \ \text{with} \ Sw = 0.$$

Such a minimizing solution can be derived using MATLAB via so-called "matrix left division" x=S\r. The following MATLAB script pseudoinverse_10.m demonstrates the algebraic reconstruction using MATLAB's matrix left division applied to the Radon transform of a 32×32 Shepp and Logan phantom and the display of the reconstructed image.

```
1:> syma=systemMatrix(32);
2:> ph=phantom(32)*64;
3:> Rph = radotra(ph,180);
4:> Rphvec=reshape(Rph',180*32,1);
5:> x=syma\Rphvec;
6:> image(reshape(x,32,32)');
7:> colormap(gray(64));
```

The matrix inversion in line 5 produces the warning:

```
Warning: Rank deficient, rank = 1023, tol = 2.0141e-11.
```

The system matrix in this example has $180 \times 32 = 5760$ lines and $32^2 = 1024$ columns, the rank could be at most 1024. But we have learned it is just 1023, therefore the dimension of the kernel is 1. As this produces the above mentioned ambiguity, we should find a basis element in the kernel. If we recall the way the system matrix was produced from Figure 10.7, we notice that for rotation angles big enough the four corner points will be outside of the image and therefore set to zero. If we take a matrix like in Equation 10.12 this will span the kernel of S, as the sums of columns are zero even if the matrix is unchanged, e.g., for $\varphi = 0$, and other small angles. If we denote the smallest vector space containing a set A by $< A >$, we have

$$\ker S = \left\langle \begin{pmatrix} 1 & 0 & \dots & 0 & -1 \\ 0 & & \dots & & 0 \\ & & \dots & & \\ 0 & & \dots & & 0 \\ -1 & 0 & \dots & 0 & 1 \end{pmatrix} \right\rangle. \tag{10.12}$$

Luckily all interesting objects tend to lie near the center of a CT slice (at least in this chapter) we therefore don't care about the ambiguity of the result and ignore the warning.

Unfortunately this kind of matrix inversion is time consuming even on modern computers. An alternative approach would be to solve the equation $Sx = p$ iteratively. Hounsfield rediscovered a method previously published by Kaczmarz for the first CT scanner. We will illustrate this method in the following. Given is a set of n-1 dimensional (hyper)planes in n-dimensional space, we want to find their intersection point. From a starting value we project orthogonally to the first plane, from there to the second and so on.

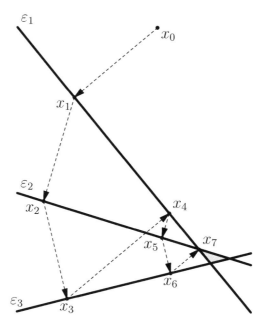

FIGURE 10.10: The Kaczmarz algorithm illustrated for three lines in the plane. The lines have no proper intersection point, nevertheless the x_i points generated by the algorithm approach the gray triangle.

This procedure is illustrated in the plane, using straight lines as (hyper)planes, in Figure 10.10. Every row of the system matrix represents a (hyper)plane in normal form, i.e., x : $(a, x) = b$, where a is a row of the matrix S and b the appropriate component of the right hand side vector r. From linear algebra we know that a is orthogonal to the plane,[3] the normalized version of a will be denoted as $n := \frac{a}{\|a\|}$. In a situation as illustrated in Figure 10.11 we want to find the projection P' of the given P.

If we take another arbitrary point Q in the plane ε we see that by definition of the inner product $(\overrightarrow{QP}, n) = (P - Q, n)$ is the length of the vector $\overrightarrow{PP'}$. Therefore $P' = P - (P - Q, n)n = P + ((Q, n) - (P, n))n$, using $(Q, n) = \frac{b}{\|a\|}$ and $n = \frac{a}{\|a\|}$, we have:

Kaczmarz Algorithm 1 (Kaczmarz S., 1937) *A set of hyperplanes in n-dimensional space is given, the planes are in normal form* $(a_k, X) = b_k$, $k = 1, \ldots m$. *The sequence*

$$x_{s+1} = x_s + \frac{b_k - (a_k, x_s)}{\|a_k\|^2} a_k$$

converges to the intersection of the planes.

In the formulation of the algorithm we omitted the interesting problem of the plane order.

---

[3]Given two points x, y in the plane we have $(a, x) = b$ and $(a, y) = b$; therefore $(a, (x - y)) = 0$ and $(x - y) \perp a$.

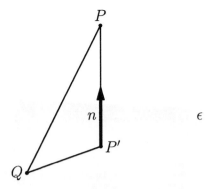

FIGURE 10.11: For Kaczmarz algorithm we have to find P' given P.

We could simply follow the line number, $k = 1, \ldots m, 1, \ldots m$, and so on; more formal $k \equiv s + 1 \mod m$, but this would hardly be optimal. Plane order influences convergence speed massively, if we think of planes ε_i being almost perpendicular or, the other extreme, nearly parallel. For instance in Figure 10.10 projecting x_0 to ε_3 instead of ε_1 would have produced an x_1 nearer to the gray triangle. In some recent papers by Herman et al. and Strohmer et al. randomly chosen planes are discussed. The MATLAB implementation of such a randomized Kaczmarz algorithm in the script `kaczmarz_randomised.m` is straightforward:

```
1:> function x = kaczmarz_randomised(A,b,cycles)
2:> [noOfLines, xlength] = size(A);
3:> x=zeros(xlength,1);     % starting value
4:> allks = ceil(noOfLines.*rand(cycles,1));
5:> for cy=1:cycles
6:>    k = allks(cy);
7:>    la = 1/norm(A(k,:))^2 * (b(k) - A(k,:)*x);
8:>    x = x + la * A(k,:)';
9:> end
```

`cycles` is the number of cycles, starting value is the vector $x = (0, 0, \ldots)$ in line three. Random line numbers are computed in the fourth line. On the CD accompanying the book a MATLAB script called `iterative_10.m` can be found that is similar to `pseudoinverse_10.m` except for line 5 which is changed to `x = kaczmarz_randomised(syma,Rphvec,10000);`.

In Figure 10.12 reconstructions for a 64×64 version of the Shepp-Logan phantom are displayed using MATLAB matrix division respectively iterative solution with 10000 steps of the randomized Kaczmarz method. Matrix inversion takes about three minutes on a 3 GHz machine whereas 10000 iterations of Kaczmarzs method are done in about three seconds.

10.4   SOME REMARKS ON FOURIER TRANSFORM AND FILTERING

The Fourier transform was introduced in Section 5.2 and used for image filtering as well as for the definition of the convolution operation. We need to know some facts about the Fourier transform and its relation to the convolution for the other reconstruction methods

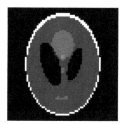 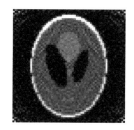 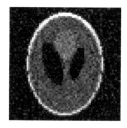

FIGURE 10.12: The left image shows the Shepp and Logan phantom of size 64×64. In the second image a reconstruction using matrix left division is shown. The image on the right was reconstructed using the 10000 steps of the randomized Kaczmarz method.

to be presented in the rest of this chapter. To make this chapter independently readable, we will repeat them in the current section.

First we recall the definition of the Fourier transform for functions of one and two variables:

$$\hat{f}(k) := \frac{1}{\sqrt{2\pi}} \int_{-\infty}^{\infty} f(x) e^{-ikx} \, dx \tag{10.13}$$

$$\hat{f}(k, s) = \frac{1}{2\pi} \int_{-\infty}^{\infty} \int_{-\infty}^{\infty} f(x, y) e^{-i\left(\frac{x}{y}\right)\cdot\left(\frac{k}{s}\right)} \, dx \, dy \tag{10.14}$$

The formulae for the inverse Fourier transform look similar, we have just to interchange f and $\hat{f}$ and to cancel the "$-$" from the exponent of the exponential function. A classical low pass filter example, cleaning a signal from high frequency noise, was given in Section 5.4.1. The Fourier transform of the disturbed function was set to zero at high frequencies and left unchanged for the others. This can also be done by a multiplication of the disturbed function's Fourier transform by a step function which is 0 at the frequencies we want to suppress, and 1 else. As this is the way the filter acts in the frequency domain we call the step function the *frequency response* of the filter. We will now write a simple MATLAB function `filt.m` that takes two arguments, the function and the frequency response of a filter. It plots the function, the absolute value of its Fourier transform, the frequency response of the filter, the product of filter and Fourier transform, and the inverse Fourier transform of this product, which is the filtered function.

```
1:> function filt(f,fi)
2:> ff=fftshift(fft(f));
3:> subplot(5,1,1);  plot(f);
4:> subplot(5,1,2);  plot(abs(ff));
5:> subplot(5,1,3);  plot(fi);
6:> subplot(5,1,4);  plot(abs(fi.*ff));
7:> subplot(5,1,5);  plot(real(ifft(...
                         ifftshift(fi.*ff))));
```

For the filtered and back-transformed signal the imaginary part is an artifact; we therefore neglect it. A sine function disturbed by a high frequency noise function can be low pass filtered as follows (to be found in the script `two_low_pass_filters_10.m`):

```
1:> x=(0:128).*2*pi/128;
```

```
2:> fi=zeros(1,129);
3:> fi(65-10:65+10)=1;
4:> filt(sin(2*x)+0.2*sin(30.*x),fi)
```

generating Figure 10.13a. In Figure 10.13b there is an example for a low pass filter with a frequency response similar to a Gaussian bell curve. The figure was produced by

```
5:> filt(sin(2*x)+0.3*sin(30.*x),...
              exp(-((x-x(65))/1.4).^2))
```

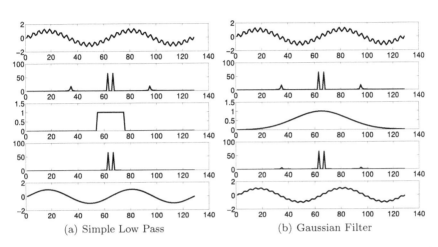

(a) Simple Low Pass   (b) Gaussian Filter

FIGURE 10.13: Filtering using the Fourier transform. The graphs in the figure show (top down) the original function, its Fourier transform, the filter's frequency response, the product of filter and the function's Fourier transform, and the filtered function transformed back to the spatial domain. In (a) a simple rectangle low pass is used, (b) uses a Gaussian filter.

As we have already seen in Section 5.2.3, linear filtering operations (convolutions) can be accomplished by a multiplication in Fourier space, Equation 10.16. A formal definition of the convolution of two functions avoiding the notation of a Fourier transform is given in Equation 10.15.

$$f \star g\,(x) := \int_{-\infty}^{\infty} f(t)g(x-t)\,dt \tag{10.15}$$

$$\widehat{f \star g} = \sqrt{2\pi}\,\hat{f}\,\hat{g} \tag{10.16}$$

For the sake of completeness we will give the simple derivation of Equation 10.16 from Equation 10.15 in the following.

$$\sqrt{2\pi}\,\widehat{f \star g} = \int_{-\infty}^{\infty}\int_{-\infty}^{\infty} f(t)g(x-t)\,dt\,e^{-ikx}\,dx = \int_{-\infty}^{\infty} f(t)\int_{-\infty}^{\infty} g(x-t)\,e^{-ikx}\,dx\,dt$$

$$= \int_{-\infty}^{\infty} f(t)\int_{-\infty}^{\infty} g(y)\,e^{-ik(y+t)}\,dy\,dt = \int_{-\infty}^{\infty} f(t)e^{-ikt}\,dt\int_{-\infty}^{\infty} g(y)\,e^{-iky}\,dy = 2\pi\hat{f}\hat{g}$$

10.5   FILTERED BACKPROJECTION

While algebraic reconstruction methods are conceptually simple they need lots of memory and processing time. A very different approach is presented in the following using the projection slice theorem, a formula that connects the Radon transform to the Fourier transform.

10.5.1   Projection slice theorem

If we want to derive a relation connecting the Radon transform to the two dimensional Fourier transform, we should find something like $\int f(x,y)d\cdots$ in Equation 10.14 as this would look similar to the Radon transform in Equation 10.6. We could start by getting rid of one of the exponentials in Equation 10.14 by setting $s = 0$:

$$\hat{f}(k,0) = \frac{1}{2\pi} \int_{-\infty}^{\infty} \int_{-\infty}^{\infty} f(x,y)e^{-\mathrm{i}xk} \, dx \, dy$$

$$= \frac{1}{2\pi} \int_{-\infty}^{\infty} \left[\int_{-\infty}^{\infty} f(x,y) \, dy \right] e^{-\mathrm{i}xk} \, dx$$

$$= \frac{1}{2\pi} \int_{-\infty}^{\infty} R_f(0,x)e^{-\mathrm{i}xk} \, dx = \frac{1}{\sqrt{2\pi}} \widehat{R_f(0,\cdot)}(k)$$

where we used the fact that $R_f(0,x) = \int_{-\infty}^{\infty} f(x,y) \, dy$, and denote $\widehat{R_f(0,\cdot)}(k)$ for its Fourier transform. Summed up we have found:

$$\hat{f}(k,0) = \frac{1}{\sqrt{2\pi}} \widehat{R_f(0,\cdot)}(k) \tag{10.17}$$

Equation 10.17 tells us that projecting (or summing up) a mass density function f along the y-axis (which is perpendicular to the x-axis) and then applying the Fourier transform is the same as taking the two dimensional Fourier transform and cutting a slice along the x-axis. The procedure is illustrated in Figure 10.14. We can also immediately verify this for the discrete Fourier transform in MATLAB, for instance in a phantom image produced by

```
1:> ff = fft2(phantom(128));
2:> r = sum(phantom(128));
3:> mean(abs(fft(r)-ff(1,:)))
ans =   9.7180e-14
```

The geometrical interpretation of Equation 10.17 motivates the name *projection slice theorem*.[4] It also holds for lines with angle φ other than zero, as we will see below.

Projection Slice Theorem 1 (Cramér, H., Wold, H., 1936) *Given a real-valued function f defined on the plane, then*

$$\hat{f}(\lambda\left(\begin{smallmatrix} \cos\varphi \\ \sin\varphi \end{smallmatrix}\right)) = \frac{1}{\sqrt{2\pi}} \widehat{R_f(\varphi,\cdot)}(\lambda) \tag{10.18}$$

---

[4]Sometimes it is called *Fourier slice theorem.*

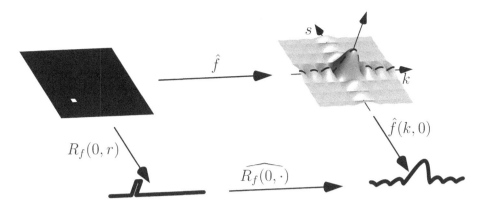

FIGURE 10.14: The projection slice theorem for $\varphi = 0$. Taking the two dimensional Fourier transform and subsequent taking the slice at $s = 0$ (which is $\varphi = 0$ if we parametrize like in Figure 10.2) is the same as taking the Radon transform at $\varphi = 0$ and the one dimensional Fourier transform of the result. The image shows absolute values of the Fourier transforms.

The proof is a straightforward integration using the substitution $\left(\begin{smallmatrix} x \\ y \end{smallmatrix}\right) = \left(\begin{smallmatrix} \cos\varphi & -\sin\varphi \\ \sin\varphi & \cos\varphi \end{smallmatrix}\right)\left(\begin{smallmatrix} a \\ b \end{smallmatrix}\right)$ and the definition of the Radon transform in Equation 10.6. We start with the two dimensional Fourier transform along the line with angle φ:

$$\hat{f}(\lambda\left(\begin{smallmatrix} \cos\varphi \\ \sin\varphi \end{smallmatrix}\right)) = \frac{1}{2\pi} \int\limits_{-\infty}^{\infty} \int\limits_{-\infty}^{\infty} f(x,y)e^{-i\lambda\left(\begin{smallmatrix} \cos\varphi \\ \sin\varphi \end{smallmatrix}\right)\cdot\left(\begin{smallmatrix} x \\ y \end{smallmatrix}\right)} dx\, dy$$

$$= \frac{1}{2\pi} \int\limits_{-\infty}^{\infty} \int\limits_{-\infty}^{\infty} f(\ldots)e^{-i\lambda\left(\begin{smallmatrix} \cos\varphi \\ \sin\varphi \end{smallmatrix}\right)\cdot\left[a\left(\begin{smallmatrix} \cos\varphi \\ \sin\varphi \end{smallmatrix}\right)+b\left(\begin{smallmatrix} -\sin\varphi \\ \cos\varphi \end{smallmatrix}\right)\right]} da\, db$$

$$= \frac{1}{2\pi} \int\limits_{-\infty}^{\infty} \left[\int\limits_{-\infty}^{\infty} f((\begin{smallmatrix} \cos\varphi & -\sin\varphi \\ \sin\varphi & \cos\varphi \end{smallmatrix})(\begin{smallmatrix} a \\ b \end{smallmatrix}))db\right] e^{-i\lambda a} da$$

$$= \frac{1}{2\pi} \int\limits_{-\infty}^{\infty} R_f(\varphi,a)e^{-i\lambda a} da = \frac{1}{\sqrt{2\pi}} \widehat{R_f(\varphi,\cdot)}(\lambda)$$

The projection slice theorem provides a new way of reconstructing the function f from its Radon transform, often called *direct Fourier method*:

1. take one dimensional Fourier transforms of the given Radon transform $R_f(\varphi,\cdot)$, for a (hopefully large) number of angles φ.

2. take the inverse two dimensional Fourier transform of the above result.

Unfortunately from Equation 10.18 above we will be able to reconstruct $\hat{f}$ only on radial lines $\lambda\left(\begin{smallmatrix} \cos\varphi \\ \sin\varphi \end{smallmatrix}\right)$, $\lambda \in \mathbb{R}$. As we have only limited data (e.g., angle steps) $\hat{f}$ will be very inaccurate far from the origin, resulting in reconstruction errors for high frequencies. We will therefore not discuss the *direct Fourier method* any further and derive another reconstruction algorithm using the projection slice theorem, the filtered backprojection algorithm.

10.5.2 Filtered backprojection algorithm

Our starting point is the inverse two dimensional Fourier transform

$$f(x,y) = \frac{1}{2\pi} \int\limits_{-\infty}^{\infty} \int\limits_{-\infty}^{\infty} \hat{f}(k,s)e^{i\left(\begin{smallmatrix} k \\ s \end{smallmatrix}\right)\cdot\left(\begin{smallmatrix} x \\ y \end{smallmatrix}\right)}\, dk\, ds \qquad (10.19)$$

From the projection slice theorem, Equation 10.18, we know $\hat{f}$ at lines through the origin $r\left(\begin{smallmatrix} \cos\varphi \\ \sin\varphi \end{smallmatrix}\right)$. We therefore transform to a polar coordinate system (r,φ):

$$\begin{pmatrix} k \\ s \end{pmatrix} = \begin{pmatrix} r\cos\varphi \\ r\sin\varphi \end{pmatrix}.$$

The determinant of the Jacobian matrix is

$$\det \frac{\partial(k,s)}{\partial(r,\varphi)} = \begin{vmatrix} \frac{\partial k}{\partial r} & \frac{\partial k}{\partial \varphi} \\ \frac{\partial s}{\partial r} & \frac{\partial s}{\partial \varphi} \end{vmatrix} = \begin{vmatrix} \cos\varphi & -r\sin\varphi \\ \sin\varphi & r\cos\varphi \end{vmatrix} = r$$

the inverse Fourier transform from 10.19 will therefore become

$$2\pi f(x,y) = \int\limits_{0}^{2\pi}\int\limits_{0}^{\infty} \hat{f}(r\left(\begin{smallmatrix}\cos\varphi\\\sin\varphi\end{smallmatrix}\right))e^{ir\left(\begin{smallmatrix}\cos\varphi\\\sin\varphi\end{smallmatrix}\right)\cdot\left(\begin{smallmatrix}x\\y\end{smallmatrix}\right)} r\, dr\, d\varphi = \int\limits_{0}^{\pi}\ldots + \int\limits_{\pi}^{2\pi}\ldots$$

$$= \int\limits_{0}^{\pi}\ldots + \int\limits_{0}^{\pi}\int\limits_{0}^{\infty} \hat{f}(r\left(\begin{smallmatrix}\cos(\varphi+\pi)\\\sin(\varphi+\pi)\end{smallmatrix}\right))e^{ir\left(\begin{smallmatrix}\cos(\varphi+\pi)\\\sin(\varphi+\pi)\end{smallmatrix}\right)\cdot\left(\begin{smallmatrix}x\\y\end{smallmatrix}\right)} r\, dr\, d\varphi$$

$$= \int\limits_{0}^{\pi}\ldots + \int\limits_{0}^{\pi}\int\limits_{0}^{\infty} \hat{f}(-r\left(\begin{smallmatrix}\cos\varphi\\\sin\varphi\end{smallmatrix}\right))e^{i(-r)\left(\begin{smallmatrix}\cos\varphi\\\sin\varphi\end{smallmatrix}\right)\cdot\left(\begin{smallmatrix}x\\y\end{smallmatrix}\right)} r\, dr\, d\varphi$$

$$= \int\limits_{0}^{\pi}\int\limits_{0}^{\infty}\ldots + \int\limits_{0}^{\pi}\int\limits_{-\infty}^{0} \hat{f}(r\left(\begin{smallmatrix}\cos\varphi\\\sin\varphi\end{smallmatrix}\right))e^{ir\left(\begin{smallmatrix}\cos\varphi\\\sin\varphi\end{smallmatrix}\right)\cdot\left(\begin{smallmatrix}x\\y\end{smallmatrix}\right)} (-r)\, dr\, d\varphi$$

$$= \int\limits_{0}^{\pi}\int\limits_{-\infty}^{\infty} \hat{f}(r\left(\begin{smallmatrix}\cos\varphi\\\sin\varphi\end{smallmatrix}\right))e^{ir\left(\begin{smallmatrix}\cos\varphi\\\sin\varphi\end{smallmatrix}\right)\cdot\left(\begin{smallmatrix}x\\y\end{smallmatrix}\right)} |r|\, dr\, d\varphi$$

we can now use the projection slice theorem 10.18 for $\hat{f}(r\left(\begin{smallmatrix}\cos\varphi\\\sin\varphi\end{smallmatrix}\right))$ in the last term obtaining the famous

Filtered Backprojection 1 (Bracewell, R.N., Riddle, A.C., 1967) *Let $f(x,y)$ describe a function from the plane to the real numbers, and $R_f(\varphi,r)$ its Radon transform, then*

$$f(x,y) = \frac{1}{2\pi} \int\limits_{0}^{\pi} \left[\frac{1}{\sqrt{2\pi}} \int\limits_{-\infty}^{\infty} \widehat{R_f(\varphi,\cdot)}(r)\, |r|\, e^{ir\left(\begin{smallmatrix}\cos\varphi\\\sin\varphi\end{smallmatrix}\right)\cdot\left(\begin{smallmatrix}x\\y\end{smallmatrix}\right)}\, dr \right]\, d\varphi \qquad (10.20)$$

Now we should justify the name of the theorem. In Equation 10.20 the expression in squared brackets is the inverse Fourier transform of the function $\widehat{R_f(\varphi,\cdot)}(r)\,|r|$ evaluated at $t := \left(\begin{smallmatrix}\cos\varphi\\\sin\varphi\end{smallmatrix}\right)\cdot\left(\begin{smallmatrix}x\\y\end{smallmatrix}\right) = x\cos\varphi + y\sin\varphi$. According to Section 10.4, this is a filtering operation of the function $R_f(\varphi, r)$ interpreted as a function of r (with a fixed angle φ) and a filter with a frequency response of $|r|$, which we will call *ramp filter* for obvious reasons (this filter is sometimes called the *Ram-Lak filter* after Ramachandran and Lakshminarayanan who re-invented the backprojection method in 1971 independent of Bracewell and Riddle). To get the value of the original function f at the point (x, y) we have to derive $R_f(\varphi, \cdot) \star \text{ramp}$ for every φ, evaluate this at $t = x \cos \varphi + y \sin \varphi$, add them up (integrate them) and then divide the result by 2π:

$$f(x, y) \approx \frac{1}{2\pi} \sum_i (R_f(\varphi_i, \cdot) \star \text{ramp})(t_i).$$

Furthermore all points on a certain line l_1 with angle φ_1 have clearly the same orthogonal distance t_1 for this line, see Figure 10.15.

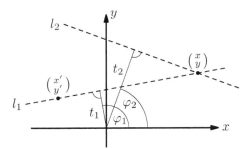

FIGURE 10.15: To compute $f(x, y)$ one has to derive the orthogonal distance $t = x \cos \varphi + y \sin \varphi$ for all lines through the point (x, y). The value $(R_f(\varphi_1, \cdot) \star \text{ramp})(t_1)$ can but used as a summand also for $f(x', y')$.

Therefore all the points on the line with parameters (φ_1, t_1) have the summand $(R_f(\varphi_1, \cdot) \star \text{ramp})(t_1)$ in common.

A geometrical method to reconstruct f would be to smear the value $(R_f(\varphi_1, \cdot) \star \text{ramp})(t)$ over the line with angle φ_1, to do this for all different radial distances t and then to proceed to φ_2 and smear $(R_f(\varphi_2, \cdot) \star \text{ramp})(t)$ over the line with angle φ_2, and all different t values, and so on. In our more discrete world of MATLAB we could do like this:

1. start with an empty matrix

2. set $k = 1$

3. for angle φ_k derive $(R_f(\varphi_k, \cdot) \star \text{ramp})(t)$, for all valid t

4. add $(R_f(\varphi_k, \cdot) \star \text{ramp})(t)$ to all the points along the lines with parameters (φ_k, t)

5. next k

As with the MATLAB implementation of the Radon transform we will rotate the matrix and add along the columns instead of adding along lines with angle φ. The MATLAB code for the filtered backprojection is the function file `fbp.m`

```
1:> function reco=fbp(r,steps,filt)
2:> reco=zeros(128);
3:> for k=1:steps
4:>    q=real(ifft(ifftshift(...
```

```
                    filt'.*fftshift(fft(r(k,:))))));
5:>    reco = reco + ones(length(q),1)*q;
6:>    reco=imrotate(reco,-180/steps,'bicubic','crop');
7:> end
8:> reco=imrotate(reco,180,'bicubic','crop');
```

The function `fbp` has three arguments, `r` is the Radon transform of a density function (or an image). The number of angle steps is given as a second argument, this is also the number of lines of `r`. As a third argument the filter function is given, this could be a simple ramp filter like in Equation 10.20 but we will also use some other filter functions in this chapter's practical lessons section, Section 10.6.

Compatible to the output of our Radon transform implementation, the lines of the matrix `r` represent the different angles, i.e., $R_f(\varphi_k, \cdot) = $ `r(k,:)`. As described above we start with an empty image `reco`, then filter the lines of `r` with the filter function in the way we have seen in Section 10.4. The filtered function is then added to the rotated `reco` image. The same function value is added to all the elements of a column. This is done by constructing a matrix that has the different $(R_f(\varphi_k, \cdot) \star \text{ramp})(t)$ values in the columns like in the example:

```
>> a=[1 2 3]; ones(2,1)*a
ans =
      1     2     3
      1     2     3
```

Our rather simple example is a slightly rotated square. We have the square rotated because in our implementation of the Radon transform (which we will use to produce `r` for lack of a real CT) the first angle is always $\varphi = 0$. This produces a discontinuous Radon transform for a square with edges parallel to the y-axis. On the other hand, projections that are not parallel to an edge of the square are continuous. Hence the filtered projection would look very different for the first and the subsequent angles. A ramp filter could be built by

```
1:> function ra=ramp(n)
2:> ra=abs((((0:127)/127-0.5)*2))';
3:> ra([1:(64-n) (65+n):128])=0;
```

The output of `ramp(n)` is a ramp of size $2 \times n$ in a vector of length 128, i.e., a ramp filter multiplied by a simple low pass filter with cut-off frequency n. In the first line of the function the absolute value is taken of a vector of size 128 with values from -1 to 1. The second line sets the elements below $64 - n$ and above $65 + n$ to zero. In Figure 10.16 we see the square, its Radon transform for $\varphi = 0$, and the Radon transform for $\varphi = 0$ after a ramp filter was applied. The latter is what we have to reproject along the lines with angle $\varphi = 0$.

If we apply `fbp` using a `ramp(64)` filter to the square and to an 128×128 Shepp and Logan phantom for three, ten, and thirty angle steps we get Figure 10.17.

The mechanism of the backprojection can be seen quite nicely by using MATLAB functions `mesh` or `surf`, as shown in Figure 10.18.

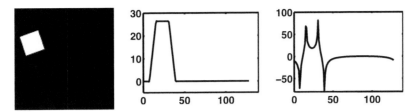

FIGURE 10.16: The left image is a slightly rotated square, the middle image shows the Radon transform for $\varphi = 0$, i.e., $R_f(0, \cdot)$. In the right image we can see this function after a ramp filter was applied.

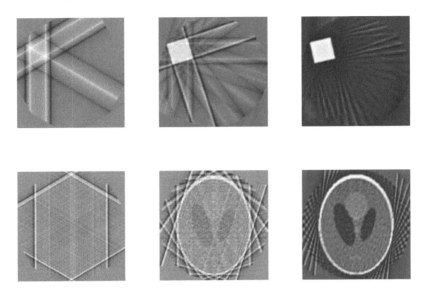

FIGURE 10.17: Filtered backprojection of the square from Figure 10.16 and a Shepp and Logan phantom with 3, 10 and 30 angle steps.

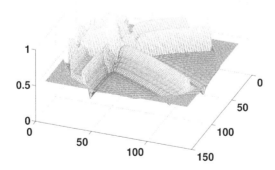

FIGURE 10.18: Mesh plot of the filtered backprojection of the square from Figure 10.16 using three angle steps.

10.6 PRACTICAL LESSONS

In this section we will apply and extend the methods we have developed above.

10.6.1 Simple backprojection

Our MATLAB implementation of the filtered backprojection accepts an argument called `filt`, a filter, which was set to `ramp(64)` because this is the filter that appears in equation 10.20. In this section we will introduce other filters and test their effect.

As the most simple filter is no filter we start with reprojection without filtering. We can simply set the filter to `ones(128,1)`, the square and the Shepp and Logan phantom would then look like in Figure 10.19. The images are massively blurred, but we can recognize the

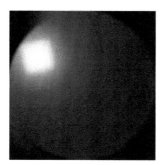 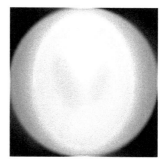

FIGURE 10.19: Simple backprojection without filtering applied to a square and the Shepp and Logan phantom. The images are windowed to see the whole range, $[1, 64] \longrightarrow [\min, \max]$.

shapes of the figures. To sharpen the image a filter amplifying the higher frequencies but retaining the lower frequencies (the structures) would be desirable. The frequency response of such a filter would increase with the frequency, in the simplest case like a straight line. On the one hand this is another motivation for our ramp filter. On the other hand we could try to do the filtering *after* an unfiltered backprojection, by a filter with a two-dimensional frequency response shaped like a cone. In the following script `conefilter_10.m` we will apply this to an 8×8 checkerboard image of size 128×128, which we create using the `repmat` function:

```
1:> tile = [zeros(16) ones(16); ones(16) zeros(16)];
2:> cb = repmat(tile,4,4);
```

Using our MATLAB functions for Radon transform and reconstruction we should not have image data outside of a circle of diameter 128, because we always crop the images after rotation. In the following lines everything out of this circle is set to zero.

```
3:> for k=1:128
4:> for j=1:128
5:>  if ((k-64.5)^2+(j-64.5)^2>64^2) cb(k,j)=0;
6:>  end
7:> end
8:> end
```

Radon transformation and unfiltered backprojection are done as expected

```
9:> rcb = radotra(cb,180);
10:> brcb = fbp(rcb,180,ones(128,1));
```

Now we need a cone to filter with. We use the MATLAB function `meshgrid` to generate the (x, y) coordinates:

```
11:> [X,Y]=meshgrid(1:128,1:128);
12:> cone=abs((X-64.5)+i*(Y-64.5));
```

Filtering is done as usual

```
13:> fbrcb=real(ifft2(ifftshift(fftshift(...
        fft2(brcb)).*cone)));
```

Figure 10.20 shows the histograms of the unfiltered backprojected checkerboard before and after a cone filter was applied. In the left histogram (before filtering) we can see a peak around 0, which is the background and a wide peak at about 10 which is the pattern. It is impossible to distinguish between black and white squares in the histogram. The second histogram (after filtering) has three sharp peaks, the first being the background, second and third are the black and white squares respectively.

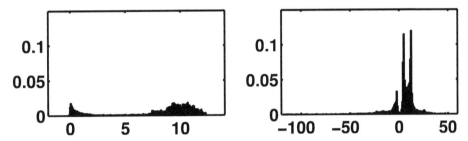

FIGURE 10.20: The histograms of the unfiltered backprojected checkerboard before and after a cone filter was applied. Axis values have been scaled appropriately.

Using the histograms we can find appropriate windows for the two images, see Figure 10.21.

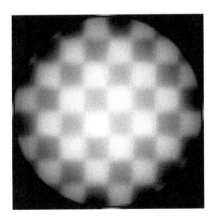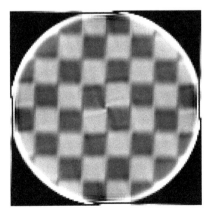

FIGURE 10.21: The unfiltered backprojection of a checkerboard, before and after application of a cone filter. Gray values were scaled appropriately.

Additional Tasks

Explain the output of `plot(sum(radotra(phantom(128),180)'))`. What happens if you change the interpolation method in `radotra`?

Change the interpolation in `radotra` to nearest neighbor and do an algebraic reconstruction using the pseudo inverse (MATLAB matrix left division) of a small test image. Explain why the result is so much better than with other interpolation methods.

10.6.2   Noise

While we have seen what the cone and the ramp filter do in Sections 10.6.1 and 10.5, we will now see the effect of filters on the image noise, especially on noise in the sinogram.

In the MATLAB script `noise_10.m` we start with the Radon transform of a phantom image and add noise.

```
1:> rim = radotra(phantom(128),180);
2:> nrim = rim + 5*rand(180,128);
```

Then we construct a Hann window (named after Julius von Hann, an Austrian meterologist)

```
3:> ha=zeros(128,1);
4:> ha(65-(1:32))= 0.5+0.5*cos(pi*(0:31)/32);
5:> ha(64+(1:32))= ha(65-(1:32));
```

Finally we reconstruct the image using the Hann window (multiplied with the ramp filter) and, for comparison, using the original ramp filter, the images are displayed in Figure 10.22.

```
6:> fbnrim = fbp(nrim,180,ha.*ramp(64));
7:> bnrim = fbp(nrim,180,ramp(64));
```

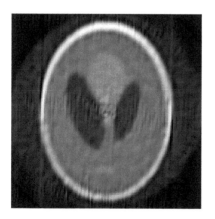 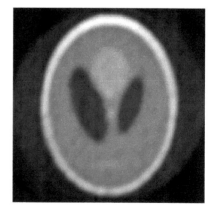

FIGURE 10.22: Backprojection of a disturbed Radon transform using the ramp filter (left image) and a ramp filter multiplied with a Hann window (right image).

Additional Task

To test different filters and their response to noise, write a MATLAB script with an output like in Figure 10.16. The script should take the Radon transform of an image (just for $\varphi = 0$, to make it faster), disturb it with noise of variable level, and then filter the disturbed function with a variable filter. Test the script with ramp and Hann filters.

10.6.3   Ring artifacts

In Section 1.5.3 we discussed different types of images artifacts for computed tomography. We will now simulate ring and streak artifacts with our MATLAB implementation of the Radon transform and reconstruction methods.

Modern CTs (second generation and newer, see Figure 1.8) have more than one detector element, and measure the attenuations of more than one beam at a time. If one of these detectors would be out of calibration, it could produce a signal lower than the others by a factor of λ.

Using the simple parallel beam CT from Figure 10.1 this can be simulated by scaling one of the columns of the (image) matrix produced by the Radon transform (we will denote the matrix by R). In Section 10.2.3 we have seen that the Radon transform of a line with equation $x \cos \varphi + y \cos \varphi = r$ is a point with coordinates (φ, r). A column in R consists of points with different φ but the same r. Changing a column of R therefore changes the original image along lines with different slope but the same normal distance r to the origin. The most prominent change will be the envelope of these lines, which is a circle of radius r and center at the origin.

In order to see this using our MATLAB code, we have to write 360° versions of radotra and fbp otherwise we would only see semi-circles. We will call them radotra360 and fbp360 and leave the implementation as an exercise to the reader. In the script ring_artefact_10.m we start with a test image consisting of random numbers:

```
1:> ti=rand(128);
2:> for k=1:128
3:>   for j=1:128
4:>     if ((k-64.5)^2+(j-64.5)^2>64^2) ti(k,j)=0;
5:>     end
6:>   end
7:> end
```

In lines 2 to 7 the image is confined to a disc. A homogeneity phantom (for instance a cylinder filled with water) would give a similar image.

```
 8:> Rti = radotra360(ti,180);
 9:> Rti(:,40)= Rti(:,40)*0.8;
10:> fbpRti=fbp360(Rti,180,ramp(32));
```

In line 10 we chose a ramp filter of length 32 because we otherwise would have artifacts due to high frequencies. Figure 10.23 shows the image fbpRti. The ring artefact caused by multiplying a column of the Radon transform by 0.8 is clearly visible.

Finding ring artifacts in an image can be of interest, for instance in quality assurance of tomography systems. Like above we think of noise (equally distributed in $[-1, 1]$) in a disc shape centered of an image. If we sum up all numbers on a circle of radius r this should

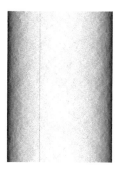 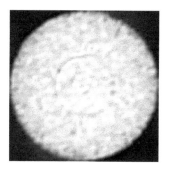

FIGURE 10.23: On the left the Radon transform of a random image is shown; column 40 is scaled by 0.8 (the small dark line). The right image shows the backprojection of this violated Radon image. A ring artifact can be seen.

vanish. Should the color values on a circle have an offset, we can expect to find them in this way (see additional tasks).

Additional Tasks

Create an image containing a disc with random numbers. The random numbers should be equally distributed in $[-1, 1]$. Then add a ring to the image at a certain radius (compute the radius like in line 4 of the code above, and round to the next integer). Summing up the gray values for every circle is the last step. The image and the sums versus radii should look like in Figure 10.24.

Apply the abovementioned method to the backprojected image `fbpRti`. The values on a circle will not cancel out, nevertheless the distribution of the values should be the same everywhere. Therefore the sums divided by the length of the circumference of the circle should always have the same value. It was column 40 of the Radon transform that we scaled, what radius do you expect?

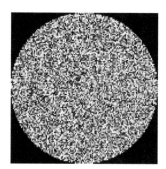 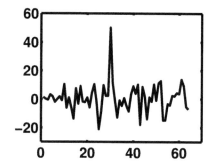

FIGURE 10.24: On the left an image filled with random numbers and an invisible circle with offset 0.2 is shown. The right image shows the sums versus the different radii. What is the radius of the circle?

10.6.4 Streak artifacts

Streak artifacts can be caused by the presence of high density metallic objects in the scan region, for instance gold fillings but also bone. As the main cause of such artifacts are metallic objects, they are often called *metal artifacts*. We will simulate the effect by adding two small areas of high density to a phantom image, the script is called `streak_artefact_10.m`:

```
1:> im=phantom(128);
2:> im(95:100,40:45)=60;
3:> im(95:100,80:85)=60;
4:> Rim = radotra(im,180);
```

These regions should act as a barrier for x-rays, we therefore use a maximum value in the Radon transform. This cup value will be the maximum of the Radon transform of the same phantom image without the two regions.

```
 5:> M=max(reshape(radotra(phantom(128),180),128*180,1))
 6:> for k=1:180
 7:>   for l=1:128
 8:>     if (Rim(k,l)>M)  Rim(k,l)=M;
 9:>     end
10:>   end
11:> end
```

A standard ramp filter is used for reconstruction.

```
12:> fbpRim = fbp(Rim,steps,ramp(32));
```

The image with streak artifacts should look like in Figure 10.25.

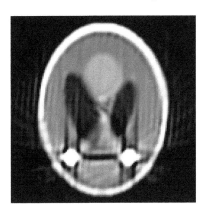

FIGURE 10.25: This image shows streak artifacts caused by two regions of high attenuation.

10.6.5 Backprojection revisited – cone beam CT reconstruction

Equation 10.20 can be used to reconstruct from more general projection geometries. Fan beam projections as they are used in a third generation CT can be *resorted* into corresponding parallel beams followed by parallel beam reconstruction.

Alternatively an algorithm for reconstruction of fan beam projections can be found by a coordinate transformation in Equation 10.20 based on the geometry of the fan beam.

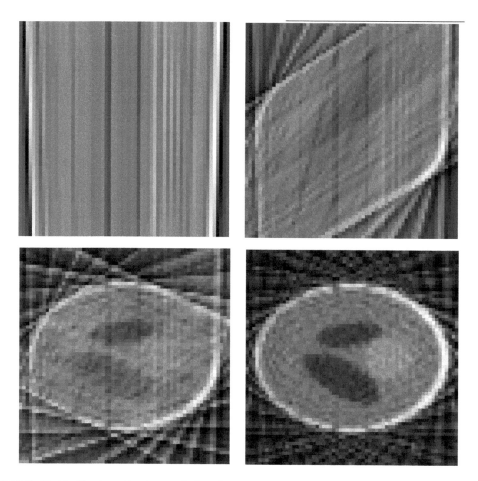

FIGURE 10.26: Backprojections of the three-dimensional Shepp-Logan phantom used in Example 10.6.5 from one, five, nine, and 25 projections.

The cone beam reconstruction by Feldkamp et al. is based on fan beam reconstructions for equidistant beams. In the following code we follow strictly the notation in Kak & Slaney, Chapter 3.6, *Three-Dimensional Reconstructions*. In the files on the CD containing this code every step is commented linking to the appropriate equation of the book. A three dimensional version of the Shepp and Logan phantom is provided in the file `SheppLogan3D_64.mat`. The dimensions of the phantom are $64 \times 64 \times 64$ pixels.

A cone beam projection function is given in the file `projection(vol, angle_rad)`. Its first argument is the volume, the second argument is the direction of the projection. The different directions are simulated by rotating the volume slice by slice around the $z-$axis using the `volrotate(vol,deg)` function. Octave users may need to replace the `imrotate` function with the `mirotate` function provided.

```
1:> function rvol = volrotate(vol, deg)
2:> [xl yl zl] = size(vol);
3:> rvol = zeros(xl,yl,zl);
4:> for k = 1:zl
5:> rvol(:,:,k) = imrotate(vol(:,:,k),deg,...
```

```
'bilinear','crop');
6:> end
```

Certain parameters defining the projection geometry are hard coded in the functions: DDE denotes the distance from the rotation axis (the origin) to the detector, DSO is the distance to the x-ray source. The projection will be returned in img. The size of the detector is 120×140 pixels. we have to find the phantom points on every ray from the x-ray source to a detector pixel (u,v). This is done stepwise in y-direction. From Figure 10.27 we derive $pu = \frac{u(DSO-y(k))}{DSO+DDE}$, the $+63/2+1$ transforms to row and column numbers in the phantom. X-rays penetrating the phantom cover different distances therein. The scaling step in line

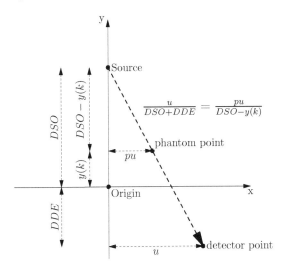

FIGURE 10.27: To find the phantom point that is projected to a certain detector point similar triangles are used.

15 takes account of this difference (see also Figure 10.27 for this factor).

```
1:>  function img = projection(vol,angle_rad)
2:> DDE=500;
3:> DSO=1000;
4:> img = zeros(120,140);
5:> [u,v] = meshgrid((0:139)-139/2,(0:119)-119/2);
6:> volr = volrotate(vol,angle_rad*180/pi);
7:> y = (0:63)-63/2;
8:> k_slice=zeros(64);
9:> for k = 1:64
10:> pu = u*(DSO-y(k))/(DSO+DDE) + 63/2 + 1;
11:> pv = v*(DSO-y(k))/(DSO+DDE) + 63/2 + 1;
12:> k_slice(:) =volr(:,k,:);
13:> img=img+interp2(k_slice,pu,pv,'linear',0);
14:> end
15:> img=img.*sqrt((DSO+DDE)^2+u.^2+v.^2)./...
(DSO+DDE);
```

The backprojection is implemented as in Kak and Slaney, 1988. The argument R is the collection of projections, its size is $64 \times 64 \times$ number of angles. vol is an empty structure for the reconstructed volume. Reconstruction is done for x, y planes at once, the plane coordinates are defined in line 6. In line 8 the detector coordinates are normalized by the factor $\frac{DSO}{DSO+DDE}$ because the algorithm in Kak & Slaney assumes an imaginary detector placed in the origin. The angle steps are assumed to be equal. A simple ramp is used as filter, in contrast to the previously used notation this ramp has the high frequency answer in the middle. The loop from line 11 to 19 is the integral over $d\beta$, line 12 inverts the step in line 15 of projection. Line 13 filters the projection using the ramp filter. In lines 14 and 15 the coordinates of the rotated points are computed. The method covers a x, y plane at once and loops over z in the loop from line 16 to 18. Line 17 is a weighted backprojection.

```
1:> function vol = fdk_backprojection(R)
2:> num_proj=length(R(1,1,:));
3:> vol=zeros(64,64,64);
4:> DDE=500;
5:> DSO=1000;
6:> [x, y]=meshgrid((0:63)-63/2,(0:63)-63/2);
7:> z=(0:63)-63/2;
8:> [p, zeta]=meshgrid(((0:119)-119/2)*DSO/...
(DSO+DDE),((0:139)-139/2)*DSO/(DSO+DDE));
9:> beta=(0:360/num_proj:359)/180*pi;
10:> filter=[1:60 60:-1:1]/60;
11:> for i=1:num_proj
12:> R_dash=R(:,:,i).*(DSO./sqrt(DSO^2+p.^2+zeta.^2))';
13:> Q = real(ifft(fft(R_dash).*(filter'*...
ones(1,140))));
14:> t=x.*cos(beta(i))+y.*sin(beta(i));
15:> s=-x.*sin(beta(i))+y.*cos(beta(i));
16:> for k=1:64
17:> vol(:,:,k)=vol(:,:,k)+ interp2(p,zeta,Q',...
t.*DSO./(DSO-s),z(k).*DSO./(DSO-s),...
'linear',0).*DSO^2./(DSO-s).^2;
18:> end
19:> end
20:> end
```

To run the Feldkamp example one has to load the phantom, to compute the projections and to put them in a three-dimensional array. Then the reprojection function can be called and the reconstructed volume may be displayed. A script for this is also provided on the CD.

10.7 SUMMARY AND FURTHER REFERENCES

CT reconstruction methods are an active field of research since the construction of the first CT by Godfrey Hounsfield. While Hounsfield used algebraic methods it soon became clear that filtered backprojection, invented by Bracewell and Riddle and independently later by Ramachandran and Lakshminarayanan, was superior. The invention of the spiral CT in 1989, and the multislice CT at about 2000 motivated research for three-dimensional reconstruction methods.

A very clear and simple introduction to pre–spiral CT can be found in the book of Kak and Slaney. Buzug's book is almost as easy to read, but presents also the latest technology. Another modern introduction is the book by GE Healthcare scientist Jiang Hsieh.

Algebraic reconstruction methods are discussed in the article by Herman and the literature cited therein. The book of Natterer and also the proceedings edited by Natterer and Herman where we cited an article by Hejtmanek as an example, present more mathematical treatments.

Literature

J.F. Barrett, N. Keat: Artifacts in CT: Recognition and avoidance, RadioGraphics 24(6), 1679-1691, 2004

R.N. Bracewell, A.C. Riddle: Inversion of fan–beam scans in radio astronomy, Astrophysical Journal, vol. 150, 427-434, 1967

R.A. Brooks, G. diChiro: Principles of computer assisted tomography (CAT) in radiographic and radioisotopic imaging, Phys Med Biol, 21(5), pp 689-732, 1976

T. Buzug: Computed Tomography, Springer, 2008

H. Cramér, H. Wold: *Some theorems on distribution functions*, J. London Math. Soc, 11(2). S. 290-294, 1936

J. Hejtmanek: The problem of reconstruction objects from projections as an inverse problem in scattering theory of the linear transport operator, in: Herman, Natterer, *Mathematical Aspects of Computed Tomography*, Springer LNMI 8, 28-35, 1981

G. Herman: Algebraic reconstruction techniques can be made computationally efficient, IEEE Trans Med Imag, 12(3), 600-609, 1993

G. N. Hounsfield: Computerized transverse axial scanning (tomography): Part I. Description of the system, Br J Radiol, 46(552):1016-1022, 1973

J. Hsieh: Computed Tomography: Principles, Design, Artifacts, and Recent Advances, Wiley, 2009

S. Kaczmarz: Angenäherte Auflösung von Systemen linearer Gleichungen, Bull. Internat. Acad. Polon. Sci. Lettres A, pages 335-357, 1937.

A.C. Kak, M. Slaney: Principles of computerized tomographic imaging, IEEE Press 1988

F. Natterer: The mathematics of computerized tomography, Wiley, New York, 1986

J. Radon: Über die Bestimmung von Funktionen durch ihre Integralwerte längs gewisser Mannigfaltigkeiten., Berichte über die Verhandlungen der königlich sächsischen Gesellschaft der Wissenschaften, Vol. 69, 262-277, 1917

G. N. Ramachandran, A. V. Lakshminarayanan: Three-dimensional reconstruction from radiographs and electron micrographs: Application of convolutions instead of Fourier transforms, PNAS 68:2236-2240, 1971

T. Strohmer, R. Vershynin: A randomized Kaczmarz algorithm with exponential convergence, J. Fourier Anal. Appl. 15(1), 262-278, 2009

L. A.. Feldkamp. L. C. Davis, J. W. Kress: Practical cone-beam algorithm, J. Opt. Soc. Am. A 1(6), 612-619, 1984.

CHAPTER 11

A Tutorial on Image-Guided Therapy

Özgür Güler and Ziv Yaniv

CONTENTS

11.1	A hands-on approach to camera calibration and image-guided therapy	371
11.2	Transformations	372
	11.2.1 Central projection	372
	11.2.2 Homography	373
11.3	Camera calibration	375
	11.3.1 Pinhole camera model	375
	11.3.2 Camera calibration with 3D object	376
	11.3.3 Camera calibration with 2D object	377
11.4	Image-Guided therapy, introduction	379
11.5	Image-Guided therapy, navigation system	381
	11.5.1 Setup and calibration	381
	11.5.2 Procedure planning	382
	11.5.3 Navigation	384
11.6	Image-Guided therapy, theory in practice	384
	11.6.1 Camera calibration	384
	11.6.2 Tracking accuracy	385
	11.6.3 Human computer interaction	385
	11.6.4 Dynamic reference frame	386
	11.6.5 Paired-Point rigid registration	387
	11.6.6 Iterative-closest point	389
11.7	Summary and further references	390

11.1 A HANDS-ON APPROACH TO CAMERA CALIBRATION AND IMAGE-GUIDED THERAPY

In this chapter, we refine some of the basic methods of camera calibration as introduced in Chapter 9. We then make ends meet – we introduce you to a domain which utilizes the technologies described throughout the book, Image-Guided Interventions (IGI) (T. Peters

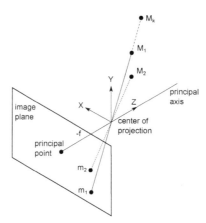

FIGURE 11.1: The pinhole camera, *camera obscura*, device creates images by projecting the light entering through a small hole at the front of the device onto a plane at the back which is at a distance f from it. Images appear upside down.

and K. Cleary 2008)[1]. As our goal is to provide you with both theoretical understanding and applied experience we provide a toy navigation system at minimal cost. The navigation system software is found on the companion website at www.crcpress.com. In addition you will need LEGO[TM] bricks to construct your "patient" and a webcam, which serves as a tracking system.

11.2 TRANSFORMATIONS

11.2.1 Central projection

Our eye, an off-the-shelf camera and an x-ray imaging device, all have one thing in common, these devices create an image by sensing the light or x-rays that pass through a single point. The transformation mapping all points along rays through a common point, namely the eye point, is called a *central projection*. Figure 11.1 illustrates this, where all world points M_i are transformed to image points m_i via rays that pass through the center of projection. The axis perpendicular to the image plane is called the principal axis or principal ray, and the point where it intersects with the image plane is the principal point. Setting the center of projection as the origin of the vector space $\mathbb{R}^3$ we see that the image plane is a projective space, $\mathbb{P}^2$, as it is comprised of the set of lines in $\mathbb{R}^3$ that pass through the origin, the definition of a projective space.

An image plane or focal plane can be defined by fixing one coordinate, e.g., $z = -f$. This represents a plane parallel to the XY-plane with an offset of f in negative z direction as illustrated in Figure 11.1. The central projection takes a point $M = (X, Y, Z)^T$ and maps it to the image plane, so that point M in space, camera center C, and the image point are collinear. Using this *camera obscura* model we obtain an image which is upside down. To obtain an image that is right side up, we model the device as if the image plane is in front of the center of projection. This is mathematically equivalent to the physical setup, as

---

[1]Synonyms for image-guided interventions that often appear in the literature include among others: computer-assisted surgery, computer-integrated surgery, computer-aided intervention, image-guided surgery, and image-guided therapy.

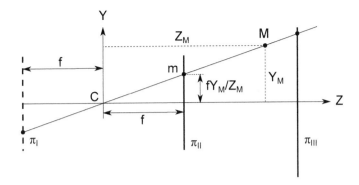

FIGURE 11.2: Mapping of world coordinates to image coordinates via similar triangles.

illustrated in Figure 11.2, with π_I corresponding to the physical setup and π_{II} corresponding to this modification. The mapping from world coordinates to image coordinates is derived using similar triangles. That is, point $(X, Y, Z)^T$ is mapped to the point $(fX/Z, fY/Z, f)^T$ on the image plane. The image of a point $M \in \mathbb{R}^3$ on the image plane has the coordinates:

$$x = f\frac{X}{Z}, \ y = f\frac{Y}{Z} \tag{11.1}$$

with x and y the 2D image coordinates.

Consider the points M_1 and M_k in Figure 11.1. Since M_k lies on the same line as M_1 which originates from the origin, the point M_k can be defined as sM_1, with s an appropriate scale factor. Note that the image of both points M_1 and M_k is m_1; moreover for all s the image is the same. Therefore $s(X_1, Y_1, Z_1)$ with the property that the projection is m_1 builds an equivalence relation. We can add an extra coordinate to account for s. Then (sX_1, sY_1, sZ_1, s) is the homogeneous representation of the point (X_1, Y_1, Z_1). Furthermore, the central projection, can be expressed as a linear mapping using homogeneous coordinates. We can thus express the central projection transformation in matrix form:

$$\begin{bmatrix} x \\ y \\ 1 \end{bmatrix} = s \begin{bmatrix} f & 0 & 0 & 0 \\ 0 & f & 0 & 0 \\ 0 & 0 & 1 & 0 \end{bmatrix} \begin{bmatrix} X \\ Y \\ Z \\ 1 \end{bmatrix}. \tag{11.2}$$

11.2.2 Homography

A homography is an invertible mapping h from a projective space, $\mathbb{P}^n$, to itself such that three points x_1, x_2, x_3 lie on the same line if and only if $h(x_1)$, $h(x_2)$, $h(x_3)$ are on the same line. That is, this transformation maps straight lines to straight lines.

A central projection relating points on a plane in $\mathbb{R}^3$ to image points is a planar homography as it maps points on the world plane $\mathbb{P}^2$ to points on the image plane, also $\mathbb{P}^2$ as shown in Figure 11.3.

A point on the world plane is defined in a local coordinate system as $[p, q, 0]$. Using homogenous coordinates this point is mapped to the image plane as follows:

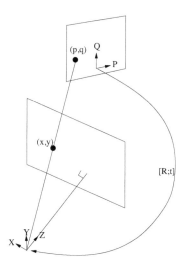

FIGURE 11.3: Central projection maps a plane in the world to the image plane. This mapping defines a homography between the two planes.

$$
\begin{bmatrix} x \\ y \\ 1 \end{bmatrix} = s \begin{bmatrix} f & 0 & 0 & 0 \\ 0 & f & 0 & 0 \\ 0 & 0 & 1 & 0 \end{bmatrix} \begin{bmatrix} r_{11} & r_{12} & r_{13} & t_x \\ r_{21} & r_{22} & r_{23} & t_y \\ r_{31} & r_{32} & r_{33} & t_z \\ 0 & 0 & 0 & 1 \end{bmatrix} \begin{bmatrix} p \\ q \\ 0 \\ 1 \end{bmatrix} \tag{11.3}
$$

where the plane's local coordinate system is related to the central projection coordinate system via a rigid transformation. After some algebra we see that the point on the world plane is related to the point on the image plane via a 3x3 invertible transformation:

$$
\begin{bmatrix} x \\ y \\ 1 \end{bmatrix} = s \begin{bmatrix} fr_{11} & fr_{12} & ft_x \\ fr_{21} & fr_{22} & ft_y \\ r_{31} & r_{32} & t_z \end{bmatrix} \begin{bmatrix} p \\ q \\ 1 \end{bmatrix} = H \begin{bmatrix} p \\ q \\ 1 \end{bmatrix} \tag{11.4}
$$

Note that this transformation has only eight degrees of freedom as it is defined up to scale.

This relationship between image points and points on the world plane can be expressed in terms of the vector cross product as $[x_i, y_i, 1] \times H[p_i, q_i, 1] = 0$ which leads to an analytic estimate for H. Defining $M_i = [p_i, q_i, 1]$, for each point pair we have:

$$
\begin{bmatrix} 0^T & -M_i^T & y_i M_i^T \\ M_i^T & 0^T & -x_i M_i^T \\ -y_i M_i^T & x_i M_i^T & 0^T \end{bmatrix} \begin{bmatrix} h^1 \\ h^2 \\ h^3 \end{bmatrix} = 0 \tag{11.5}
$$

with h^i the i-th row of H.

The three equations are linearly dependent, thus each pair of points contributes two linearly independent equations:

$$
\begin{bmatrix} 0^T & -M_i^T & y_i M_i^T \\ M_i^T & 0^T & -x_i M_i^T \end{bmatrix} \begin{bmatrix} h^1 \\ h^2 \\ h^3 \end{bmatrix} = 0 \tag{11.6}
$$

With four points in general configuration, no three are collinear, we obtain an exact solution. Remember that H is defined up to scale so we can either arbitrarily set one entry $H_{ij} = 1$, or solve the system of equations subject to the constraint that the solution's vector norm is one.

In Section 11.3.3 we describe a refined camera calibration method similar to the direct linear transform from Section 9.6 which takes advantage of the fact that the mapping between points on a world plane and points on the image plane is a homography.

11.3 CAMERA CALIBRATION

A camera takes an image of the world, whereby it projects the real world scene onto an image plane. This mapping follows certain rules, such as straight lines remain straight in the image. Although parallel lines in the world will often intersect in the image. Modeling this mapping from world to image, taking the above observations and constraints into account, opens the door to interesting applications. Camera calibration is the task of estimating the parameters for a mathematical model, which describes the transformation between an object in 3D space and its projection to a 2D image.

The initial use of camera calibration was in photogrammetry, where it was used to extract metric information from images, making measurements from photographs. With known camera parameters and multiple views the motion of the camera or the motion of objects in the scene can be estimated. Additional applications include estimation of object shape using stereo images or series of images which show the same scene from different views. In the field of computer vision camera calibration is used to augment real video scenes with 3D graphics, also known as augmented reality. Similarly, in image-guided therapy (Section 7.5) structures of interest such as vessels, nerves, or a tumor can be superimposed onto x-ray images or endoscopic video. In addition, knowledge of the projection properties of x-ray devices is used in 2D/3D registration (see Section 9.7.2).

The following model is principally designed for standard off-the-shelf cameras, head-mounted displays or endoscopes, but it is also applicable to other devices where you have a point source, such as X-ray images.

11.3.1 Pinhole camera model

We use the *pinhole camera model* to describe the relation between the physical world scene and its projection onto an image plane. This model is based on the central projection transformation described above.

In general the pixel coordinates of a digital image are based on a different coordinate system than that of the central projection model, such, that the image origin is not the principal point but the top left corner of the image with +x-axis going from left to right and +y-axis going from top to bottom. Taking this into account, the more general mapping is expressed as follows: $(X, Y, Z)^T \mapsto (fX/Z + p_x, fY/Z + p_y)^T$ where $(p_x, p_y)^T$ are the coordinates of the principal point. In homogeneous representation we now have:

$$K = \begin{bmatrix} f & 0 & p_x \\ 0 & f & p_y \\ 0 & 0 & 1 \end{bmatrix} \tag{11.7}$$

we can write,

$$m = K[I|0]M_{cam} \tag{11.8}$$

The homogeneous 4-vector M_{cam} is expressed with respect to the camera coordinate

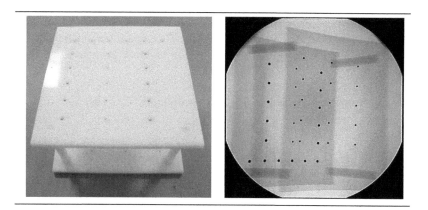

FIGURE 11.4: A custom calibration object constructed with high precision and its x-ray image.

frame. The matrix K represents the intrinsic calibration parameters of the camera. The intrinsic parameters are geometric properties of the device. There are cases when the pixels of our imaging device are not square. If we want to express image coordinates in pixel coordinates, we have to take this into account introducing scale factors m_x and m_y. Finally for a more general form of our camera we cannot assume that the coordinate axis are perpendicular as they may be skewed. We thus introduce a skew factor s resulting in the following camera model:

$$K = \begin{bmatrix} \alpha_x & s & x_0 \\ 0 & \alpha_y & y_0 \\ 0 & 0 & 1 \end{bmatrix} \qquad (11.9)$$

with $\alpha_x = fm_x$ and $\alpha_y = fm_y$ representing the focal length in pixel dimensions in x and y direction, respectively. Here m_x and m_y are pixel per unit distances in x and y directions. Likewise, the principal point in terms of pixel coordinates is $\tilde{m}_0 = (x_0, y_0)$ with $x_0 = m_x p_x$ and $y_0 = m_y p_y$.

In general, points in physical space are expressed in a coordinate system which differs from the camera's coordinate system, and thus we need to transform them to the camera coordinate system prior to applying the projection matrix. This leads to the formula:

$$m = K[R|t]M = PM \qquad (11.10)$$

with P a 3×4 homogeneous camera projection matrix or *finite projective camera*.

Camera calibration is performed by combining knowledge about the scene the camera is observing and measurements acquired on the image. Depending on the structure of the observed scene, calibration methods can be classified as 3D, 2D, 1D or self calibration. We next describe camera calibration methods using 3D and 2D calibration objects.

11.3.2 Camera calibration with 3D object

Camera calibration with 3D calibration objects require construction of objects whose geometry is known with high precision. Often these are constructed from two or three planes with checker board pattern orthogonal to each other. For x-ray calibration there are other calibration object structures that enable accurate identification of image points corresponding to unique object points, such as that shown in Figure 11.4. The advantage of using a 3D object for calibration is that only one image of the calibration object is sufficient to perform camera calibration.

Recall Equation 11.10. Points M in world coordinate frame are projected applying P, to their corresponding image points m. We have a set of n pairs of points m_i and the associated 3D points M_i. Our goal is to estimate P. A simple algorithm to achieve this is the *Direct Linear Transform* (DLT), which is easily formulated using homogeneous coordinates; a 3D coordinate M is transformed by a 3×4 matrix P as:

$$m = PM \tag{11.11}$$

This relationship can be expressed in terms of the vector cross product as $m_i \times PM_i = 0$ which enables a simple linear solution for P. Given m_i in homogenous coordinates, $m_i = (x_i, y_i, w_i)^T$, for each correspondence $M_i \leftrightarrow m_i$ the following relationship exists:

$$\begin{bmatrix} 0^T & -w_i M_i^T & y_i M_i^T \\ w_i M_i^T & 0^T & -x_i M_i^T \\ -y_i M_i^T & x_i M_i^T & 0^T \end{bmatrix} \begin{bmatrix} P^1 \\ P^2 \\ P^3 \end{bmatrix} = 0 \tag{11.12}$$

with P^i the i-th row of P.

Since the three equations are linearly dependent we can omit the third one.

$$\begin{bmatrix} 0^T & -w_i M_i^T & y_i M_i^T \\ w_i M_i^T & 0^T & -x_i M_i^T \end{bmatrix} \begin{bmatrix} P^1 \\ P^2 \\ P^3 \end{bmatrix} = 0 \tag{11.13}$$

That in turn means that one point correspondence contributes two equations. From n point correspondences we obtain a $2n \times 12$ matrix. Since a projection is defined up to scale the projection matrix P has 11 degrees of freedom. For an exact solution we thus need $5\frac{1}{2}$ point correspondences, which means that we require at least 6 points. If we have more than six points, we can augment the matrix from Equation 11.13 by adding more rows; let us call this matrix A. Equation 11.13 becomes a homogeneous system of equations

$$A \begin{bmatrix} P^1 \\ P^2 \\ P^3 \end{bmatrix} = 0 \tag{11.14}$$

whose solution is obtained using a *linear least squares* method. Example 9.9.6 demonstrates this.

11.3.3 Camera calibration with 2D object

If you take an image of a flat surface, then we can use the knowledge that all image points that belong to that surface are projections of points lying on a plane in the world. This constrains the projective mapping, which in turn allows us to estimate the camera parameters. This observation is at the heart of the camera calibration approach which we describe in the next subsections, and is due to (Z. Zhang 2000). This approach has several attractive characteristics. The calibration object is a plane and thus easy and cost effective to create. For a visible light camera the pattern can be printed using a standard printer. Image acquisition is flexible, requiring two or more images of the plane in general poses relative to the camera. This allows us to either move the phantom or the camera.

In Section 11.3.1 we constructed the model relating points in an arbitrary, world, coordinate system to the image plane as described by Equation 11.10. When our object consists of a plane we can arbitrarily decide that it coincides with the local XY plane such that all points have a Z-coordinate value of zero.

If we denote the ith column of the rotation matrix R by r_i. From 11.10, we have

$$s \begin{bmatrix} u \\ v \\ 1 \end{bmatrix} = K \begin{bmatrix} r_1 & r_2 & r_3 & t \end{bmatrix} \begin{bmatrix} X \\ Y \\ 0 \\ 1 \end{bmatrix} = K \begin{bmatrix} r_1 & r_2 & t \end{bmatrix} \begin{bmatrix} X \\ Y \\ 1 \end{bmatrix} \tag{11.15}$$

Given $\tilde{M} = [X, Y, 1]^T$ a point on the world plane. There is a homography, H, which maps all points on this plane to the image:

$$sm = H\tilde{M} \tag{11.16}$$

The 3×3 matrix H is defined up to a scale factor and can be directly estimated using four or more corresponding points in the image and calibration phantom plane as described in Section 11.2.2. This mapping is equal to the mapping described by Equation 11.15, which means:

$$H = K \begin{bmatrix} r_1 & r_2 & t \end{bmatrix} \tag{11.17}$$

Given that r_1 and r_2 are the first two columns of a rotation matrix we know that $r_1^T r_2 = 0$ and $r_1^T r_1 = r_2^T r_2$ providing us with the following constraints on the intrinsic camera parameters:

$$h_1^T K^{-T} K^{-1} h_2 = 0 \tag{11.18}$$
$$h_1^T K^{-T} K^{-1} h_1 = h_2^T K^{-T} K^{-1} h_2 \tag{11.19}$$

where h_i are the columns of H.

We obtain the camera calibration parameters by first estimating the intrinsic parameters (K) and then estimating the extrinsic ones.

Let

$$B = K^{-T} K^{-1} = \begin{bmatrix} B_{11} & B_{12} & B_{13} \\ B_{21} & B_{22} & B_{23} \\ B_{31} & B_{32} & B_{33} \end{bmatrix} \tag{11.20}$$

B is symmetric and defined by the following vector:

$$b = \begin{bmatrix} B_{11} & B_{12} & B_{13} & B_{22} & B_{23} & B_{33} \end{bmatrix}^T \tag{11.21}$$

Using the columns of matrix H we have:

$$h_i^T B h_j = v_{ij}^T b \tag{11.22}$$

where

$$v_{ij} = [h_{i1}h_{j1}, h_{i1}h_{j2} + h_{i2}h_{j1}, h_{i2}h_{j2},$$
$$h_{i3}h_{j1} + h_{i1}h_{j3}, h_{i3}h_{j2} + h_{i2}h_{j3}, h_{i3}h_{j3}]^T$$

We now combine Equations 11.18 and 11.19 into a single equation system:

$$\begin{bmatrix} v_{12}^T \\ (v_{11} - v_{22})^T \end{bmatrix} b = 0 \tag{11.23}$$

Using n views of the plane we create the following equation system:

$$Vb = 0 \tag{11.24}$$

where V is a $2n \times 6$ matrix.

For $n \geq 3$ we can obtain a unique solution for b, up to a scale factor. The solution of this equation system is obtained as the right singular vector of V associated with the smallest singular value.

Once b is estimated, we compute the camera intrinsic parameters as follows. Matrix B is estimated up to scale, i.e, $B = \lambda K^{-T} K^{-1}$ with λ an arbitrary scale. Extract the intrinsic parameters from matrix B using:

$$\begin{aligned}
v_0 &= (B_{12}B_{13} - B_{11}B_{23})/(B_{11}B_{22} - B_{12}^2) \\
\lambda &= B_{33} - [B_{13}^2 + v_0(B_{12}B_{13} - B_{11}B_{23})]/B_{11} \\
\alpha &= \sqrt{\lambda/B_{11}} \\
\beta &= \sqrt{\lambda B_{11}/(B_{11}B_{22} - B_{12}^2)} \\
\gamma &= -B_{12}\alpha^2\beta/\lambda \\
u_0 &= \gamma v_0/\beta - B_{13}\alpha^2/\lambda
\end{aligned} \tag{11.25}$$

Once K is known the extrinsic parameters for each image are computed as follows. From 11.17 we have

$$r_1 = \lambda K^{-1}h_1, \; r_2 = \lambda K^{-1}h_2, \; r_3 = r_1 \times r_2, \; t = \lambda K^{-1}h_3 \tag{11.26}$$

with $\lambda = 1/ \parallel K^{-1}h_1 \parallel = 1/ \parallel K^{-1}h_2 \parallel$.

11.4 IMAGE-GUIDED THERAPY, INTRODUCTION

Reducing procedure invasiveness and increasing interventional accuracy have been shown to improve clinical outcomes. As a consequence, direct visual feedback, available in open surgery, has been replaced with imaging and mental inference of the spatial relationships between anatomical structures and instruments. In turn, this increases the dependency of a favorable outcome on the physician's ability to interpret the images, recreate the underlying spatial relationships, and transfer a plan into action. IGI systems facilitate improved understanding of the spatial structures and increase accuracy by integrating medical images and other sources of information, such as position and orientation of tracked instruments or robotic devices.

Most of the technologies involved in IGI were described throughout the book, including:

1. Medical imaging (Chapters 1 and 10).

2. Data visualization (Chapters 4 and 8).

3. Segmentation (Chapter 6).

4. Registration (Chapter 9).

5. Tracking systems (Chapter 7).

Two technologies which are relevant for IGI and which we did not cover are human computer interaction (Shneiderman et al. 2009) and robotics (Rosen et al. 2010). The interested reader can find additional information about these subjects in the referenced textbooks.

The cost of clinical image-guided navigation systems is typically between tens of thousands of US dollars to several hundred thousands. Obviously, this limits access to such systems. As a result, hands on experience with IGI systems is most often limited to clinicians or research laboratories. In the next section we introduce a simplified navigation system that provides many of the functions available in clinical navigation systems, yet is all but free. "How is this possible?" you ask. The answer is, by providing open access to CT scans of a "reproducible patient", and by developing the system using open source software.

We provide instructions for building a LEGO^{TM} phantom which serves as our patient. Given that LEGO^{TM} blocks are manufactured with a high tolerance (knob tolerance is 0.02mm [The LEGO^{TM} Group]), we are ensured that the phantom you build is all but identical to the one we scanned. The cost of these blocks is the main expense associated with our hands-on approach. To complete our setup all we need is a tracking system and the software to perform planning and navigation. We provide a suite of programs that allow you to: turn a camera into a tracking device (e.g., your laptop computer's webcam), plan an "intervention", and perform it.

All of the software was developed using open source toolkits written in C++, primarily the Image-Guided Surgery Toolkit (IGSTK) (Cleary et al. 2009). Figure 11.5 shows the software architecture and lists all of the toolkits.

IGI Tutorial						
Camera Calibration	Pivot/Pointer Calibration	Planning	Navigation	Digitizer	Remote Control	Tracker Data
IGSTK						Qt
ITK	VTK	OpenCV	ArUco			

FIGURE 11.5: The suite of programs comprising the IGI tutorial was developed using a variety of free open source C++ toolkits. It is primarily based on the Image-Guided Surgery Toolkit (IGSTK) and Qt for the graphical user interface. IGSTK in turn uses the Insight Segmentation and Registration Toolkit (ITK), the Visualization Toolkit (VTK), the Open Source Computer Vision toolkit (OpenCV), and the ArUco augmented reality library. The set of programs marked in gray provide the functionality required by our simplified navigation system. The remaining programs are used to illustrate various other concepts in IGI.

Before we can start our practical lessons you will have to install the software from the book's website at www.crcpress.com. We provide three binary distributions, Windows 7, Linux Ubuntu, and Mac OS X[2] If you are unsure of how to interact with an application you can always access its help information, by clicking the question mark icon. For our more adventurous readers we also provide the C++ source code which you can compile on your own and modify as you see fit.

---

[2]The remote control application is only available on the Windows platform.

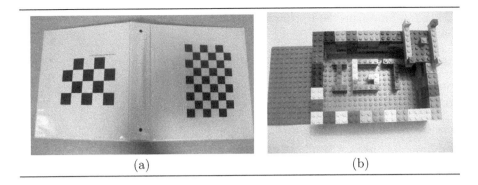

$$(a) \qquad\qquad\qquad\qquad\qquad (b)$$

FIGURE 11.6: (a) The patterns used for camera calibration and calibration evaluation attached to the two sides of a binder, and our simple LEGO^{TM} phantom (b).

11.5   IMAGE-GUIDED THERAPY, NAVIGATION SYSTEM

Now that you have installed the software we will walk you through a navigated intervention. From here on we assume the tutorial was installed in a directory named IGITutorial, the programs are in IGITutorial/Programs, and the data is found in IGITutorial/Data. The procedure we simulate is a needle biopsy, a procedure in which a needle is used to take fluid or cell samples from a suspicious lesion. The goal of the navigation system is to guide you so that you can insert the needle tip into an internal structure without puncturing critical structures along the way.

Before we can start you should gather the following materials: a pencil, a metric ruler, scissors, clear tape or glue, a hardcover book or binder, a webcam, and enough LEGO^{TM} blocks to build our phantom (see IGITutorial/Data/Print/legoPhantomInstructions.pdf). We divide this hands-on exercise into three steps:

setup and calibration

procedure planning

navigation.

11.5.1   Setup and calibration

Before you can use the webcam you will have to disable its autofocus, if it has this functionality. This is done using the camera control software which comes with the device. If you are unable to do this, you can still continue with the tutorial, just try to work at about the same distance from the camera at all times.

Our next step is to print out all of the patterns used in the tutorial and the instructions for building the phantom. Go to the Data/Print subdirectory and print all of the files. Using the ruler, check that the ValidationGrid and markers files were printed at the correct size (specified in the files). Attach the CalibrationGrid and ValidationGrid printouts to a rigid planar surface. Two sides of a hard cover book or a binder should do nicely, as illustrated in Figure 11.6(a). To complete the setup, all we need to do is build the phantom, shown in Figure 11.6(b), using the instructions you just printed.

We now calibrate our camera, transforming it from a qualitative device to a quantitative one, a tracking system. Run the IGICameraCalibration application found in the `Programs` directory and shown in Figure 11.7(a):

1. Press the "Start Camera" button and you should see the live video stream.

2. Capture five or more images of the calibration grid (saved to the `Programs/tmp` sub-directory).

3. Press the "Calibrate" button and select the images you want to use for calibration. The resulting calibration file is written to `Configuration/camera.yml` or you will get an error message informing you that calibration failed.

4. Position the validation pattern so that it is visible to the webcam and press the "Validate" button. A window with the image should open and the estimated length of two edges should be displayed, it should be approximately 60 mm as shown in Figure 11.7(b). We have empirically seen that estimation errors of less than 2 mm are sufficiently accurate for our purposes.

Once we have our tracking system we need to construct our tracked "needle". Select one of the markers, cut it out along the dotted line and glue it to the pencil. Our calibrated camera tracks the position and orientation of the printed marker, but we are interested in the location of the tool's tip. To determine the location of this point relative to the tracked coordinate system we need to calibrate the tool. Note that the orientation of the marker attached to the tool is unimportant, but that the tracking of the tool tip is more accurate if the distance between the marker and tip is shorter.

We will determine the tool tip location relative to the marker by pivoting. That is, we rotate the tool in all directions while keeping its tip in a fixed location, as illustrated in Figure 11.8(a). Run the IGIPivotCalibration application found in the `Programs` directory and shown in Figure 11.8(b). You will now:

1. Setup the system for calibration: select the marker attached to the tool from the program's dropdown menu, select the number of transformations (the default works well, but you can increase it), and press the "Initialize tracker" button.

2. Check that the tracked marker is visible in the location where you want to pivot (check camera view), and calibrate. You have 5s between pressing the calibrate button till data acquisition starts. The results are displayed in the application window, with the quality of the calibration given by the root mean square error (RMSE). For our purposes an RMSE of 3mm or less is sufficient.

This concludes our setup, we are ready to plan the intervention.

11.5.2 Procedure planning

To plan our procedure we use the IGIPlanning application. We specify the required information in three steps: (1) navigation system setup; (2) tracked marker selection; and (3) registration fiducials and target points localization. Figure 11.9 shows the corresponding application tabs.

We start by providing the system with the following information:

1. The directory containing the CT scan we want to use for navigation (we provide one in `Data/CT/LegoPhantom`).

2. The camera calibration file (`Configuration/camera.yml`).

3. The pointer tool calibration file (`Configuration/ToolTip.xml`).

4. The pointer tool 3D model file (`Data/MeshModels/ball.msh`).

Obviously we are assuming that you have already calibrated the camera and pointer tool as described in the previous section, as you need to select the files created by these calibration procedures.

Once you have selected the CT scan it is displayed using the reformatting technique described in Chapter 7. In our case, we use the standard radiological views: (trans-)axial, sagittal, and coronal; and an additional 3D view displaying all three reformatted images in their spatial locations. You can now modify the display's intensity mapping using the window/level approach as described in Chapter 4. Your choice of window/level values is recorded and will later be used during navigation.

To represent our pointer tool in the navigation system we use a sphere. A cylinder is a more appropriate representation for a needle like tool, but in our case we should not use it. The reason being that the pivot calibration procedure only provides us with the location of the tool's tip and not its orientation. Consequentially, using a cylinder at an arbitrary orientation can result in unrealistic feedback. That is, the cylinder tip will be displayed at the correct location but the orientation will not correspond to that of the tool in the physical world.

In the next step you will select tracked markers, one attached to the tool and one attached to our phantom. The latter is referred to as a Dynamic Reference Frame (DRF), see Figure 11.10. This coordinate system is rigidly attached to the phantom, and becomes the center of our world. That is, all spatial relationships will be described relative to this coordinate system. The main advantage of defining our world relative to the phantom is that we can freely move the phantom or tracking system and all of the spatial relationships remain valid. Without the DRF the spatial relationship between the tracking system and the patient must remain fixed, once we perform the physical space to image registration. Which brings us to our third and final step in the procedure planning, identifying and localizing fiducial points and target points.

To perform navigation we need to obtain the rigid transformation between the physical space, our DRF, and the image space, our CT. We will estimate this transformation using the paired-point rigid registration algorithm due to B.K.P. Horn and described in Chapter 9. This algorithm requires that we localize corresponding points in the image and on the phantom. You can choose any set of three or more non-collinear points. A convenient choice is the set of points shown in Figure 11.10. In the planning stage we localize our fiducials in the image. Start by identifying them, scroll through the axial slices, find the bounds of the fiducial configuration, and identify the fiducials based on their relationship with the phantom walls. To accurately localize each fiducial in the image you can zoom (press right mouse button and drag) and pan (press middle mouse button and drag) the axial slice. You can optionally specify target point(s). The distinction being that these are points which are not used for registration. To indicate that a set of points will serve as targets uncheck the "Registration Points" checkbox. Localization of the targets is done the same way as fiducials.

All that remains to be done is save the configuration and move to the navigation step. The configuration files are saved in the `IGITutorial/Configuration` directory in XML format, which is viewable in any text editor.

11.5.3 Navigation

To navigate to our target you will use the IGINavigation program. Start by loading the configuration file generated in the planning phase. The CT data is displayed using the previously selected window/level settings, and the tracker is activated. You can browse through the image data, see that the fiducials and target(s) are in the expected locations and ensure that the phantom is positioned in physical space so that the DRF is visible in the camera view.

The final step before navigation is to register the image and physical spaces so that the information displayed on screen matches the physical world. In the previous step we obtained the fiducials in image space, we now need to obtain the corresponding fiducials in physical space. To digitize a fiducial location you need to place the tip of the tracked tool on the fiducial and "accept" it. The program will automatically move to the next fiducial once the previous one is digitized (order corresponds to that defined in the planning stage). Once you acquire three or more non-collinear fiducials you can perform registration. Figure 11.11 shows the physical setup and corresponding screen captures of the navigation program before and after registration.

If registration succeeds we report the fiducial registration error and save the transformation to file, `Configuration/RegistrationResult.xml`. We remind you that FRE does not reflect the quality of registration, as noted in Chapter 9. It should only be used to validate that the spatial relationship between the fiducials is unchanged [3]. From here on the display is updated based on the location of the tracked tool's tip. That is, the tip location is coincident with the displayed axial, sagittal and coronal planes. Move the pointer around and the display should update accordingly. Depending on the quality of your camera you will visually experience the effects of tracking noise. That is, the display will jitter even when the pointer and phantom are motionless. These effects are much less perceptible when using a commercial tracking system.

To truly evaluate the quality of registration we are interested in the target registration error. In the planning phase you specified one or more targets, you can now assess the quality of registration using these points. Place the tip of the tracked tool on the visible target and press the specific target's button. The TRE is displayed. These numbers do indicate the quality of registration. This type of evaluation is only relevant in a laboratory setting where the targets are visible. In the clinical setting we can only reach the target after navigation as it is not directly accessible.

At this point you should have a good grasp of the technologies used in IGI and how they are integrated into a navigation system. In the next section we use these programs to further enhance your understanding of various theoretical concepts.

11.6 IMAGE-GUIDED THERAPY, THEORY IN PRACTICE

11.6.1 Camera calibration

As we learned in the introductory parts of this chapter the camera parameters estimated using Zhang's (Z. Zhang 2000) calibration algorithm are invariant to uniform scaling of the pattern. We will now see this in practice. Remember that the calibration pattern file is

---

[3]Most likely you'll be happier to see a smaller FRE even though this is irrelevant to the task at hand.

found in the `Data/Print` subdirectory. Simply print two copies of the pattern at different scales. This is easily done, by switching from landscape to portrait and indicating that the print size should fit the page.

Now that we have our two calibration patterns, run the IGICameraCalibration program and perform calibration and validation as described in Section 11.5.1. Using the validation pattern, the estimated distance will be (almost) the same irrespective of the pattern you used.

11.6.2   Tracking accuracy

For many tracking systems accuracy and precision vary in space. That is, the performance reported by the manufacturers is most often an average of the measurements acquired throughout the system's working volume. In most cases this variability can be ignored by the user, though in some cases it does merit further scrutiny (Hummel et al. 2005). When using a webcam as our tracking device we fall into the latter category. In this exercise we will evaluate the quality of tracking in a spatial region.

Start by calibrating your camera using the IGICameraCalibration program. Then, print the `TwoMarkerConfiguration.pdf` file. This file contains two markers with a known transformation between them. Attach the markers to a rigid planar surface, a thicker piece of paper such as construction paper works well. We will acquire transformations for the two markers at multiple locations inside the tracking system's workspace using the polar grid shown in Figure 11.12(a). At each location we acquire data at three different heights. Before moving on to data acquisition you should construct the LEGO^{TM} holder for our markers. The build instructions are found in the `legoTowerInstructions.pdf` file.

At each of the 27 grid locations in the work volume we acquire transformation data from the tracking system to each of the markers. Acquisition is done with the IGITrackerData program, which saves the transformations to files. Each row in a file corresponds to a single rigid transformation with rotation parameterized using a unit quaternion as described in Section 7.3.4. The file format is: "time $t_x\, t_y\, t_z\, q_1\, q_2\, q_3\, q_0$" ($q_0$ is the scalar part of the quaternion).

At each location you have multiple transformations from the tracking system to each of the markers, the two files containing the transformations. This yields N estimates of the transformation between the two coordinate systems per location. For each estimate you will compute the TREs for eight vertices of a cube centered on the origin of the marker ($[-10, -10, -10] \ldots [10, 10, 10]$):

$$\|T_{estimate,i}\mathbf{p}_j - T_{known}\mathbf{p}_j\|, \; i = 1 \ldots N, \; j = 1 \ldots 8$$

For each location we now have 8N measurements. Compute the max, median, and standard deviation of the TRE at each spatial location. What is the spatial region in which tracking is most accurate?

In clinical practice we position the tracking system so that the targeted anatomy is inside the tracker's spatial region which is most accurate.

11.6.3   Human computer interaction

Human computer interaction (HCI) plays a significant role in the integration and acceptance of navigation systems in the clinical setting. In this subsection we briefly discuss HCI and point out issues that are specific to intra-operative interaction.

Two unique constraints imposed by the intra-operative domain are that the physician can only interact with devices that have been sterilized, and that the working environment has limited space. As a result it is not uncommon to see physicians interact with a system via proxy. That is, they direct another person in performing the desired interactions. At first glance this seems to be a reasonable solution. Unfortunately, this is sub-optimal and can be extremely time consuming. Case in point, Grätzel et al. report observing a single mouse click taking seven minutes and involving four people.

While there are many approaches to solving this issue, most of them require introducing additional hardware into the workspace. As we noted earlier, the operating environment has limited space making such solutions less desirable. Ideally we utilize existing hardware. In our case, tracking devices which are already part of navigation systems can also provide HCI functionality. High level gesture based interaction can be implemented using the existing hardware in a similar manner to the interactions offered by the popular Microsoft Kinect gaming device. Simpler methods of interaction have been commercially available. Trigger like input devices have been incorporated into tracked tools, or in a stand-alone manner such as the foot switch for the Polaris system from Northern Digital Inc. shown in Figure 11.13(a). For more complex interactions Visarius et al. introduced the concept of a tracked virtual keypad as shown in Figure 11.13(b). Key press events are triggered based on the proximity of a tracked tool to the virtual buttons. Both keyboard and tracked tool are sterilizable.

We will now see how we can use our webcam based tracking system as an HCI component. We have implemented a simplistic remote control program, IGIRemoteControl (only available for the Windows operating system). Our remote control sends specific key-press events, to the program that currently has focus, based on the visibility of tracked markers. For a marker to trigger an event it must be visible to the tracking system for a specific length of time (we arbitrarily chose 2s). Figure 11.14 shows our remote control interface. If you run this program in conjunction with a Power Point presentation you will be able to remotely advance and move backwards in your slide presentation.

11.6.4 Dynamic reference frame

In our tutorial above we used a DRF. If you did not move your phantom during navigation you may have missed the importance of using this patient centered coordinate system. We now explicitly show why navigation systems use a DRF. For this exercise we assume that you have completed the tutorial above (Section 11.5).

We now perform navigation. Remember that the DRF must be attached to the phantom. Once you have registered the phantom, go to a target point and obtain the target registration error as you previously did in the tutorial. Now move the phantom several centimeters in an arbitrary direction. Obtain the TRE again. The two values are similar, the quality of the guidance is maintained even when the phantom is moved. This conclusion is not completely valid as we are assuming that the tracking accuracy is constant throughout the tracking device's work volume. This is often not the case (see previous exercise).

Now, detach the DRF from the phantom and repeat the process. The TRE prior to moving the phantom is similar to the previous two TREs. The TRE after moving the phantom is much higher. That is, the guidance has become inaccurate. Finally, perform registration again and obtain the TRE for the target point. It is again similar to the results obtained with the DRF and to the result prior to motion. The patient mounted DRF allowed us to maintain a valid registration between the patient and image-spaces even when the patient has moved. It should be noted that the DRF also allows us to freely move the tracking system. This is an advantage in the operating room, where one would prefer to have the flexibility of moving equipment around even after registration.

At this point, we hope to have convinced you that using a DRF is the correct approach, as it will maintain registration throughout a procedure even when the patient is moved. What we have neglected to discuss is the bigger picture. Attaching a DRF to a patient is not the same as snapping two pieces of LEGO^{TM} together. In many cases this is an invasive procedure which can potentially lead to clinical complications. Thus, the decision whether to use a DRF or rely on patient immobilization is procedure specific. If the clinical procedure does guarantee that the patient and tracking system will not be moved we can dispense with the DRF. An example illustrating this is the clinical study described in (Ilsar et al. 2007), showing that for fixation of femoral neck fractures the DRF is not necessary.

11.6.5 Paired-Point rigid registration

In this section we experiment with key properties of paired-point rigid registration as described in Chapter 9. Our intention is to bring theoretical discussions, many of which are due to Prof. J. M. Fitzpatrick, to life. We start by experimenting with fiducial configurations and then empirically see that fiducial registration error is not correlated with target registration error.

Fiducial Configurations

One of the first publications to discuss the effects of various fiducial configurations on TRE was (West et al. 2001). They conclude that near-collinear configurations are best avoided. It is easy to see that with a collinear fiducial configuration we cannot resolve the rotation around the axis defined by the fiducials as rotations around the axis will have no effect on fiducial location. When the fiducials are nearly collinear we resolve this rotation, but it is inaccurate.

Identifying that we are primarily dealing with errors in rotation, we remind ourselves that unlike errors in translation, the effect of rotation depends on the center of rotation. Simply stating that we have a x^o error is meaningless as we cannot judge its effect on the location of the target. In the extreme, the center of rotation is at the target point or very far from it. In the former case rotational errors have no effect on the TRE, in the later case small rotational errors can result in a large TRE. This is often referred to as the "lever effect". After this exercise we expect that whenever encountering a sentence such as "the rotation error was x^o..." you will immediately ask "Where is the center of rotation?"

We now turn our attention to the practical exercise at hand. You will use a nearly collinear set of fiducials provided by us (`nearlyCollinearFiducials.xml`) to perform registration. Assuming you have completed the tutorial above you should have an xml configuration file, `IGIConfiguration.xml`. Go to the `Configuration` directory and edit it. You will need to replace the current location specified by the "FiducialSetFile" tag with the location of our fiducial xml file. After you have saved the modified configuration file place your DRF in a position similar to that shown in Figure 11.15. This figure also shows the fiducial positions. Now run the IGINavigation program and perform registration. We expect similar results to those illustrated in Figure 11.15. That is, the farther you move the pointer tool from the DRF in a direction perpendicular to the fiducial axis the larger the error in the display. The longer the lever, the larger the effect of the rotational error.

A key assumption in paired-point rigid registration is that the points are paired correctly. Human beings are highly adept at this, even when the fiducial configuration is ambiguous. We are able to uniquely identify the markers by relating their positions to other structures that are easily identifiable. The down side to this approach is that when we localize a specific fiducial we need to explicitly indicate which one it is. Ideally, a clinician should be able to localize the fiducials in any order without any constraints, including deviating from a fixed order chosen preoperatively. In other words, we want fiducials to be matched automatically.

A specific category of fiducial configurations that cannot be matched automatically is the set of rotationally symmetric configurations. The reason being that these configurations can be matched in multiple ways. One would think that we can easily avoid such configurations. Two factors can lead us to make the mistake of using such a configuration: (1) human beings find symmetry pleasing and thus have a natural tendency to design symmetric objects, and (2) we intentionally design a symmetric configuration to improve performance of automated identification in an image. In this case symmetry improves detection robustness as we can rule out potential fiducials that do not have symmetric counterparts.

To experiment with such configurations we use the fiducials defined in the tutorial as shown in Figure 11.10. In our case we will only use fiducials 1-4. At this point you should plan the intervention using the IGIPlanning program and then run the IGINavigation program. Our next step is to register the image and physical spaces. We first register after digitizing the fiducials in the correct order. This will result in a reasonable FRE and TRE, as expected. Now digitize the fiducials in an order corresponding to an in plane rotation of 180° ($1 \rightarrow 3, 2 \rightarrow 4, 3 \rightarrow 1, 4 \rightarrow 2$). This simulates an incorrect, yet valid matching which can potentially result from an automatic matching. This will yield a reasonable FRE, but the TRE is extremely high.

FRE and TRE are Uncorrelated

The experiments in this section are based on the examples given in (Fitzpatrick 2001). We remember that the paired-point rigid registration solves a least squares formulation, minimizing the sum of distances between the points. Once we have obtained a solution it is only natural that we look at the FRE. It is always good to know that when you intend to minimize a quantity it is indeed reduced. What we will observe in our experiments is that the FRE does not inform us about the quality of our registration, the TRE.

We start by removing the fiducial configuration we used in all of our experiments, obtaining the phantom structure shown in Figure 11.16. If you have previously planned a procedure you should have an xml configuration file, `Configuration/IGIConfiguration.xml`. Otherwise plan the procedure using the IGIPlanning program and create a dummy fiducial and target files, specify an arbitrary point in each of them. Now edit the configuration file. Replace the fiducial points, "FiducialSetFile" tag, and the target points, "TargetSetFile" tag, with the files we provide: `FREunCorrelatedWithTREFiducials.xml`, `FREunCorrelatedWithTRETarget.xml`.

We can now run the IGINavigation program and start experimenting. In our first experiment we introduce a consistent error to all fiducials. Instead of digitizing the correct location with our pointer, we touch points that are three knobs to the left, as shown in Figure 11.16(a). After registration we see that the reported FRE is small. Now obtain the TRE by positioning the pointer tool on the target and pressing the target button in the navigation program. You can see that we have a large TRE, even though the FRE is small.

In our second experiment we introduce errors in the fiducial localization that are accounted for by the least squares formulation, resulting in a correct solution. Instead of digitizing the correct locations, for fiducials one and two we touch three knobs to the right, and for fiducials three and four we touch three knobs to the left, as shown in Figure 11.16(b). After registration we see that the reported FRE is large. Now obtain the TRE. You can see that we have a small TRE, even though the FRE is large.

Input: point set P_l, point set P_r, initial transformation T_0, improvement threshold $\tau > 0$, maximal number of iterations n

0. Initialization:

   (a) Set cumulative transformation to T_0, and apply to points.

   (b) Pair closest points and compute the root mean square error (RMSE) of the distances $(\sqrt{\frac{\sum_{i=1}^{n} \|T(P_{l,i}) - P_{r,match(P_{l,i})}\|^2}{n}})$

1. Iterate:

   (a) Compute incremental transformation using the current correspondences (Horn's algorithm), update cumulative transformation and apply to points.

   (b) Find closest points and compute distance RMSE.

   (c) If improvement in RMSE is less than τ, or number of iterations has reached n terminate.

TABLE 11.1   Iterative Closest Point algorithm.

While the localization errors in these two experiments are artificial, similar scenarios can occur in practice. A phantom containing a fiducial configuration which is unintentionally moved, introducing a consistent error to all fiducials, or skin adhesive fiducials that change location due to skin elasticity.

11.6.6   Iterative-closest point

A relatively straightforward extension of the paired-point rigid registration algorithm is the Iterative-Closest Point (ICP) method described in Chapter 9 and summarized in Table 11.1. In this exercise you will implement the ICP algorithm and experiment using your implementation. We explore three characteristics of the ICP algorithm:

1. Its sensitivity to the initial user provided transformation.

2. Its sensitivity to outliers.

3. The computational complexity associated with the matching step.

We provide three files containing point clouds corresponding to the exterior faces and bottom of our phantom. *Note that the bottom of the phantom is modeled as a flat surface, points are not on the knobs.* The files are simple text files where each row represents a single point's coordinates (x, y, z). Each of the files corresponds to the same surfaces sampled at different resolutions. The base resolution is found in `legoPhantomSampledPoints.txt`. An order of magnitude larger sampling is found in `legoPhantomSampledPointsX10.txt`, and another order of magnitude in `legoPhantomSampledPointsX100.txt`. These point sets are similar to the results obtained from a segmentation of the phantom's CT image. Figure 11.17(a) shows a visualization of the base resolution point cloud.

To register these point clouds to the physical world using the ICP algorithm we need to digitize points in the world. We provide you with a program that allows you to do just that, IGI3DDigitizer. This program allows you to manually acquire a point cloud using a tracked pointer. You can either use it with a DRF, recommended, or without, if you are sure your phantom will not move during the point acquisition process. Figure 11.17(b) shows the program's interface after point cloud acquisition. Once you save the manually acquired point cloud you will register it to the point sets we provided using different initial transformations.

The ICP algorithm receives as input an initial transformation, T_0. In many cases when we have no prior information we set $T_0 = I$. A successful end result is highly dependent upon this initialization. In our case the point cloud data we provide describes a rotationally symmetric phantom, a box. As a consequence the ICP algorithm may be successful in minimizing the distances between the two point clouds but the resulting transformation may be incorrect (180^0 rotation around the phantom's center). To see the effect of the initial transformation we will experiment with the ICP algorithm using the base resolution point cloud we provide, `ForeDevelopers/legoPhantomPoints.txt`, and the manual point cloud you acquired.

First, register the two point clouds using the identity transformation. How many iterations were required until the algorithm converged? Did it converge to the correct solution? Compare to a result obtained using the paired-point registration obtained by the IGINavigation program, see the `RegistrationResult.xml` file. Now initialize using a rough estimate obtained via paired-point registration, this will increase the chances of a correct and accurate registration. By rough estimate we mean that you digitize points near the actual fiducial locations and not the exact ones. How many iterations were required in this case? Did the algorithm result in a correct solution?

As the ICP algorithm is based on paired-point registration which uses a least squares formulation we know that it is sensitive to outliers. We now ask that you add outliers to the point cloud which you digitized by editing the file. Do this in an incremental manner and evaluate the results each time. Select a set of target points and evaluate the TRE using the estimate without outliers as compared to with outliers. Plot the mean TRE $\left(\frac{\sum_{i=1}^{n} \| T_{noOutliers}(P_i) - T_{outliers}(P_i) \|^2}{n} \right)$ as a function of the percentage of outliers. What is the breakdown point, percentage of outliers, of the ICP algorithm?

Another important aspect of the ICP algorithm is the computational complexity of the matching step. To experience the effect of point cloud size on the running time of the algorithm, repeat the experiments above using the higher resolution point clouds we provide (`ForDevelopers/legoPhantomPointsX*.txt`). How does the resolution affect the running time? Note that if you implemented a naive matching approach your answer will be different than if you used a spatial data structure such as an Octree (Samet 1990).

11.7 SUMMARY AND FURTHER REFERENCES

We hope these hands-on exercises have enhanced your understanding of the basics of image-guided interventions and several other related concepts taught throughout the book. It is also appropriate at the end of this book to point out that each of the subjects covered in the various chapters is a broad domain onto itself. Thus, while we have provided you with a wide set of tools which can be combined into a clinically useful system, this is only the beginning of your journey into medical image analysis and image-guided interventions.

Literature

K. Cleary, P. Cheng, A. Enquobahrie, and Z. Yaniv, eds., *IGSTK: The Book*, Signature Book Printing, 2009.

J. M. Fitzpatrick, "Detecting failure, assessing success", In J. V. Hajnal, D. L. G. Hill, and D. J. Hawkes eds., *Medical Image Registration*, CRC Press, 2001.

C. Grätzel, T. Fong, X. Grange, and C. Baur, "A non-contact mouse for surgeon-computer interaction", *Technol. Health Care*, 12(3):245–257, 2004.

J. B. Hummel, M. R. Bax, M. L. Figl, Y. Kang, C. R. Maurer Jr., W. Birkfellner, H. Bergmann, and R. Shahidi, "Design and application of an assessment protocol for electromagnetic tracking systems", *Med. Phys.*, 32(7):2371–2379, 2005.

I. Ilsar, Y. A. Weil, L. Joskowicz, R. Moshieff, and M. Liebergall, "Fracture-table-mounted versus bone-mounted dynamic reference frame tracking accuracy using computer-assisted orthopaedic surgery - a comparative study", *Comput. Aided Surg.*, 12(2):125–130, 2007.

T. Peters and K. Cleary, eds., *Image-Guided Interventions Technology and Applications*, Springer-Verlag, 2008.

J. Rosen, B. Hannaford, and Richard M. Satava, eds., *Surgical Robotics Systems, Applications, and Visions*, Springer, 2010.

H. Samet, *The Design and Analysis of Spatial Data Structures*, Addison-Wesley, 1990.

B. Shneiderman, C. Plaisant, M. Cohen, and S. Jacobs, *Designing the User Interface: Strategies for Effective Human-Computer Interaction*, Addison-Wesley, 2009.

H. Visarius, J. Gong, C. Scheer, S. Haralamb, and L. P. Nolte, "Man-machine interfaces in computer assisted surgery", *Comput. Aided Surg.*, 2(2):102–107, 1997.

J. B. West, J. M. Fitzpatrick, S. A. Toms, C. R. Maurer Jr., and R. J. Maciunas, "Fiducial point placement and the accuracy of point-based, rigid body registration", *Neurosurgery*, 48(4):810–817, 2001.

Z. Zhang, "A Flexible New Technique for Camera Calibration", *IEEE Trans. Pattern Anal. Machine Intell.*, 22(11): 1330-1334, 2000.

The LEGO group: A short presentation, 2012. Last accessed January 1 2013 http://aboutus.lego.com/en-us/news-room/media-assets-library/documents/.

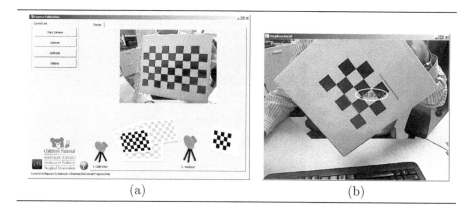

(a)   (b)

FIGURE 11.7: Camera calibration application (a) acquisition of calibration pattern images, and (b) evaluation of calibration using validation pattern with known size (ellipse highlights estimated size).

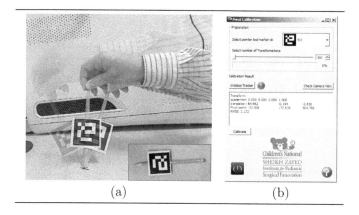

(a)   (b)

FIGURE 11.8: (a) Pivoting the tracked pointer tool (insert), X marks the fixed rotation point (b) application for determining the tool tip location relative to the tracked marker.

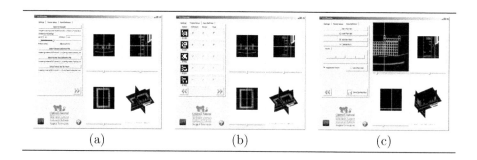

(a)   (b)   (c)

FIGURE 11.9: The three steps required by our procedure planning (a) system setup; (b) tracked marker selection; and (c) registration fiducials and target points specification.

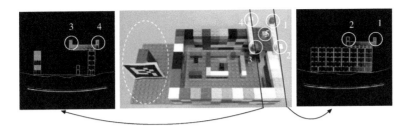

FIGURE 11.10: Use fiducials that are easily identifiable in physical space and image spaces. Fiducials indicated by solid circles, numbers indicate correspondences in image and physical spaces. DRF is inscribed by the dashed ellipse.

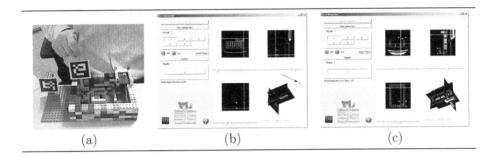

FIGURE 11.11: Use of the navigation program (a) physical setup, touching the target point, top left knob of the letter I; (b) corresponding display before registration does not reflect the physical world, arrow shows tool tip location; and (c) after registration display correctly reflects the tool tip location.

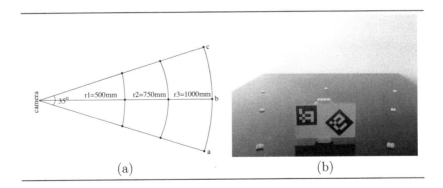

FIGURE 11.12: Evaluate the accuracy of our tracking system at multiple locations in the work volume: (a) locations on polar grid and (b) picture acquired by tracking system for polar grid location r1-b-height1. At each location data is acquired at three heights.

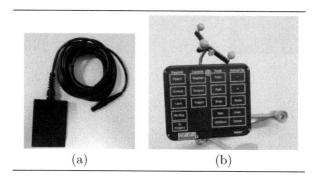

(a)   (b)

FIGURE 11.13: Human computer interaction devices (a) foot switch for the Polaris tracking system from NDI; and (b) tracked virtual keypad (courtesy N. Glossop).

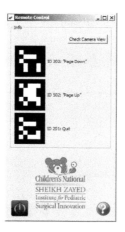

FIGURE 11.14: Our remote control application sends "page up" and "page down" events to the program that currently has focus.

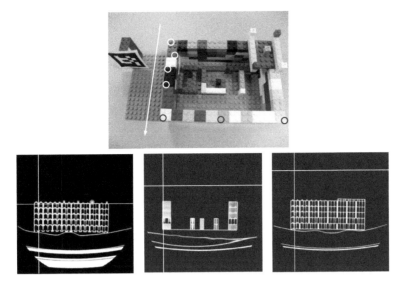

FIGURE 11.15: The result of using a nearly collinear fiducial configuration. Fiducials are highlighted by white circles. The angular error is highest around the main axis of the fiducial configuration. The transformation is relative to the DRF, with its origin at one of the marker corners. The tracked pointer is placed at each of the locations marked by a black circle. The farther we are from the origin the larger the effect of the rotational error as illustrated by the location of the cross hairs, corresponding to the tool tip location, overlaid onto the axial slice.

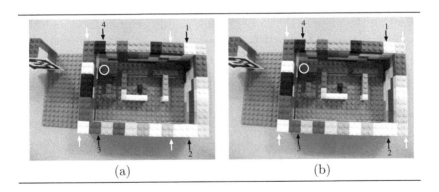

(a) (b)

FIGURE 11.16: Two examples of localizing fiducial points. Black arrows correspond to the fiducials, white arrows to their localization. The target is marked by the white circle (top left knob of the I). The erroneous localizations result in (a) FRE < TRE, all localizations were acquired to the "left" of the actual fiducials, and (b) FRE > TRE, two localizations were acquired to the "left" and two to the "right".

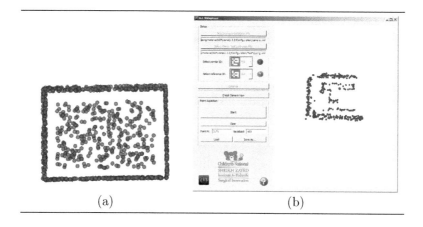

(a) (b)

FIGURE 11.17: Data for experimentation with the ICP algorithm (a) visualization of point cloud representing the phantom. The points are on the exterior faces and bottom of the phantom; and (b) manually acquired points using our digitization program and a tracked pointer.

CHAPTER 12

A Selection of MATLAB® Commands

CONTENTS

12.1   Control structures and operators 397
12.2   I/O and data structures 398
12.3   Mathematical functions 399
12.4   Further references 401

As already stated in the foreword, this book is not an introduction to MATLAB programming; rather than that, we used MATLAB or Octave as some sort of vehicle for executing scripts that illustrate the basic concepts of image processing algorithms. The drawback of this approach is the poor performance of some of the scripts. The advantage, on the other hand, lies in the fact that virtually no knowledge of MATLAB or a more sophisticated programming environment is necessary.

Here, we have collected all commands, control structures and mathematical functions used in the scripts from the `LessonData` folder. While this selection is by no means representative of the capabilities of MATLAB, it may serve as some resource if a command in the scripts is unclear. You may, of course, also use the `help` command in the MATLAB shell.

12.1   CONTROL STRUCTURES AND OPERATORS

`for`: A loop structure that executes a sequence of commands for a given number of times. The command sequence is delimited by the **end** keyword.

`while`: A loop structure that repeats a sequence of commands until a logical condition is met. The command sequence is delimited by the **end** keyword.

`if`: A decision structure that executes a sequence of commands if a logical condition is met. The command sequence is delimited by the **end** keyword.

`*`: Matrix multiplication; if the operands are scalar, this is the standard multiplication operator.

`.*`: Component-wise multiplication of matrix elements; the matrices have to have the same dimension.

^: The power-operator. We only use it for computing powers of scalar values.

>: *greater than* operator.

<: *less than* operator.

>=: *greater or equal* operator.

<=: *less or equal* operator.

~=: *not equal* operator.

&: logical AND operator. This operator can also be used as a *short circuit* operator &&.

|: logical OR operator. This operator can also be used as a *short circuit* operator ||.

(:): The colon operator can be used to assign rows and columns in total. While this is a very powerful tool in MATLAB for fast matrix operations, it also tends to obfuscate the code. We therefore only used it to maintain the shape of a matrix when assigning a stream of data.

@: This operator de-references a call to a function; it is, for instance, used for calling a merit function to be optimized.

12.2   I/O AND DATA STRUCTURES

;: Suppresses output in the MATLAB console.

cd: Changes the working directory of MATLAB.

image: Shows a graphical representation of an arbitrary matrix. The numerical entries in the matrix are shown as colored dots. The assignment of colors can be defined by the colormap command.

colormap: Choose a lookup table for the image command. Since medical images do usually not feature color, we mainly use the gray scale lookup table of MATLAB which features 64 shades of gray.

imshow: A more sophisticated command from the image processing toolbox for directly displaying images; a similar command is also available in Octave. Usually, we do not use this functionality; rather than that, the image command is used.

plot: A command to display a functional relationship from data stored as vectors or matrices.

ylim: This command sets the range of the y-axis in a plot.

bar: Plots a bar chart from a vector or matrix data.

surf: Generates a surface plot from a matrix.

fopen: Opens a file for read or write access, which is defined by the additional 'r' or 'w' attribute. If the file exists, a structure – the file pointer – for reading from or writing to the file is assigned. If the operation fails, fopen returns a value -1.

fseek: A function that moves the file pointer in a file by a given number of bytes. The starting position for this incremental procedure can be defined. Here, we only used 'bof', which stands for *beginning of file*.

fread: A function that reads a given number of bytes from a file using the file pointer.

fclose: This functions stops the access to a file and forces data to be written to disk.

imread: A function that reads the content of more complex image file formats and saves the content in matrix. A similar command exists for Octave.

imwrite: Another function that allows for saving matrices as images in common file formats such as JPG. A similar command with a slightly different syntax exists for Octave.

save: A command for writing a matrix to a file from MATLAB.

load: A command for reading matrix data from a file.

sprintf: This function returns a string, or a vector of characters from other characters or numbers.

fprintf: This function writes binary data for a file using the file pointer.

\n: A non-printable character – the line break.

input: This function is used for reading input from the console. We only use it to stop program execution until a key is pressed.

char: The 8 bit integer datatype of MATLAB.

short: The 16 bit integer datatype of MATLAB.

uint8(...): 'uint8' stands for an unsigned 8 bit integer datatype. Calls of this type force a typecast on a number – it is therefore possible to change the datatype of a variable. A similar call would be **double(...)**.

zeros: This function generates a matrix of arbitrary dimension, filled with zeros.

eye: This function returns an identity matrix; only one argument is required since the number of columns and rows in an identity matrix is identical.

12.3 MATHEMATICAL FUNCTIONS

function: This keyword allows for definition of custom functions in MATLAB. In order to keep the sample code simple and compact, we did not use this possibility to a large extent.

transpose: The transposition operation switches rows and columns in a matrix. We use this operation frequently, especially since MATLAB may show a flipped version of images sometimes. Applied to a vector, it changes a row vector to a column vector and vice versa.

max: This function returns the maximum element of a vector. If it is applied to a matrix, it returns a vector of the maximal element in each column.

min: This function returns the minimum value; otherwise, its behavior is identical to max.

size: Returns the dimension of a matrix or a vector.

mean: Returns the average value of all entries in a vector; if applied to a matrix, it returns a vector of the averages from each column.

median: Returns the median value of all entries in a vector.

std: Returns the standard deviation of all entries in a vector.

sort: Returns a vector with sorted vector entries.

round: Returns a rounded integer value if applied to floating point number.

floor: Returns the next smallest integer value if applied to floating point number.

log: The logarithm.

exp: The exponential function.

sin: The sine.

cos: The cosine.

fft: Returns a complex-valued vector which represents the Fourier transform stored in a vector.

ifft: The inverse Fourier transform, which maps from k-space to the spatial domain.

fft2: The two-dimensional fast Fourier transform.

ifft2: The inverse two-dimensional fast Fourier transform.

fftshift: A phase shift for aligning images in a symmetrical manner when applying the DFT.

ifftshift: The inverse phase shift, necessary before transforming an image back to the spatial domain.

abs: The absolute values of a scalar or of matrix components. The length of a vector is computed by calling the norm function.

real: Returns the real part of a complex number.

mod: Returns the modulus of a division.

inv: The inverse of a matrix.

det: The determinant of a matrix.

lsqlin: Solves a system of equations using the method of linear least squares. It is part of the Optimization toolbox of MATLAB.

eig: Returns the eigenvalues and eigenvectors of a matrix.

fminsearch: The MATLAB version of the Nelder-Mead algorithm . It is part of the Optimization Toolbox. The same function does not perform very well in Octave.

`cross`: The outer product of two vectors.

`dot`: The scalar product of two vectors.

`pi`: ... approximately 3.14159.

12.4 FURTHER REFERENCES

S. Attaway: MATLAB: A Practical Introduction to Programming and Problem Solving, Butterworth-Heinemann, (2009)

R. C. Gonzalez, R. E. Woods, and S. L. Eddins: Digital Image Processing Using MATLAB, Gatesmark Publishing, (2009)

Glossary

AC: Alternating Current.

ACR: American College of Radiologists.

Analyze 7.5: A file format for medical volume data; it is derived from the older releases of the *Analyze* software and consists of two files, a `....hdr` file containing information on image size, depth and other metadata, and the image data file `....img` itself.

API: Application Programmers Interface, a library of routines to be linked to a program.

ASCII: American Standard Code for Information Interchange – a standard for encoding characters.

BMP: BitMaP, an image file format.

CAD: Computer Aided Design.

CBCT: Cone-Beam Computed Tomography.

CCD: Charge Coupled Device, a common type of image detector.

CNR: Contrast to Noise Ratio.

COC: Center of Curvature.

CR foils: Computed radiography foils, a replacement technology for radiographic films.

CT: Computed Tomography.

DC: Direct Current.

DCT: Discrete Cosine Transform.

DFT: Discrete Fourier Transform.

DICOM: Digital Imaging and Communications in Medicine – a common standard for storage and exchange of radiological image data.

DICOM-RT: An extension of the DICOM standard for storage of planning data in radiotherapy.

DICOMDIR: A file that organizes single image files in a DICOM study.

DLT: Direct Linear Transform, a method to derive projection geometry from image data.

dof: degrees-of-freedom.

DQE: Detector Quantum Efficiency, the conversion ratio of quanta imparted vs. generated signals.

DRR: Digitally rendered radiograph, a perspective volume rendering from CT simulating an x-ray.

DSA: Digitally subtracted angiography, a radiological method for visualization of vessels after application of contrast agents.

EBCT: Electron Beam Computed Tomography.

EPI: Electronic Portal Image, an attenuation image of γ-quanta used in radiotherapy.

EPID: Electronic Portal Image Detector.

EPS: Encapsulated PostScript, an image file format.

FDG: Fluordeoxyglucose, a PET tracer.

FEM: Finite Element Modelling.

FFT: Fast Fourier Transform.

FID: Free Induction Decay, a quantity measured in MR imaging.

FITS: Flexible Image Transport System, a 16 bit image file format popular in astronomy.

FLE: Fiducial Localization Error.

FOV: Field-of-View.

FRE: Fiducial Registration Error.

GIMP: GNU Image manipulation program.

GUI: Graphical User Interface.

Gy: Gray, a unit for measuring *physical dose*.

HU: Hounsfield Unit, a range of possible gray values used in CT; $\rho \in \{-1024 \ldots 3072\}$.

ICP: Iterative Closest Point algorithm.

IGES: Initial Graphics Exchange Specification, a file format for triangulated surface data.

ITF: Intensity Transfer Function.

JPEG: Joint Photographics Expert Group, a collection of standards for image file compression.

JPG: see *JPEG*.

Kerma: Kinetic Energy Released in MAtter, a unit for deployed energy in radiation physics.

kV: KiloVolt.

LINAC: LINear ACcelerator, the common source of high energy radiation in external beam radiation therapy.

LOR: Line Of Response, a term from PET technology.

LUT: LookUp Table, a table of translations for numerical values to color.

mAs: milliAmpereseconds.

MIP: Maximum Intensity Projection, a volume rendering technique.

MR: Magnetic Resonance.

MRI: Magnetic Resonance Imaging.

MTF: Modulation Transfer Function.

NEMA: National Electrical Manufacturers Association.

NifTI: Neuroimaging Informatics Technology Initiative, a medical volume data format derived from the *Analyze 7.5* format.

NIR: Near Infrared Imaging.

NMI: Normalized Mutual Information, a popular measure for intermodal image registration.

OCT: Optical Coherence Tomography.

OpenGL: Open Graphics Language, an API for 3D visualization.

PACS: Picture Archiving and Communications System, an abbreviation for the infrastructure and standards for the administration of radiological image data.

PCA: Principal Component Analysis.

PDE: Partial Differential Equation.

PDF: Probability Density Function.

PET: Positron Emission Computed Tomography.

PGM: Portable GrayMap, a simple image file format.

PM: PhotoMultiplier, a device for conversion of single photons to an analog current.

PNG: Portable Network Graphics, an image file format.

PSD: Photoshop Document, the file format for Adobe Photoshop images.

PSF: Point Spread Function.

rad: Radiation Absorbed Dose, an older unit for physical dose.

RF: Radio Frequency.

RGB: Red – Green – Blue, a color model.

RLE: RunLength Encoding, a compression technique.

ROI: Region of Interest.

SNR: Signal-to-Noise Ratio.

SPECT: Single Photon Emission Computed Tomography.

STEP: Standard for the Exchange of Product Model Data, a file format for triangulated 3D surface data.

STL: Surface Tesselation Language or Standard Triangulation Language, a very common format for triangulated 3D surface data.

Sv: Sievert, a unit for biological dose.

TFT: Thin Film Transistor.

TIFF: Tagged Image File Format. Another image file format.

TRE: Target Registration Error.

US: UltraSound.

XCF: eXperimental Computing Facility, the native image file format of GIMP.

YCbCr: Yellow – Chroma Blue – Chroma Red, a color model.

List of MATLAB sample scripts

`dsa_3.m`: A demonstration of digital subtraction angiography as an example for algebraic operations on images.

`OpenDICOM_3.m`: Opening a single DICOM file and saving it in another image file format.

`ConvertColorImage_3.m`: Reading a color JPG image and storing it as a grayscale image.

`BetterConvertColorImage_3.m`: Same as `ConvertColorImage_3.m`, but in more decent MATLAB programming style.

`SNRExample_3.m`: Determination of x-ray dose compared to the signal-to-noise ratio in a series of x-ray images.

`LinearIntensityTransform_4.m`: Simple linear intensity scaling from arbitrary depth to six bit.

`ComposeColorImage_4.m`: Composing a color image from three single black-and-white photographs.

`LogExample_4.m`: The logarithm of image gray values as an example of a non-linear intensity transform.

`SigmoidIntensityTransform_4.m`: An example of generalized non-linear intensity transfer functions.

`Histogram_4.m`: Computation of an image histogram with arbitrary bin width.

`OptimizeContrast_4.m`: Automated contrast optimization based on histogram operations.

`SimpleLowPass_5.m`: Convolution with a low-pass filter or blurring kernel in the spatial domain.

`NumericalDifferentiation_5.m`: Introduction of the concept of numerical differentiation in one dimension.

`ForwardDifference_5.m`: A simple differentiation kernel for partial derivatives of images.

`Sobel_5.m`: Computing the absolute value of the total differential using Sobel-kernels, which results in an edge image.

`UnsharpMask_5.m`: Linear combination of filtering kernels; in this case, unsharp masking is presented as an example.

`MedianFiveTimesFive_5.m`: The median filter as an example of a non-linear filter.

`Sine_5.m`: A simple demonstration of bandpass-filtering in the Fourier domain on a onedimensional function.

`ChordSpectrum_5.m`: Another demonstration of the Fourier transform - the computation of power spectra for a musical chord played on three instruments.

`Rect_5.m`: Reconstruction of a onedimensional rectangle function including a demonstration of the Gibbs phenomenon.

`WallFourier_Y_LP_5.m`: Directional band pass filtering in Fourier space on a 2D image.

`MouseSpectrum_5.m`: Power spectrum of a 2D image.

`Simpleconvolution_5`: A demonstration of the convolution operation of onedimensional functions.

`FourierDiffRect_5.m`: Differentiation of simple functions in Fourier space.

`BetterFourierDiffRect_5.m`: An improved version of `FourierDiffRect_5.m`.

`MouseFourierLP_5.m`: Blurring images in the Fourier domain.

`MouseConvolve_5.m`: Application of the convolution theorem to a 2D image.

`ComputeMTF_5.m`: A real-life example of measuring the resolution of a γ camera with a point source.

`Hough_5.m`: Computation of the Hough transform on a binary image.

`DistanceMap_5.m`: Demonstration of the distance transform on a binary image.

`ROIExample_6.m`: Evaluation of pixel intensities in a region-of-interest as a direct correlate of activity from a nuclear medicine tracer.

`ROIExampleWithJPGs_6.m`: A variation of `ROIExample_6.m` demonstrating that image depth is indeed of importance in image processing.

`Threshold_6.m`: Segmentation by intensity thresholding.

`RegionGrowing_FourConnected_6.m`: A simple implementation of region growing.

`RegionGrowing_WanderingStaticSeed_6.m`: A simple demo of the problems connected to 3D region growing.

`SimpleSnakeSeeds_6.m`: An initial, naive implementation of an active contour algorithm.

`BetterSnakeSeeds_6.m`: A variation of `SimpleSnakeSeeds_6.m` featuring an additional, more sophisticated energy term.

`BetterSnakeSeedsConstrained_6.m`: Another improved version of `SimpleSnakeSeeds_6.m`.

`MorphologicalOps_6.m`: Erosion of a binary shape.

`Hausdorff_6.m`: Computation of the Hausdorff-distance between two contours.

`Dice_6.m`: Computation of a Dice-coefficient for two binary regions.

`StepOne_Hough_6.m`, `StepTwo_DilateHough_6.m` as well as `StepThree_Threshold_6.m` are used in `BrachyCleanup_6.m` as parts of a more complex segmentation example on a multi-exposure x-ray.

`Preprocessing_6.m` and `BetterSnakeSeedsConstrainedTwo_6.m` are parts of another more complex segmentation example showing the influence of appropriate preprocessing on active contours.

`Simple2DRotation_7.m`: Naive implementation of image rotation in 2D.

`NNInterpolation_7.m`: Image rotation of a 2D image using a not-so naive version of nearest neighbor interpolation.

`BiLinearInterpolation_7.m`: An example of bilinear interpolation on a low-resolution image.

`BinaryPCA_7.m`: Application of the principal axis transform on a binary segmented shape.

`Conesects_7.m`: A geometrical example on 3D spatial transforms and reformatting – the computation of conic sections.

`ReformattingSmall_7.m`: 3D spatial transforms and reformatting on a small volume dataset.

`ReformattingBig_7.m`: Same as `ReformattingSmall_7.m` on a bigger dataset.

`ThreeDConvolutionSmall_7.m`: With reformatting at hand, we can also demonstrate that convolution, for instance with an edge-detection filter, also works in 3D.

`ThreeDConvolutionBig_7.m`: Same as `ThreeDConvolutionSmall_7.m` with a high-resolution version of the volume.

`Perspective_8.m`: A simple projection example using homogeneous coordinates and a projection operator.

`Raytracing_8.m`: A simple orthogonal rendering example.

`RaytracingRotated_8.m`: Same as `Raytracing_8.m` with additional 3D spatial transforms applied to the volume dataset.

`Splatting_8.m`: An alternative rendering method based on a projection operator in homogeneous cooridnates.

`BetterSplatting_8.m`: A more sophisticated version of `Splatting_8.m`.

`VolumeSplatting_8.m`: Volume rendering using color encoding of voxel grey values.

`DepthShading_8.m`: A simple surface rendering technique where the distance of a surface voxel to the image plane is encoded.

`SurfaceShading_8.m`: Example of a more common surface rendering technique employing a simple shading model.

`Triangulation_8.m`: A simple implementation of the cuberille algorithm producing a STL-file from a segmented voxel volume dataset.

`BetterShadingII_8.m`: A script that demonstrates shading for surface rendering of voxel volumes.

`CC2DRegistration_9.m`: Demonstration of a merit function based on cross correlation for intramodal registration.

`More2DRegistration_9.m`: Same as `CC2DRegistration_9.m`, but for quasi-intramodal registration.

`JointHistogram_9.m`: Computation of a joint histogram for an image compared to a rotated copy of the same image.

`MultimodalJointHistogram_9.m`: Same as `JointHistogram_9.m` but with a multimodal pair of images showing the same subject.

`PlotMutualInformation2D_9.m`: Computation of the mutual information measure for multimodal images.

`DTChamfermatch_9.m` and `PlotChamferMatch2D_9.m`: An example of chamfer matching, a gradient based technique.

`SimpleOptimization_9.m`, `spike.m` and `strangeSine.m`: An illustrative example on the pitfalls of numerical optimization.

`Optimize2D_9.m` and `MI2D.m`: Examples on optimization for registration.

`DirectLinearTransform_9.m`: An example of camera calibration using the direct linear transform.

`MarkerRegistration_9.m`: Analytical solution to the point-to-point registration problem.

`mirotate.m`: Replacement for the `imrotate` function of MATLAB for Octave users.

`radotra.m`: Computes the Radon-transform of a given image.

`systemMatrix.m`: Computation of a system matrix for algebraic reconstruction.

`pseudoinverse_10.m`: Algebraic reconstruction using inversion of the system matrix.

`kaczmarz_randomised.m`: An implementation of Kacmarz algorithm.

`iterative_10.m`: Algebraic reconstruction using Kacmarz algorithm.

`filt.m`: A function that plots the single steps in a filtering operation.

`two_low_pass_filters_10.m`: An illustration of `filt.m`.

`ramp.m`: A ramp filter.

`conefilter_10.m`: Application of a conefilter after unfiltered backprojection.

`noise_10.m`: Illustration of filtering effects on image noise.

`radotra360.m`: 360 degree version of `radotra.m`

`fbp360.m`: 360 degree version of `fbp.m`

`ring_artefact_10.m`: Example of the origins of ring artifacts.

`streak_artefact_10.m`: Illustration of streak artifacts generated by high attenuation.

`volrotate.m`: Rotates a volume around the z-axis.

`projection.m`: Cone-beam projection using `volrotate.m`.

`fdk_backprojection.m`: Cone-beam backprojection using the method of Feldkamp. Notation, etc., from Kak & Slaney.

`demo_fdk.m`: The demo script loads a 3D phantom file, computes cone-beam projections and then applies `fdk_backprojection`.

Epilogue

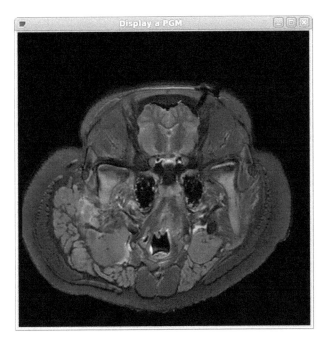

FIGURE A.1: Compiling the `displaypgm.cpp` code from the `LessonData` folder should give you something like this.

Once you have reached this chapter, you have made it. You made acquaintance with the most important basic methods and algorithms in medical image processing. If you want to go further, you may find a plethora of advanced textbooks and research articles to guide you. However, one problem remains. MATLAB is a fantastic tool for experimenting and teaching, but it is not necessarily the right environment for advanced programming, especially when it comes to managing the memory requirements of really large datasets. Here begins the domain of high-level languages such as C++, C#, Java and so on. The good news is that the basic algorithms do not really change when you switch to such an environment, and most of our examples are indeed basically C-code transported to MATLAB.

The only challenge is to display the images, something we usually accomplished by the `image` command of MATLAB. When using a compiled language, things may become slightly more cumbersome. At this point I would like to introduce one of the many platform-independent toolkits for programming graphical user interfaces - *wxWidgets*, a C++ toolkit available for all major platforms. It is in the public domain and can be obtained from `http://www.wxwidgets.org/`. Once you have installed and configured this library properly, you may try to compile[1] the `displaypgm.cpp` file which can also be found in the `LessonData` folder. This program of 68 lines length reads the PGM-file `PIG_MR.pgm` generated by the `OpenDICOM_2.m` from Chapter 3. The looks may vary for different platforms.

So if you are inclined to use C++ or another high-level language, you may now go on your own. Finally, you should be aware that medical image processing is an applied field. The best ideas from research emerge from discussions with physicians and other end users. Listen to them.

---

[1]On my Linux operating system, the line in question reads `g++ displaypgm.cpp -o displayPGM` `'wx-config -libs' 'wx-config -cxxflags'`

Index

T_2^*, 22
T_1, 20
T_2, 22
γ camera, 34, 164
(:) (MATLAB), 398
* (MATLAB), 397
.* (MATLAB), 397
; (MATLAB), 398
< (MATLAB), 398
<= (MATLAB), 398
> (MATLAB), 398
>= (MATLAB), 398
& (MATLAB), 398
^(MATLAB), 398
\n (MATLAB), 399
~= (MATLAB), 398
ComputeMTF_5.m, 164
WallFourier_Y_LP_5.m, 156
180° pulse, 22
26-connected neighbors, 124, 181, 260, 261
2D/3D registration, 55, 255, 321
3D ultrasound, 29, 31
3DSlicer, 54, 81, 112
4-connected neighbors, 124, 181
6-connected neighbors, 124, 181
8-connected neighbors, 124, 181
90° pulse, 20

A-mode ultrasound, 29
abs (MATLAB), 400
absorbed dose, 39
AC, 403
ACR, 71, 403
active contours, 184, 199, 209
addition of complex numbers, 133
affine transformation, 224, 301
algebraic reconstruction, 339, 345
aliasing artifacts, 277
amplitude, 132
Analyze 7.5, 73, 245, 403
AnalyzeAVW, 72, 73, 128, 179, 182, 195, 208, 245, 257–259, 262, 271, 273, 300, 301

anisotropic diffusion filter, 128
annihilation radiation, 8, 35
anode, 3
API, 221, 261, 403
ASCII, 403
attenuation correction, 36
attenuation of US, 29
augmented matrix, 223
augmented reality, 263
AVW, 73

B-mode, 29
B-spline, 302
bar (MATLAB), 398
barrel distortion, 267
bas-relief kernel, 122
base functions, 130, 131, 134, 140
beam hardening, 15
Beer – Lambert law, 7, 340
BetterSnakeSeeds-
ConstrainedTwo_6.m, 211
Better_SnakeSeeds-
Constrained_6.m, 202
BetterFourierDiffRect_5.m, 160
BetterShadingI_8.m, 292
BetterShadingII_8.m, 294
BetterSnakeSeeds_6.m, 201
BetterSplatting_8.m, 274
bilinear interpolation, 216, 217, 219, 237, 238
BiLinearInterpolation_7.m, 237
binary numbers, 64
BinaryPCA_7.m, 240
Blender, 291
blurring, 8
blurring kernel, 118
BMP, 67, 403
BrachyCleanup_6.m, 207
Bremsstrahlung, 4
Butterworth filter, 138

CAD, 70, 261, 262, 265, 403
camera calibration, 316, 375

capture range, 302
Cartesian coordinate system, 128, 133, 141, 222, 229, 285, 316
cavitation effects in US, 33
CBCT, 16, 228, 403
CC2DRegistration_9.m, 323
CCD, 116, 403
cd (MATLAB), 398
central difference, 123
centroid, 178, 222, 240
chamfer matching, 310, 328
char (MATLAB), 399
characteristic x-radiation, 4
checkerboard visualization, 55
chemical shift artifacts, 25
ChordSpectrum_5.m, 152
closing, 187, 204
CNR, 403
COC, 116, 403
coincidence detection, 35
collimator, 34
collision detection, 263, 264
color Doppler US, 31
color flow mapping US, 31
colormap (MATLAB), 398
ComposeColorImage_4.m, 100
complex conjugate, 133
complex numbers, 132, 133
complex plane, 133, 134
complex unit, 133
component-wise multiplication, 63, 159, 178, 220, 397
compound scan, 29
Compton effect, 7
computer aided surgery, 229
cone beam CT, 14, 54, 365
cone sections, 242
Conesects_7.m, 243
conjugate algorithm, 314
connectedness, 124, 125, 181
Continuous wave Doppler US, 31
contrast agent, 75, 179, 182, 253
contrast optimization, 107
convergence range, 302
ConvertColorImage_3.m, 85
convex scan heads, 29
convolution, 118, 125, 137, 138, 158, 186, 247, 351, 353
convolution in k-space, 137

cos (MATLAB), 400
cosmic radiation, 42
cost functions, 302
Covariance, 225
CR foils, 138, 403
CR plates, 6
cross (MATLAB), 401
cross product, 260, 285, 401
CT, 10, 46, 119, 179, 182, 183, 186, 212, 245, 255, 264, 271, 283, 297, 300, 319, 403
CT-generations, 11
cuberille algorithm, 263, 287, 292
cubic interpolation, 219
curved reformatting, 229
cycles over range, 139, 159

DC, 403
DCT, 69, 140, 403
deconvolution, 138
deformable registration, 54
demodulation, 31
depth shading, 256, 258, 259, 280, 291
DepthShading_8.m, 280
det (MATLAB), 400
determinant, 220
deterministic damage, 40
DFT, 69, 135, 137, 400, 403
Dice coefficient, 189, 205
Dice_6.m, 205
DICOM, 45, 71, 73, 190, 191, 403
DICOM header, 71
DICOM-RT, 71, 403
DICOMDIR, 71, 73, 403
differentiation, 121
differentiation in k-space, 137, 159
digital subtraction angiography, 75
digital volume tomography, 17
digitally rendered radiograph, 51
dilation, 186, 188, 204, 207, 209, 312
direct Fourier method, 355
direct linear transform, 318, 335, 377
direct piezo effect, 29
DirectLinearTransform_9.m, 335
discretization artifacts, 215, 221, 253
displacement field, 301
distance transform, 142, 172, 310, 312
DistanceMap_5.m, 172
dithering, 98
DLT, 318, 377, 403

dof, 299, 301, 403
Doppler effect, 30
Doppler US, 30
dose, 3
dosimetry, 39
dot (MATLAB), 401
dot product, 128, 401
DQE, 7, 403
DRR, 253, 254, 256, 264, 277, 404
DSA, 75, 404
DTChamfermatch_9.m, 328
dynamic range, 92, 125
dynode, 34

EBCT, 37, 404
echo time, 23
edge artifacts in MR, 25
edge detection, 47, 121, 247, 310
eig (MATLAB), 400
eigenfunction, 137, 222
eigenvalue, 222, 225, 337, 400
eigenvector, 222, 225–227, 241, 337, 400
electrical impedance tomography, 3
electromagnetic tracking, 230, 232
electron, 8
electron beam CT, 37
endoscope, 3, 266
endoscopy, 38, 66
energy dose, 39
energy window, 36
EPI, 404
EPID, 3, 15, 16, 404
EPS, 70, 404
equivalent, 40
erosion, 186, 188, 203, 204
Euler angles, 222, 226
Euler's formula, 133
evaluation of registration, 315, 322
exp (MATLAB), 400
expectation value, 225, 240
extrinsic image features, 299
eye (MATLAB), 399

fclose (MATLAB), 399
FDG, 35, 404
featurelet, 302
FEM, 263, 302, 404
FFT, 135, 404
fft (MATLAB), 400
fft2 (MATLAB), 400

fftshift (MATLAB), 400
FID, 20, 22, 23, 404
fiducial marker, 178, 299, 319
fiducial registration error, 315
field inhomogeneity in MR, 25
field of view, 24
filtered backprojection, 24, 339, 354, 356
filtering, 116
finite difference, 121
finite element models, 263, 302
fisheye effect, 267
FITS, 74, 404
flat panel detectors, 7
flat shading, 260, 266, 283, 292
FLE, 322, 404
floor (MATLAB), 400
fluorescence imaging, 3
fminsearch (MATLAB), 400
focal spot, 3
focusing cup, 4
fopen (MATLAB), 398
for (MATLAB), 397
forward difference, 122, 146
ForwardDifference_5.m, 147
Fourier Series, 131
Fourier slice theorem, 354
Fourier transform, 24, 25, 47, 128, 131, 134,
        137, 150, 222, 312, 351, 356, 400
FourierDiffRect_5.m, 159
FOV, 24, 404
fprintf (MATLAB), 399
frameless stereotaxy, 229
FRE, 315, 322, 404
fread (MATLAB), 399
free induction decay, 20
frequency, 132, 134
frequency response, 352
fseek (MATLAB), 399
function (MATLAB), 399

gamma curve, 102
gamma radiation, 3
gamma value, 92
Gaussian, 121, 137, 140, 162, 164, 222, 225,
        293, 305
genetic algorithms, 314
geometric primitives, 260, 261, 263
Gibbs phenomenon, 162
GIF, 70
Gimbal lock, 226

GIMP, 70, 92, 102, 181, 186, 204, 206, 207, 210, 292, 293, 329, 404
global optimization algorithm, 313, 314
Gouraud shading, 266, 267, 292
gradient based merit functions, 303, 310
gradient field, 27
Gray, 39
gray scale conversion, 84
GUI, 404
Gy, 39, 404
gyromagnetic ratio, 20

half life, 192
Hamming filter, 138
Hann filter, 138, 362
Hausdorff distance, 188, 202, 205
Hausdorff_6.m, 205
head-mounted display, 316
Heel effect, 206
helical CT, 12
Hesse normal form, 141, 142, 170, 341
HF-tracking, 231
histogram, 49, 257, 305, 309, 361
histogram bins, 96
histogram equalization, 97
Histogram_4.m, 105
histology, 38, 66
homogeneous coordinates, 223
hormesis, 41
Horn's algorithm, 319
Hough transform, 141, 167, 207, 209
Hough_5.m, 167
Hounsfield units, 46
HU, 11, 64, 93, 179, 180, 182, 274, 275, 404

ICP, 320, 321, 404
identity matrix, 220, 399
if (MATLAB), 397
ifft (MATLAB), 400
ifft2 (MATLAB), 400
ifftshift (MATLAB), 400
IGES, 70, 266, 404
IGSTK, 291
IGT, 319, 322
image (MATLAB), 398
image addition, 63
image averaging, 63
image based tracking, 231
image blending, 63
image blurring, 138, 143, 161, 293

image color, 64
image depth, 63
image differentiation, 310
image driven rendering, 253
image file formats, 66
image fusion, 297
image intensity transforms, 91
image interpolation, 215
image inversion, 100
image registration, 297
image resolution, 215
image rotation, 233
image sharpening, 118, 138, 143
image smoothing, 118
image-guided therapy, 54, 229, 316, 375
ImageJ, 81, 108, 112, 145
imaginary part of complex numbers, 133
imaginary unit, 227
imread (MATLAB), 399
imrotate (MATLAB), 339
imshow (MATLAB), 398
imwrite (MATLAB), 399
index, 209
inertial tracking, 231
inhomogeneities of the magnetic field, 22
inner product, 128, 134, 219, 260, 285, 401
inner product for functions, 130
input (MATLAB), 399
intensification screens, 6
intensity based merit functions, 303
intensity clipping, 253
intensity histograms, 95, 105
intensity transform, 179, 210
intensity windowing, 93
Interfile, 74
intermodal registration, 300
internal radiation exposition, 42
interpolation, 12, 49, 216, 236, 253, 302
intramodal registration, 300, 304
intrinsic image features, 299
inv (MATLAB), 400
inverse matrix, 220, 224
inverse piezo effect, 29
inverse square law, 281
iodine-123, 33
iterative closest point algorithm, 320
ITF, 92, 102, 404
ITK, 291
ITK SNAP, 185

Jacobi decomposition, 241
Jacobian matrix, 356
joint histogram, 305, 325, 327
joint PDF, 304
JointHistogram_9.m, 325
JPEG, 69, 404
JPG, 69, 140, 192, 399

k-space, 134, 135, 400
Kaczmarz algorithm, 350
Kerma, 39, 404
Kitware, 291
Kronecker function, 129
Kullback-Leibler distance, 309
kV, 5, 404

Lambert's law, 260
Lambertian shading, 260
Larmor frequency, 19, 20, 24
law of radioactive decay, 191
law of reflection, 116
law of refraction, 116
level set method, 48, 183, 185
Levenberg-Marquardt algorithm, 314
lighting model, 253, 260, 284
LINAC, 3, 299, 404
line drawing algorithms, 346
line integral, 253
line of response, 36
linear accelerator, 54
linear algebra, 128
linear elastic models, 302
linear filtering, 353
linear intensity transforms, 98
linear least squares method, 318, 336, 377, 400
linear scan heads, 29
LinearIntensityTransform_4.m, 98
linearity of the Fourier transform, 137
live wire segmentation, 184
load (MATLAB), 399
local optimization algorithm, 313, 314
local thresholding, 179
log (MATLAB), 400
LogExample_4.m, 102
Logistic function, 93
longitudinal relaxation, 20
lookup tables, 64
LOR, 36, 404
lsqlin (MATLAB), 400

LUT, 64, 79, 98, 398, 404

magnetic moment, 18
Manhattan metric, 329
marching cubes, 265, 291
marching squares, 264, 265
MarkerRegistration_9.m, 337
mAs, 5, 405
MATLAB, 62
matrix multiplication, 219
max (MATLAB), 399
maximum filter, 150
mean (MATLAB), 400
mean free path, 34
mechanical tracking, 230
median, 126
median (MATLAB), 400
median filter, 126, 149
MedianFiveTimesFive_5.m, 149
merit function, 301, 302, 313, 316, 323
metal artifacts, 16
MI, 309
MI2D.m, 333
microscopy, 3
microtome, 38
min (MATLAB), 400
minimum filter, 150
MIP, 253–255, 269, 271, 272, 274, 280, 405
mirroring in US, 30
mod (MATLAB), 400
More2DRegistration_9.m, 324
morphological operations, 174, 185, 187, 203
MorphologicalOps_6.m, 203
motion artifacts, 15
motion artifacts in MR, 25
MouseConvolve_5.m, 162
MouseFourierLP_5.m, 161
MouseSpectrum_5.m, 157
MR, 17, 23, 46, 74, 179, 212, 228, 298, 315, 319, 405
MR aliasing artifacts, 25
MR artifacts, 25
MR tissue contrast, 23
MR/PET, 315
MRI, 3, 405
MTF, 75, 139, 141, 162, 164, 405
multi-detector CT, 14
MultimodalJointHistogram-Translation_9.m, 327
MultimodalJointHistogram_9.m, 327

multiple reflections in US, 30
multiplication of complex numbers, 133
multiscale optimization, 316
mutual information, 304, 309, 327, 334

nabla operator, 122
NaI, 33
near infrared imaging, 3, 37
nearest neighbor interpolation, 236
Nelder-Mead algorithm, 313, 400
NEMA, 71, 405
neuronavigation, 229
neutron, 18, 34
NifTI, 73, 405
NIR, 37, 405
NMI, 300, 301, 310, 405
NNInterpolation_7.m, 236
noise, 8, 118, 137, 185
noise artifacts, 15, 145
noise in US, 30
non-rigid registration, 301
nonlinear filters, 126
nonlinear intensity transforms, 104, 182, 210
norm of complex numbers, 133
normal vector, 261
normalized mutual information, 310
nuclear magnetic resonance, 20
nuclear medicine, 33, 178, 185, 190
numerical differentiation, 121, 145
numerical integration, 131
NumericalDifferentiation_5.m, 145
Nyquist-Shannon theorem, 137

oblique reformatting, 229, 231, 247
OCT, 3, 36, 405
Octave, 62
OpenDICOM_3.m, 76
OpenGL, 221, 261, 405
opening, 187, 204
optical computed tomography, 36
optical ray tracing, 116
optical tracking, 230, 233
optical tracking system, 232
optimization algorithm, 313, 329, 400
Optimize2D_9.m, 333
OptimizeContrast_4.m, 108
orthogonal matrix, 221
orthogonal projection, 252, 254, 269
orthogonal reformatting, 229, 245, 248
orthogonal rendering, 276, 283

orthonormal functions, 128
OSLO, 116
outer product, 260, 285, 401

PACS, 71, 73, 405
pair production effect, 7
parametric representation, 141, 243
ParaView, 291, 292
Parsevals theorem, 137
partial derivative, 121
partial volume effect, 15
Parzen window method, 310
pattern intensity, 304
PCA, 184, 224, 226, 240, 242, 405
PDE, 128, 185, 405
PDF, 304, 309, 315, 328, 405
Pearson's correlation coefficient, 224, 225,
    301, 323
permanent magnets, 27
perspective projection, 252, 255, 267, 272
Perspective_8.m, 267
PET, 3, 8, 34, 180, 215, 216, 237, 298, 315,
    319, 405
PET-CT, 38, 54
PET-MR, 54
PET/CT, 298, 315
PGM, 67, 80, 292, 293, 405
phase, 132, 138, 312
Phong shading, 266, 295
photo multiplier, 34
photoelectric effect, 7, 34
photomultiplier, 33
photon, 2
pi (MATLAB), 401
piecewise rigid registration, 302
piezo effect, 29
pitch factor, 13
pixel, 49, 59, 95, 118, 124, 135, 215, 221,
    240, 242, 253, 256, 261, 304, 305
plot (MATLAB), 398
PlotMutualInformation2D_9.m, 327
PM, 34, 405
PNG, 69, 70, 405
point-to-point registration, 231, 319, 337
Poisson distribution, 8
polar coordinates, 141
positron, 8
Powell's method, 314
power spectrum, 137, 157
precession, 18, 19

Preprocessing_6.m, 210
principal axis transform, 224, 240
principal component analysis, 224
probability density function, 304
progressive saturation, 23
projection matrix, 223, 252, 258, 272, 274, 316
projection slice theorem, 354, 356
propagation speed of waves, 134
proton, 18, 34
PSD, 70, 405
PSF, 75, 118, 121, 139, 141, 162, 164, 405

quantum noise, 8
quaternions, 226, 231, 337

rad, 39, 405
radiation absorbed dose, 39
radiation protection, 39
radiographic film, 6
Radon transform, 339, 340, 342, 346, 354, 362
Ram – Lak filter, 357
ramp filter, 357, 358
rapid prototyping, 263
RAW, 67
ray clipping, 256
raycasting, 252, 253, 258, 269, 283
Raytracing_8.m, 269
RaytracingRotated_8.m, 271
real (MATLAB), 400
real part of complex numbers, 133
real time rendering, 263
real- and imaginary operator, 133
receiver bandwidth, 24
Rect_5.m, 154
reflection of ultrasound, 28
reformatting, 49, 50, 228, 242, 245, 251
ReformattingBig_7.m, 245
ReformattingSmall_7.m, 245
refraction of ultrasound, 28
region growing, 48, 181, 184, 192, 195, 196
RegionGrowing_
FourConnected_6.m, 193
RegionGrowing_
WanderingStaticSeed_6.m, 195
registration, 54, 230
registration to physical space, 319
relaxation times, 22
rendering, 180, 229, 231, 252

repetition time, 23
resonance frequency, 20
RF, 20, 405
RF transmission system, 27
RGB, 65, 280, 405
rigid body transformation, 224, 299
rigid registration, 54
ring artifacts, 15, 36, 363
RLE, 68, 405
ROI, 63, 178, 185, 190, 222, 256, 405
ROIExample_6.m, 190
rotation, 219
rotation matrix, 219, 222, 231, 240, 272
round (MATLAB), 400

safety aspects in US, 32
saturation, 20
save (MATLAB), 399
scalar image addition, 63
scalar image multiplication, 63, 99
scalar product, 128, 401
scaling matrix, 224
scaling property in k-space, 137
scatter event, 36
scatter radiation, 8, 41
scattering of ultrasound, 28
scintigraphy, 3, 33
scintillator, 33
sector scan heads, 30
segmentation, 48, 262
segmentation evaluation, 188
series expansion, 128
shading, 253, 291
shadowing in US, 30
Shannon's entropy, 306–308
shape models, 183, 184
shear-warp rendering, 258
Shepp – Logan phantom, 345, 351, 360
shim coils, 27
short (MATLAB), 399
Sievert, 40
Sigmoid function, 93, 210
SigmoidIntensityTransform_4.m, 104
signal spectrum, 132
similarity measures, 302
Simple2DRotation_7.m, 233
Simpleconvolution_5.m, 158
SimpleLowPass_5.m, 143
SimpleOptimization_9.m, 330
SimpleSnakeSeeds_6.m, 199

simplex algorithm, 313
simulated annealing, 314
simulator images, 51, 255
sin (MATLAB), 400
Sine_5.m, 150
singular matrix, 220
sinogram, 11, 342
size (MATLAB), 400
slice selection in MR, 24
slip ring, 13
snakes, 48, 184, 199
Snell's law, 116
SNR, 15, 27, 74, 86, 119, 405
SNRExample_3.m, 87
Sobel filter, 48, 125, 207, 210, 264, 310–312
Sobel_5.m, 148
sort (MATLAB), 400
spatial domain, 135, 164, 400
spatial localization in MR, 23
spatial transform, 54
special matrix, 221
speckle in US, 30, 31
SPECT, 3, 15, 34, 180, 228, 298, 319, 405
spherical aberration, 116
spherical mirror, 116
spike.m, 330
spin, 18
spin echo, 23
spin-echo sequence, 23
spin-echo signal, 23
spin-lattice relaxation, 20
spin-spin relaxation, 22
spiral CT, 12
splat rendering, 258, 272, 274
Splatting_8.m, 272
spline, 218
sprintf (MATLAB), 399
standard deviation, 225
statistical shape model, 48
std (MATLAB), 400
STEP, 266, 406
StepOne_Hough_6.m, 207
StepThree_Threshold_6.m, 207
StepTwo_DilateHough_6.m, 207
stereolithography, 54, 187, 263, 265
stereotactic surgery, 229
stimulated luminescence, 7
STL, 70, 265, 266, 290, 291, 406
stochastic radiation effects, 40

strangeSine.m, 330
sum of squared differences, 304
summed voxel rendering, 253, 254, 256, 272, 273, 277
superconducting magnets, 27
surf (MATLAB), 398
surface models, 54, 184, 187, 260, 261, 264, 287
surface registration, 320
surface rendering, 50, 51, 253, 258, 262, 267, 280, 281
SurfaceShading_8.m, 283
surgical simulation, 263
Sv, 40, 406
system matrix, 346

target registration error, 315
Technetium 99m, 33
temperature effects in US, 33
terrestrial radiation sources, 42
Tesla, 20
textures, 253, 266
TFT, 7, 406
thinning, 174
ThreeDConvolutionSmall_7.m, 247
ThreeDConvolutionBig_7.m, 247
Threshold_6.m, 192
thresholding, 49, 178–180, 184, 192, 206, 207, 209, 210, 254, 283, 310–312
TIFF, 69, 74, 406
time-of-flight PET, 36
tomographic reconstruction, 56, 339
tracer method, 33
tracking systems, 227, 229, 322
transfer function, 256–258, 262, 280
translation, 219
translation in k-space, 137
translation matrix, 223
transmitted bandwidth, 24
transpose (MATLAB), 399
transverse relaxation, 22
TRE, 315, 322, 406
triangulation algorithm, 263, 287, 292
Triangulation_8.m, 287
trilinear interpolation, 217, 218, 247
true coincidence, 35
tube potential, 5

uint8(...) (MATLAB), 399
ultrasonic tracking, 231

ultrasound, 28
ultrasound scan head, 29
unit quaternions, 226
unit vectors, 128, 260, 290
unsharp masking, 125, 148, 207
UnsharpMask_5.m, 148
US, 28, 29, 298, 321, 406

VBH mouthpiece, 319
vector, 128
vertex, 261
virtual endoscopy, 266, 268
viscous fluid models, 302
visualization, 215, 229, 230, 251, 265
volume compositing, 257
volume driven rendering, 258
volume regularization, 216
volume rendering, 51, 55, 253, 256
volume transformation matrix, 224, 300, 318
VolumeSplatting_8.m, 276
voxel, 49, 59, 73, 96, 124, 135, 218, 224, 229, 258, 260, 261, 280, 283, 291, 305
VTK, 291

watershed transform, 184
wave number, 134, 161
wavelength, 134
Wehnelt electrode, 4
while (MATLAB), 397
window center, 94
window width, 94
windowing, 46, 112, 182, 251
wobbling US scanheads, 31
wrap-around artifact, 135, 136

x-ray, 3, 264, 316
x-ray detectors, 6
XCF, 70, 406

YCbCr, 69, 406
ylim (MATLAB), 398

zeros (MATLAB), 399
ZIP, 69